SOCIAL PSYCHOLOGY OF HEALTH AND ILLNESS

SOCIAL PSYCHOLOGY OF HEALTH AND ILLNESS

edited by

GLENN S. SANDERS
JERRY SULS
The State University of New York at Albany

Routledge
Taylor & Francis Group
LONDON AND NEW YORK

First published 1982 by Lawrence Erlbaum Associates. Inc.

Published 2011 by Routledge
4 Park Square, Milton Park, Abingdon, Oxon OX14 4RN
605 Third Avenue, New York, NY 10017

Routledge is an imprint of the Taylor & Francis Group, an informa business

Library of Congress Cataloging in Publication Data
Main entry under title:

Social psychology of health and illness.

Bibliography: p.
Includes index.
1. Social medicine. 2. Medicine and psychology.
I. Sanders, Glenn S. II. Suls, Jerry M. [DNLM: 1. Psychology, Social. 2. Community psychiatry. WM 30.6 S677]
RA418.S6426 362.1'042 82-1465
AACR2

ISBN 13: 978-1-138-17994-3 (hbk)
ISBN 13: 978-0-8058-0554-3 (pbk)

Contents

Preface

This volume is intended to illustrate the social arena in which physical health and illness compete for existence. The competition itself is so engrossing that it is easy to overlook the importance of its context. Yet the ''distant'' influences of socialization practices, interpersonal relationships, and social organization can often be as crucial as blood counts and X-rays in determining whether health or illness will emerge the victor. Our essays describe some of the pathways through which these social influences are exerted and also offer suggestions as to how these influences can be tilted in the direction of good health. The broader aim of this volume is to make it clear that a social psychological orientation is a useful conceptual tool for the analysis of health and illness.

We do not mean to imply that this work is a pioneering effort with respect to the aforementioned goals. In recent years there has been an upsurge in many areas of applied social psychology, and the union of medical and social concerns has been a primary focus. Most of our chapters are devoted in part to a review of previous ideas and findings. This volume was created not as a first step, but as a crystalization of earlier undertakings. Heretofore, relevant studies have been dispersed without clear pattern through a vast and diverse literature. It is hoped that bringing this research together in a systematic and accessible manner will reveal the existence and the value of a *field* of medical social psychology, as opposed to isolated attacks on highly specific problems.

In the same spirit, we have not attempted a comprehensive treatment of all relevant subject matter. Beyond the intimidating physical bulk of such an endeavor, it would be difficult to retain a coherent sense of the outlines of a medical social psychology—a field that we believe both differs from and adds to the somewhat more established subjects of medical sociology and general medical psychology. Again, our main intention is to convince the reader that there *is* a social psychology of health and illness and that it is a subject well worth the difficulties of development and application.

A complementary intention is to maintain the writing style at a level understandable and interesting to the three groups of readers on whom progress in this field depends—sociomedical researchers, health care delivery professionals, and advanced undergraduate and graduate students in relevant disciplines. In order to find common ground among such a varied readership, psychological, medical, and statistical jargon is kept to a minimum. Emphasis is put wherever possible on concrete exemplars of health care and health maintenance. Yet the style is by no means popularized, glib, or superficial. Research is faithfully chronicled in sufficient detail to permit informed analyses of weaknesses and implications. Speculative comments are clearly labeled as such and are confined largely to cases in which they suggest means of addressing questions raised by current findings. As should become clear, solid contributions in medical social psychology require genuine interaction and cooperation among researchers and students with varied backgrounds. We hope this volume demonstrates that a common language, which generates comprehension, excitement, and respect, is possible.

The organization of this book highlights the four areas that we feel offer the greatest potential for medical social psychology. Part I explores the question of whether certain personality traits are systematically related to the maintenance of health and to coping with illness. Both implicit and explicit in much of the discussion is the contribution of socialization practices and interpersonal reinforcements to the development of these personalities.

In the first paper of this part, "The Hardy Personality: Toward A Social Psychology of Stress and Health," Suzanne Kobasa discusses the personality characteristics of those persons who remain healthy despite stressful life events. Kobasa also examines how personality-based stress resistance may be developed in different work contexts.

Whereas Kobasa defines the hardy personality, Charles Carver and Charlene Humphries discuss a personality style that is a significant risk factor in the development of illness, specifically coronary heart disease (CHD). In the "Social Psychology of the Type A Coronary-Prone Behavior Pattern," the authors examine recent social psychological and medical research on the Type A. Their discussion emphasizes how social and situational influences may interact with the Type A style to contribute to the etiology of CHD.

In recent years much consideration has been given to the individual's sense of control and its effects on performance, emotion, and health. Inspired by Rotter's ground-breaking efforts on locus of control, Kenneth and Barbara Wallston developed a scale to assess peoples' beliefs that their health is controlled by internal versus external factors. In "Who Is Responsible for Your Health? The Construct of Health Locus of Control," the Wallstons review the theoretical framework of their efforts, suggest a health locus of control typology, and review evidence linking health outcomes and medical compliance among persons differing in their health locus of control orientation. Overall, this work emphasizes that attention to health-related personality styles and/or beliefs may aid psychological and medical professionals in identifying those persons likely to adhere to their medical regimens or take preventive actions.

Part II turns from idiosyncratic approaches to a broader concern with the general cognitive strategies used by laypeople to make decisions relevant to health and illness. The underlying thread in these articles is the role of other people both in shaping the information-processing strategies and in supplying the information itself on which these strategies operate.

J. Skelton and James Pennebaker in "The Psychology of Physical Symptoms and Sensations" are interested in the psychological processes mediating the perception and evaluation of bodily information. What cognitive mechanisms and situational influences affect the intensity of symptoms and what are the sources of these mechanisms and influences? These questions are pursued by the authors who review previous evidence, related work in cognitive psychology, and their own recent research. Along the way, Skelton and Pennebaker discuss how a cognitive approach can account for such diverse phenomena as placebo effects, mass psychogenic illness, and medical student's disease.

The second chapter in this part, "Social Comparison and Perceptions of Health and Illness" by Glenn Sanders, considers the incidence, dynamics, and effects of relying on nonexpert opinions to assess health-related questions. Sanders reviews the literature and draws implications both for laypersons and health care professionals.

Perhaps the most directly "social" aspect of this volume is to be found in Part III. The chapters therein deal with both typical and preferred modes of interaction between health care professionals and their clients. These contributions illustrate how our understanding of interpersonal behavior can be enlisted in the service of more effective and satisfying professional care.

In "The Doctor and the Patient: A Psychological Perspective," Steven Mentzer and Melvin Snyder describe important social psychological factors that enter into doctor–patient interactions, particularly with reference to their initial encounter in the diagnostic interview. Special attention is given to the role of self-disclosure, nonverbal communication, the reluctance to give bad news, and a variety of cognitive biases that may complicate diagnosis and doctor–patient rapport.

Howard Leventhal and Robert Hirschman focus on "Social Psychology and Prevention." The authors describe the traditional biomedical view of disease prevention, its positive features, and its limitations. They then review studies to identify underlying themes and problems biomedical research has yet to solve. In a concluding section, Leventhal and Hirschman emphasize how the institutionalized efforts in prevention can benefit from a personalized self-regulation orientation.

In recent years, it has become increasingly clear that people pursuing health care careers such as doctors, nurses, and social workers face emotionally charged contacts with their clients. As Christina Maslach and Susan Jackson spell out in "Burnout in Health Professions: A Social Psychological Analysis," this emotional stress can lead to a syndrome of emotional exhaustion, depersonalization, and reduced personal accomplishment. The resulting state can impair professionals' performance and the effectiveness of the health care organization in which they work and, of course, their relationships with their needy clients. In this chapter the authors discuss their measure of burnout and the factors that facilitate its development. Special attention is given to features of the situation and social psychological processes that contribute to the burnout phenomenon. In a final section, the authors describe ways that health care professionals may cope effectively with burnout.

Part IV brings a social psychological orientation to its most general domain—the issue of the impact of social structures on the health and illness of individuals living within them. The contributors explore pieces of the vast question of whether and in what ways social planners should create environments that maximize physical well-being.

In "Social Support, Interpersonal Relations, and Health: Benefits and Liabilities," the first chapter in this part, Jerry Suls offers an analysis of the effects of social support on health outcomes. Working from the social psychological literature, Suls argues that there has been a tendency to emphasize the positive aspects of informal social supports, but the potentially harmful effects of being firmly implanted in a social network have been overlooked.

Andrew Baum, Wallace Deckel, and Robert Gatchel, in "Environmental Stress and Health: Is There a Relationship?" are concerned with crowding and noise and their impacts on health. The authors review empirical evidence linking these environmental stressors to aversive psychological and physiological outcomes. The current popularity of designing social systems to minimize noise and crowding is questioned by the authors, as they point to considerable ambiguity in the existing data.

In "Healthy, Wealthy, and Wise? Health Care Provision for the Elderly from a Psychological Perspective," Robert Kastenbaum discusses three widely held lethal assumptions regarding health care of the aged and social policies that adversely affect the elderly. He then goes on to consider what attitudes and actions by individuals, social organizations, and society at large could improve the health and lives of the aged, and how the social scientist can be of practical assistance.

As mentioned earlier, we selected topics, data, and ideas that would hopefully generate interest in pursuing the full-scale development of medical social psychology. Inevitably, this selectivity involved a certain degree of arbitrariness, both in our typology of four areas of concentration and in the assignment and ordering of chapters to and within these areas. Our typology was created for heuristic value and to impart a sense of coherence, but we do not intend the categories to be viewed either as rigid or as mutually exclusive. Indeed, most of the entries in any one section have numerous implications for contributors in other sections. When readily apparent, these links among chapters have been made explicit. Medical social psychology will fulfill its potential only when full use is made within each area of material generated by the other approaches. That is, the integration of personality research will enrich our understanding of information-processing strategies; work on improving professional–patient relationships will benefit from an understanding of the health-related environmental features surrounding the relationships; and so forth. Communication among various research emphases is just as important as the dialogue between researchers and practitioners.

We would like to close this preface by acknowledging the encouragement and helpful advice of our publisher, Larry Erlbaum. Jeannette Pusz, Anne Ruth, and Irene Farruggio were of great assistance in typing, copying, and proofing portions of the manuscript. And finally, we would like to dedicate this book to our parents—Belle and Herbert Sanders, and Abraham and Leah Suls—for their constant love and nourishment of our intellectual curiosity.

Glenn S. Sanders
Jerry Suls

SOCIAL PSYCHOLOGY
OF
HEALTH AND ILLNESS

I

HEALTH-RELATED PERSONALITY TRAITS

1 The Hardy Personality: Toward a Social Psychology of Stress and Health

Suzanne C. Kobasa
University of Chicago

For social psychologists, the pioneer work on stressful life events and illness onset was provocative yet frustrating. Holmes and Rahe (e.g., Rahe, 1968) found environmental correlates of illness that identified disease as proper subject matter for social science. By demonstrating that the occurrence of life events that cause change and readjustment (e.g., job transfer, death of parent, marriage) increases the likelihood of one's falling sick, Holmes, Rahe, and their colleagues forced our conceptualization of disease beyond physiological and biochemical processes to psychological and sociological processes. But, given their epidemiological orientation, these early investigations never specified the nature of the psychosocial dimensions. Countless studies were done that simply counted the number of stressful life events that subjects checked off on a standardized list, while weighing each event in terms of its objective or consensually defined stressfulness weight. The total stress score was then significantly correlated with some indicator of illness like self-report of symptoms, time of hospitalization, or amount of medication requested. Nothing was said about those psychosocial variables that served either to strengthen or weaken the positive correlation. Individual differences in response to stress were ignored.

The second source of frustration was stress investigators' insistence on a fundamentally passive and reactive view of human behavior. Although attaching to an individual's life-event score a numerical likelihood of getting sick in the near future (e.g., a score above 300 means that one has an 80% chance of falling ill), stress reports portrayed persons as mere victims of the changes in their environment. Working with only some parts of Selye's model of the general adaptation response (Selye, 1956), Holmes (Holmes & Masuda, 1974) maintained that both positive and negative, minor and serious events would evoke:

"adaptive efforts by the human organism that are faulty in kind or duration, lower 'bodily resistance' and enhance the probability of disease occurrence [p. 68]." Left out of this formulation was Selye's recognition that there are some human organisms so constituted as to seek out stress without risk. For social psychologists, the pessimistic equation of stress with that which simply happens to and damages the person calls into question those psychological orientations that emphasize human initiative and resilience. A diversity of social psychological theories, from James (1911) on strenuousness, Fromm (1947) on the productive orientation, and Allport (1955) on propriate striving, through White (1959) on competence, to Bandura (1978) on self-efficacy and Brehm (1966) on reactance assume that persons create as well as react to the stressful life events in their lives and thrive on as well as tolerate stressful situations.

But the research on stress and illness also provided opportunities for the psychological researcher. To the social psychologist interested in personality, it offered a way of taking situational characteristics seriously. In the wake of the person-situation debate sparked by the publication of Mischel's (1968) *Personality and Assessment* and fueled by many personality and social psychologists, researchers found themselves looking for occasions in which they might observe individual predispositions for acting, thinking, and feeling in particular ways (person variables) in transaction with the components of the environment (situation variables). Stressful life events presented themselves as important and measurable situation variables.

According to Holmes and Rahe (1967), a life event can be called stressful if it causes change in, and demands readjustment of, an average person's normal routine. This definition was founded in their empirical demonstration that there is a general consensus in our culture about which particular life occurrences cause change and readjustment, and the degree to which they do so. Holmes and Rahe used the consensus data to develop a standardized list of stresses (the Schedule of Recent Life Events) and a set of stressfulness weights (the Social Readjustment Rating Scale). If a subject is given a total stress score of 300, for example, this means that he or she experienced either a few stresses that our culture would consider very severe (e.g., death of a parent, divorce, job demotion) or several stresses thought to be moderate by the majority (e.g., job transfer, marriage of a child, etc.). With this consensual or extrapersonal stress score in hand, the social personality psychologists can then turn the investigation to the characteristic psychological processes of the subject under study. The psychologist expands the research question from whether or not there is a link between stress and illness to how effectively individual predispositions either buffer or facilitate the impact of stressful life events. This elaborated research question contributes to two fields. It helps the effort within social psychology to look more closely at those characteristics relevant to interactions between individuals and their environment and fills one of the major gaps in the stress research enterprise.

A second opportunity provided by stress research to social psychologists was the chance to test some of their more optimistic interpretations of human functioning. Staying healthy in the face of stressful life events is easily seen as an indicator of adjustment and even optimal behavior. It is highly unlikely that one will be able, in the near future, to live a productive life in the full complexity of modern, urban, and technological society without encountering a number of stressful life events. Given this, one can argue that the determination of those characteristics that keep persons healthy under stress furthers the understanding of human development and well-being.

The identification of the determinants of stress resistance may also provide an immediate public service. The early work on stress and illness was quickly and loudly taken up by the popular media. Countless magazines, newspapers, and radio and television broadcasts proclaimed the message: Avoid stress if you want to stay healthy. This message was both discouraging (stress avoidance might include giving up positive changes like a job promotion) and unrealistic (one might postpone taking on a new mortgage, but how does one avoid a parent's death?). Reports on the existence of persons who stay healthy despite stress and descriptions of their distinguishing characteristics in a form that facilitates emulation should provide more optimistic and realistic information.

I began a series of studies in the mid-1970s in response to previous stress research and in the hope of advancing a personality and social psychology with both disciplinary and social relevance. This chapter summarizes the three stages through which this research has developed. The first stage was devoted to determining the personality characteristics of those who remained healthy despite recent stressful life events. The second and prospective stage established that these traits also guarded future health from the effects of stress. The third stage involved a consideration of how personality interacts with other stress-resistance resources (e.g., social support) to keep persons healthy. The results of these studies are also considered in terms of implications for the practice of social psychology. It is easy to argue that the enterprise of stress research has significantly benefited from the perspective of social psychologists. A more difficult, but equally interesting, question is what social psychology has gained as a discipline from its preoccupation with matters of health and illness. Some possible answers to this question are offered in closing.

THEORETICAL ORIENTATION

From a variety of psychosocial mediators relevant to the stress and illness connection—including perceived social supports (e.g., Cobb, 1976), early childhood experiences (e.g., Luborsky, Todd, & Katchen, 1973), and norms governing illness behavior (e.g., Mechanic & Volkart, 1961)—personality was selected for emphasis. The basic notion throughout the research has been that persons' general orientations toward life or characteristic interests and motivations would influence how any given stressful life event was interpreted and dealt with and, thereby, the event's ultimate impact on the physiological and biological organism. The personality emphasis has sought to determine the conscious psychological processes by which persons efficiently recognize and act on their situations. The research goal is thereby distinguishable from that of both early psychosomatic researchers intent on elaborating an unconscious psychodynamic structure associated with disease (e.g., Alexander, 1939) and from some researchers of Type A behavior pattern and coronary heart disease (see Carver & Humphries, Chapter 2, this volume) who draw a direct parallel between psychological and organic states (e.g., Zyzanski, Jenkins, Ryan, Flessas, & Everist, 1976).

An existential theory of personality (cf. Kobasa & Maddi, 1977) has been central in this research. This theory has emerged as more relevant to an interest in stress than more traditional theories of personality on at least two counts. Existentialism's emphasis on persons as beings-in-the-world (e.g., Heidegger, 1962; Sartre, 1956) who do not carry around a set of static internal traits, but rather continuously and dynamically construct personality through their actions, suits the personality-in-situation emphasis of the personality and stress question (cf. Mischel, 1973). Second, existentialism portrays life as always changing and therefore inevitably stressful. The mission of existentialists has been to describe how best to confront, utilize, and shape this life. Unfortunately, more space has been devoted to depicting how persons have failed in the struggle rather than succeeded (cf. Sartre, 1956). But it is recognized, on philosophical and psychological grounds, that persons can rise to the challenges of their environment and turn stressful life events into possibilities or opportunities for personal growth and benefit. Three existential concepts appear especially relevant to this optimistic orientation: commitment, control, and challenge. Together these comprise the personality style of stress resistance or hardiness.

Commitment is the ability to believe in the truth, importance, and interest value of who one is and what one is doing (cf. Maddi, 1967, 1970) and thereby the tendency to involve oneself fully in the many situations of life, including work, family, interpersonal relationships, and social institutions. Both the inner- and other-directed aspects of commitment are hypothesized to ward off the illness-provoking effects of stress. Commitment to self provides an overall sense of purpose that mitigates the perceived threat of any given stressful life event in a specific life area. Even if the stressful life event is a threat to one's view of self (e.g., an executive who sees himself as hardworking and productive in a job he is dedicated to is suddenly fired), commitment serves as a buffer. The committed person knows not only what he or she is involved in but also *why* the involvement was chosen. A stressful life event like being fired may negate the former but not the latter. With commitment comes the recognition of one's distinctive goals and priorities and the appreciation of one's ability to make decisions and hold values. This kind of self-understanding supports and revitalizes that internal structure and strength that White (1959) and other theorists (cf. Coelho, Hamburg, & Adams, 1974) deem essential for the accurate assessment and competent handling of any life situation.

But commitment is more than self-esteem or personal competence because it is based in a sense of community—what existentialists call being-with-others. Committed persons benefit from both the knowledge that they can turn to others in stressful times if they need to and the sense that others (both specific persons like a spouse and social groups like the customers one serves) are counting on their not giving up in times of great pressure. Committed persons have both the skill and the desire to cope successfully with stress. Antonovsky (1979) calls this sense of community or accountability to others the most fundamental interpersonal resource for successful coping with stress.

Control refers to the tendency to believe and act as if one can influence the course of events. Persons with control seek explanations for why something is happening not simply in terms of others' actions or fate but also with an emphasis on their own responsibility. The efficacy of control in warding off the harmful effects of stress has been suggested in a range of laboratory and field studies (e.g., Averill, 1973; Glass, Singer, & Friedman, 1969; Lefcourt, 1978; Rodin & Langer, 1977; Seligman, 1975; Weiss, 1971). Control allows persons to perceive many stressful life events as predictable consequences of their own activity and, thereby, as subject to their direction and manipulation. The executive who appreciates the role she has played in bringing about her recent job transfer also recognizes the influence she has over its effects on her work and family life. But even those events that a person is not likely to have caused (e.g., death of a parent) are also best confronted in a spirit of control. Averill (1973) concludes from his laboratory investigations that control involves the possession of a coping repertoire (i.e., a variety of effective behavioral responses to stressful life events). Moving closer to an existential perspective, Averill also identifies decisional and cognitive dimensions of control. In the face of any stressful life event, persons in control should benefit from both autonomy and intention. They feel capable of acting effectively on their own. Further, they can interpret and incorporate various sorts of events into an ongoing life plan and transform these events into something consistent and not so jarring to the organism.

Challenge is based on the belief that change, rather than stability, is the normative mode of life (cf. Berlyne, 1964; Csikszentmihalyi, 1975). From the perspective of challenge, much of the disruption associated with the occurrence of a stressful life event can be anticipated as an opportunity and incentive for personal growth, rather than a simple threat to security. Challenge leads persons to be catalysts in their environments and to practice responding to the unexpected. Because of their search for new and interesting experiences, persons who welcome challenge have explored their surroundings and know where to turn for resources to aid their coping with stress. Further, they are characterized by an openness or cognitive flexibility and tolerance of ambiguity. This allows them to integrate and appraise effectively the threat of even the most unexpected stressful life events (cf. Moss, 1973).

As the descriptions make clear, there are both similarities and differences among commitment, control, and challenge. They can be viewed as interlocking parts of an overall orientation or style of stress resistance—a style that can be termed *hardiness*. The overarching hypothesis examined in this chapter is that when life is stressful, hardiness decreases the number and severity of illness reports.

THE PERSONALITY DISTINCTIVENESS OF STRESSED BUT HEALTHY PERSONS

The Executive Study

The initial form of the personality and stress investigation (Kobasa, 1979) was retrospective: How are persons who have lived very stressful but healthy lives (high stress/low illness) different from those who have gotten sick under comparable stress (high stress/high illness)? In the hope of maximizing the chance of observing individuals high in stressful life events with a range of illness scores, this question was first directed to middle- and upper-level business executives.

Within 3 months of each other, two composite questionnaires were mailed to the management personnel of a public utility. The first included measures of stressful life events and illness symptoms having taken place over the previous 3 ½ years (from January, 1972 to July 1975), and the second provided measures of the three components of hardiness and a variety of demographic characteristics. Response rates for the two questionnaires were 81% and 86%, providing a final sample of 324 male executives with the following modal characteristics: 40 to 49 years of age, white, married with two children, on the middle-management level and having been there for more than 6 years, graduated from college, and Protestant, attending services very or fairly often. Those 86 executives above the median score for total stress and below the median score for total illness made up the high stress/low illness group. High stress/high illness executives (n = 75) showed scores above the median for both stress and illness. Discriminant function analysis determined which of the personality and demographic variables measured in the second questionnaire significantly discriminated between the two kinds of executives. To insure the generalizability of results, the procedure was first run on 40 cases from each of the groups and then cross-validated on the remaining "holdout sample."

The measure of stress was an adaptation of the familiar Holmes and Rahe (1967) Schedule of Recent Life Events. The original schedule lists numerous positive (e.g., job promotion), negative (e.g., illness of family member), frequent (e.g., minor traffic violation), and rare (e.g., death of a child) occurrences, with a stressfulness weight based on the consensus of Holmes' and Rahe's numerous judges provided for each event. In evaluating this test, stress investigators (e.g., Dohrenwend, Krasnoff, Askenasy, & Dohrenwend, 1978; Hough, Fairbank, & Garcia, 1976) appear to agree on the problem of its occasional ambiguity and the need to supplement it with events peculiar to the distinctive population under study (Holmes and Rahe did most of their early work with U.S. Navy personnel). For the executive testing, ambiguous items were deleted or replaced by less ambiguous versions (e.g., "change in financial state" was changed to "improvement in financial state" and "worsening of financial condition"), and 15 new life events were added on the basis of pilot administration with management personnel of the utility company not subsequently used as subjects. Some stress investigators (e.g., Johnson & Sarason, 1978) have also advocated the replacement of the consensus weights for stress items by idiosyncratic, subjective weights. However, the opposite view was adopted in this study. As Dohrenwend et al. (1978) have pointed out, subjective weights represent the confusing combination of the effects of environmental changes, the stressed individual's personality and other predispositions, and his or her evaluation of the consequences of the stressful event. It was more advantageous, for the purposes of this study, to determine the effects of consensually defined stressfulness of events separately from the idiosyncratic effects of personality dispositions on health and illness and, thereby, obtain both independent person and situation effects.

Illness scores were obtained through the Seriousness of Illness Survey (Wyler, Masuda, & Holmes, 1971), a self-report checklist of 126 commonly recognized physical and mental diseases. In the development of this instrument, a general severity weight for each disorder was obtained by asking a large sample of physicians and laypersons to rate each of them. Their ratings reflect prognosis, threat to life, duration, and degree of disability and discomfort. A highly significant mean rank order correlation was found among the various samples, and a system of weights was accordingly constructed.

Both the Wyler et al. illness scale and the Schedule of Recent Life Events have been frequent tools in stress studies. They have, in fact, provided much of the basis for the claim by the popular media that stress causes illness (cf. Wolfe, 1972). But these two scales have also provided extremely variable stress and illness scores with standard deviations as large as eight times the size of the mean. The range of correlations obtained in bringing the two scales together has also been very wide, with the majority of correlations falling below .30, and frequently around .12 (cf. Rabkin & Struening, 1976). These results suggest some association between stressful life events and illness onset. But they also indicate that there are subjects with high stress scores who are not getting sick, and they provide questions about what other sorts of variables explain illness variance.

The composite questionnaire designed to assess the possible distinctiveness of the high stress/low illness executives contained four standardized and two newly constructed personality instruments, as well as questions about demographic characteristics including age, job level, and time at job level.

The *commitment* dimension of hardiness was measured through the Alienation Test (Maddi, Kobasa, & Hoover, 1979). This test yields negative indicators of commitment (i.e., alienation scores) in five areas of functioning (work, social institutions, family, interpersonal relationships, and self). Sample items from the Alienation Test are: "I try to avoid close relationships with people so that I will not be obligated to them," "I long for a simple life in which body needs are the most important things and decisions don't have to be made," and "I find it hard to believe people who actually feel that the work they perform is of value to society."

The *control* dimension was measured negatively through the Internal–External Locus of Control scale (Rotter, Seeman, & Liverant, 1962) and the Powerlessness (vs. Personal Control) and Nihilism (vs. Meaningfulness) scales of the Alienation Test (Maddi et al., 1979). It was measured positively through the Achievement scale of the Personality Research Form (Jackson, 1974). Sample control items include: "No matter how hard you work, you never really seem to reach your goals" (powerlessness), "Most of life is wasted in meaningless activity" (nihilism), and "I often set goals that are very difficult to reach" (achievement).

The *challenge* dimension was measured negatively through the Vegetativeness (vs. Vigorousness) and Adventurousness (vs. Responsibility) scales of the Alienation Test (Maddi et al., 1979), the Security Orientation scale of the California Life Goals Evaluation Schedules (Hahn, 1966), and the Cognitive Structure scale of the Jackson test (1974). Challenge was measured positively through the preference for Interesting Experiences scale of the Hahn test (1966) and the Endurance scale of the Jackson form (1974). Sample challenge items include: "I find it difficult to imagine enthusiasm concerning work" (vegetativeness), "I don't like situations that are uncertain" (cognitive structure), "A satisfying life is a series of problems; when one is solved, one moves on to the next problem" (interesting experiences), and "If I want an answer to a certain question, I sometimes look for it for days" (endurance).

Stress scores ranged from 0 to 2239, with a mean of 399 and a standard deviation of 162. Illness scores had a low of 0 and a high of 6900, with a mean of 913 and a standard deviation of 1115. A Pearson product moment correlation of .24 ($p < .025$) was obtained between the total stress and total illness scores, a figure consistent with that in most stress reports (Rabkin & Struening, 1976).

Neither analysis of unweighted stress events and illnesses nor canonical correlations of selected stresses with selected illnesses significantly improved the correlation. A sizable group of executives scored above the median stress score of 306 and below the median illness score of 550.

Discriminant function analysis established that the high stress/low illness executives are significantly different from the high stress/high illness subjects in hardiness (see Table 1.1). Demographic characteristics, however, failed to provide any discrimination between the two groups. Taking into account those variables that make the greatest contribution to the discriminant equation and that produce significant mean differences between the groups, the high stress/low illness executives are distinguished by their commitment to self, their control (indexed by an internal locus of control and a sense of meaningfulness), and their challenge (indexed by their sense of vigorousness). The intercorrelations among these variables are significant and in the expected direction, supporting the conceptualization of hardiness as a style of interlocking parts. A few indices of hardiness contribute to the discriminant equation without yielding significant group mean differences. For at least one of these three, the scale employed may

TABLE 1.1
Differences Between High Stress/Low Illness[a] and High Stress/High Illness Executives[a]

Variable	*High Stress/ Low Illness*		*High Stress/ High Illness*		*t*	*Standardized Discriminant Function Coefficient*
	M	*SD*	*M*	*SD*	*Value*	
Commitment						
Alienation from self	102.35	117.24	219.15	185.77	3.36[b]	1.04
Alienation from work	181.67	122.04	223.73	175.09	1.22	.43
Control						
Nihilism	196.05	133.61	281.02	169.86	2.49[b]	.73
External locus of control	5.92	4.10	7.90	4.61	2.03[c]	.22
Powerlessness	301.15	188.93	388.47	188.44	2.11[c]	—
Challenge						
Vegetativeness	155.50	140.24	216.27	160.94	1.98[c]	.99
Security	21.11	6.33	22.19	8.60	0.34	.35
Cognitive structure	13.25	2.81	14.10	2.85	1.10	.21

Note: For all variables, the higher the number, the greater the degree of the variable observed and the *weaker* the hardiness. A subject's alienation scores have a possible range of 0 to 1200. Nihilism, powerlessness, and vegetativeness may range from 0 to 1500. External locus has a low of 0 and an upper limit of 23. Security may range from 0 to 60. Cognitive structure may have a minimum value of 0 and a maximum of 20.

[a] $n = 40$.

[b] $p < .05$.

[c] $p < .01$.

not be clearly measuring the intended component of hardiness. Cognitive structure does not correlate with its companion challenge scales, nor does it significantly correlate with any but one of the other hardiness indices. Although it is risky to interpret the coefficients of this and the other weak variables, it is important to note that the direction of difference is in general consistent with the hypothesis concerning hardiness as an insulation against illness.

As a check on the generalizability of the findings, the unstandardized discriminant coefficients were applied to the raw data of the holdout cases showing that 35 executives (77%) with high stress/low illness scores and 21 executives (60%) with high stress/high illness scores were correctly classified ($p < .05$).

Hardiness in Other Groups

This investigator found hardiness to be important in the stress resistance of other groups as well. One hundred and fifty-seven male general practice lawyers completed stress, illness, and personality instruments (with the exception of challenge scales) similar to those used in the executive study (Kobasa, 1981). In addition, lawyers filled out a checklist of strain symptoms. This was a list of 16 physical and mental symptoms commonly associate with stress reactions (e.g., difficulty concentrating, palpitations, change in gastrointestional peristalsis, and trouble sleeping). Although lawyers showed no correlation between stressful life events and the diagnosable illnesses of the Wyler et al. scale (1971), they did manifest a significant association between stress and strain symptoms ($r = .29$, $p < .001$). But this association is in turn significantly mitigated by hardiness. Although lawyers' strain scores are increased by stressful life events, they are decreased by the personality characteristics of commitment and control. In a regression analysis of strain, personality produces a significant change in the R^2 ($F = 49.08$, $p < .001$) above and beyond that contributed by stressful life events alone.

Both the executive and lawyer projects were done with male samples. To test the generalizability of hardiness and stress resistance to women, a group of 100 gynecology outpatients—the majority being white, 25 to 35 years of age, middle class, employed full time, and married—were tested on stress, psychiatric symptomatology as indexed by the Hopkins Symptom Checklist (Derogatis, Lipman, Rickels, Uhlenhuth, & Covi, 1974), and personality (Kobasa & Hill, 1981). Those 40 women classified as high in stress but low in psychiatric symptoms (depression, anxiety, obsessive compulsiveness, somatization, and interpersonal sensitivity) reported significantly more commitment to work, family, and self, more personal control, and more of the vigor of challenge than the 60 women high on both stressful life events and psychiatric symptomatology.

Other investigators, working with similar psychological constructs, provide comparable results. Johnson and Sarason (1978) obtained from their college student subjects retrospective measures of stressful life events, depression, anxiety, and internal versus external locus of control. They found that students believing in an internal locus of control showed a lower correlation between stressful life events and illness than did subjects who reported an external orientation. In another study, Smith, Johnson, and Sarason (1978) found that only students low in sensation seeking showed a significant correlation between the number of stressful events experienced and a measure of neuroticism. The locus of control and sensation-seeking findings parallel Kobasa's emphasis on control and challenge, respectively.

PERSONALITY, STRESS, AND FUTURE HEALTH

All of the aforementioned studies employed retrospective designs, so it is possible that hardiness scores result from, rather than promote, health under stress. An executive may be so impressed by his ability to go through 3 ½ years of stressful life events and stay relatively symptomfree that he now presents himself as committed, in control, and interested in challenge. Even more likely, the executive who has suffered both high stress and high illness and has therefore realized a blow to his self-understanding may respond to a personality questionnaire in a manner that reflects his psychological debilitation. Presumably, according to this alternative explanation, he was not alienated, powerless, and uninterested in challenge before his illnesses occurred. Certainly, one would expect some change in personality as a result of an experience like a heart attack or cancer. But it is crucial for the stress, personality, and illness health model employed in this research to maintain that some significant absence of hardiness characterized the individual executive *before* he confronted the stressful events of his life and subsequently became ill.

Only a partial and tentative empirical answer to this criticism is found in the retrospective data. If it is the case that undergoing illness in the wake of a number of serious stressful life events alters an executive's personality so as to lessen hardiness, then one would predict that illness following only low levels of stress would debilitate self-evaluation even further, producing even weaker commitment, control, and challenge. However, those low stress/high illness executives show personality scores midway between those of the high stress/low illness and high stress/high illness groups (Kobasa, 1979). Their lower scores on alienation from self, nihilism, external locus of control, and vegetativeness that distinguish them from the high stress/high illness cases suggest that personality questionnaire responses indicative of lack of hardiness are not merely a response to illness.

An even better answer to the problem of the chronological status of personality was provided in a prospective extension of the executive study described earlier (Kobasa, Maddi, & Kahn, 1982). Two hundred and fifty-nine executives from whom stress, personality, and illness data had been collected in 1975 provided yearly stress and illness reports for the following 2 years. In the later administration, executives completed the same measures of stressful life events and illness symptoms used at the beginning of the research. Throughout, subjects provided good response rates (80% for the 1976 data collection and 78% for that in 1977). On demographic characteristics, including age, marital status, ethnic ties, job level, and length of time at job level, the final sample of 259 closely resembled the initial pool of all of the management personnel at the utility company.

The research period between the retrospective study and the initiation of the prospective testing was given to the construction of a better measure of hardiness. Although the majority of the scales used to index hardiness served to distinguish the high stress/low illness executives, their administration was excessively time consuming. It was decided to create a shorter version of the personality composite for use in any future personality testing as well as any further analysis of already collected data. Those scales that had proven to be the most effective in discriminating between high stress/low illness and high stress/high illness subjects and that were, in interaction with stressful life event scores, the best predictors of illness across the whole executive group were included in the composite. Alienation from Self and Alienation from Work from the Alienation Test (Maddi et al., 1979) were selected as negative indicators of commitment. The dimension of control was also measured negatively through the Internal External locus of Control scale (Rotter et al., 1962) and the Powerlessness scale of the Alienation Test (Maddi et al., 1979). Finally, challenge was measured negatively by the Security scale of the California Life Goals Evaluation Schedule (Hahn, 1966). The intercorrelations among the five chosen scales were found to be significant and in the expected direction. In a principal components factor analysis, a first factor (accounting for 46.5% of the variance) emerges that is interpretable as hardiness. To provide a single personality hardines score for each executive, *z* scores were computed for the five measures. As the challenge dimension was indexed by only one scale (Security), its scores were doubled. This weighted security score was added to the other four scores. It is this composite hardiness that was evaluated in the prospective study as one of the contributors to future health.

Executives' illness scores from the later data collections were summed in such a way as to insure at least a month and up to 2 years time lag between personality self-reports and the onset of any illness. With this total illness as the dependent variable, an analysis of covariance was run. The hardiness composite and stressful life event reports from the time period concurrent with that of illness were entered as independent variables. Executives' illness scores from the retrospective study, covering 1972–1975, served as the covariate, which had the effect of controlling for prior illness. Hardiness was thereby put to the test of predicting *changes* in executives' stress-provoked illness scores.

TABLE 1.2
Analysis of Covariance on Illness Using a Prospective Estimate of Hardiness and a Concurrent Estimate of Stressful Life Events with Prior Illness Controlled

Classification	*Mean Illness*	*n*	*F*
High-stress executives			
High hardiness	552.89	65	
Low hardiness	1254.20	64	
Low-stress executives			
High hardiness	368.34	65	
Low hardiness	387.29	65	
Covariate: prior illness			65.71[a]
Main effect: stressful life events			13.17[a]
Main effect: hardiness			5.35[b]
Interaction: stress × hardiness			7.84[a]

[a] $p < .001$.
[b] $p < .02$.

Table 1.2 presents the results of this prospective analysis. Prior work is both confirmed and elaborated. Even when prior illness is controlled for, stressful life events are linked with an increase and hardiness with a decrease in illness reports. The significant stress and hardiness interaction demonstrates that it is especially crucial for one's health to be hardy when one is undergoing an intensely stressful time.

PERSONALITY AND OTHER STRESS-RESISTANCE RESOURCES

Although the personality style of hardiness has been emphasized in the research presented in this chapter, it has never been thought to be the only crucial stress-resistance resource (cf. Antonovsky, 1979). One would expect that a variety of psychosocial processes as well as sociocultural (e.g., income) and physiological (e.g., genetic background) factors either facilitate or hinder the debilitating effects of stress. Evidence exists for the separate effectiveness of each of the following in reducing the likelihood of stress-provoking illness: psychological needs for sensation and arousal seeking (e.g., Smith et al., 1978), private self-consciousness or attending to one's internal somatic and psychological processes (Mullen & Suls , 1982) , absence of Type A personality dimensions (e.g., Friedman, Rosenman, & Carroll, 1958), fit between person and work role (e.g., French, 1973), coping strategies (e.g., Lazarus & Cohen 1977), intelligence (e.g., Antonovsky & Bernstein, 1977), social supports (e.g., Gore, 1978), norms governing illness behavior (e.g., Mechanic & Volkart, 1961), marital status (Myers, Lindenthal, & Pepper, 1975), income (e.g., Luborsky et al., 1973), social class (e.g., Antonovsky, 1968), health practices such as exercise (e.g., Alterkrause & Wilmore, 1973), absence of certain diseases in one's blood relatives (e.g., Weiner, 1977), and immunological mechanisms (e.g., Burnet, 1971).

These stress-resistance resources represent only a partial listing of those factors found to be effective on their own, and one should expect a significant extension of this list in the near future. It is fair to say that the current preoccupation in the stress and illness enterprise is with the identification of mitigating variables. But very little of this work has been turned to the examination of several resistance resources in interaction with each other. It would appear truer to the nature of things to consider how a set of psychological, social, and constitutional factors work together to keep persons healthy under stress. Such a concern should also serve to clarify some of the points of dispute and ambiguity in the relevant research literature.

Personality and Constitutional Predisposition

What is actually specified about the physiological and biological organism in models that link stressful life events to illness onset varies from one investigator to another. But most assume that a person's basic constitution acts like a filter that shapes both the initial organismic response to stress and the eventual degree of physical breakdown in the aftermath (e.g., Rahe, 1974). At least two mechanisms have been suggested for this influence. One mechanism relates to the differential ability of various organs and systems to withstand the ravages of stress reactions. Individuals are thought to differ in the resilience of their various constitutional components. The theory (e.g., Selye, 1956) suggests that stress-provoked illness occurs in the weakest organ or system. The other proposed mechanism emphasizes the management of stress reactions by immunopotentiating and immunosuppressing processes (e.g., Pelletier, 1977). These processes cause some persons to react with excessive physiological intensity to stressful life events, others with an overly inhibited response that leaves the organism vulnerable to debilitation, and still others with an optimally energizing yet protective reaction. There is evidence for at least a partial genetic determination of these mechanisms (cf. Wiener, 1977). Among disorders where proof of a genetic link is strongest are peptic ulcer, essential hypertension, and various allergic reactions such as bronchial asthma. These illnesses run in families and occur in persons whose blood relations have extensive and varied illness histories and early deaths.

A measure of constitutional predisposition was obtained by the investigator and her co-workers from executives' medical records kept at their company

(Kobasa, Maddi, & Courington, 1981). In family medical histories, subjects have answered standardized questions about the kind and frequency of illnesses suffered by their natural parents. These histories were completed prior to the initiation of the stress research discussed in this chapter. A simple count was taken of those illnesses thought to indicate a kind of genetic frailty. For control purposes, the raw frequency was divided by the sum of parents' ages at the time the medical history form had been filled out. This measure of constitutional predisposition was certainly simple, minimal, and justified in light of the available literature (e.g., Weiner, 1977) on constitutional factors. This constitutional score was examined, alongside stressful life events for the period 1972–1975 and the hardiness composite, for its influence on illness reported in 1976 and 1977.

As a first step in the analysis of these data, correlations were run between various demographic characteristics, stressful life events, hardiness, and constitutional predispositions. The correlations between the demographic and independent variables were found to be low enough (on the average, .07) to insure that any effects of stress, personality, and constitution on illness cannot be explained away as merely reflective of demographics. In addition, stressful life events, hardiness, and constitutional predisposition scores are independent of each other. Stressful life events correlated .07 and .03 with hardiness and parents' illness, respectively. The correlation between hardiness and parents' illness was .06.

TABLE 1.3
Analysis of Variance on Illness Using Constitutional Predisposition and Prospective Estimates of Stressful Life Events and Hardiness as Predictors

Classification	*Mean Illness*	*n*	
High-stress executives			
High hardiness	652.54	65	
Low hardiness	976.89	65	
Low constitutional predisposition	663.85	60	
High constitutional predisposition	944.03	70	
Low-stress executives			
High hardiness	348.22	65	
Low hardiness	574.63	64	
Low constitutional predisposition	382.20	70	
High constitutional predisposition	553.49	59	
Main effect: stressful life events			5.84[a]
Main effect: hardiness			5.01[b]
Main effect: constitutional predisposition			3.77[c]

[a] $p < .01$.
[b] $p < .02$.
[c] $p < .05$.

Analysis of variance was used to evaluate the contribution of hardiness and constitutional predisposition to the stress-illness relationship. Table 1.3 presents the results of this analysis. Conforming to prediction, both stressful life events and constitutional predisposition increase illness, whereas personality-based hardiness decreases illness. Because only the main effects, and not the interaction terms, are significant, it would appear that hardiness, constitutional predisposition, and stressful life events have an additive impact on illness symptomatology.

Even those most biased in favor of environmental explanations of human doings should not be surprised that the kind of body one inherits has something to do with adulthood illness experience. In their concern with psychological factors and illness, stress investigators were not intent on replacing physiological and biological explanations of illness, but only on supplementing them.

Personality and Social Support

A stress-resistance resource of perhaps more interest to the social psychologist is social support. The available literature on social supports, stressful life events, and illness is extensive and varied, yet fairly characterized as solidly behind the idea that social support keeps persons healthy in times of stress. Looking at a variety of stressful life events in a wide range of environmental contexts, investigators have generally found that social supports lessen the likelihood of a number of different illnesses (see Cassell, 1976; Cobb, 1976 for reviews of this literature). Ambiguity does enter the picture as the reader searches for definitive statements about what social support is and how, exactly, it has its health-promoting effect.

For some investigators (e.g., Myers, Lindenthal, & Pepper, 1975), social support is defined from a sociological or structural perspective as a matter of social centrality versus social marginality. Those persons who are not integrated into the mainstream of their society by virtue of being too poor, not married, or without a job are said to be marginal (i.e., without social support). Other investigators (e.g., Caplan, 1972) take a more psychological perspective. For them, a subject can be said to have social support if he or she experiences good relations with other persons at work or in other social contexts. What is deemed minimal for social support to have its stress-resistance effect can also differ from study to study. Some investigators suggest that the mere presence of others is sufficient (e.g., Bovard, 1959) and that those who live alone are at greatest risk for disease in stressful times. Others require that social support has a certain quality and intensity before it can buffer stress. Lowenthal and Haven (1968), for example, have studied the importance of a single intimate relationship or a confidant for the aged and demonstrated its benefit over and above that of simple social interaction.

The variety in definition is matched in the literature by diversity in investigators' construals of the function of social support. Although neither their absolute nor relative importance has been established empirically, a number of behavioral consequences of social support have been suggested as keys to the health promotion associated with social support. When social support is present, at least one or more of the following are thought to be operative: (1) others actually pitch in and help to resolve the stressful situation; (2) others remind the stressed person of good health practices and reinforce their performance in stressful periods (e.g., drinking too much and skipping dinner may be harder for the executive living with spouse and children than it is for the executive living alone); (3) others offer the rewards of recognition and interpersonal closeness, which simply make one feel better psychologically. This diversity in explanatory links is generally tolerated, but it does turn into a debate around the issue of main versus interaction effects for social support. For some investigators, social support is technically a buffer against stressful life events. In other words, one expects to find its impact on health status only when it interacts with conditions of high stressful life events. Nuckolls, Cassel, and Kaplan (1972), for example, demonstrate that social supports alone have no influence on the number of pregnancy and childbirth complications suffered by women. But they find that the interaction of social support and stress explains a significant amount of illness variation: Among women who have been highly stressed, those without social support report three times the complications of the supported women. For other investigators, however, social support is less a buffer than a general good. Gore (1978), for example, reinterprets the Nuckolls et al. and other relevant data and presents her own to argue that social support has a main effect on stress. She finds that even those in low-stress conditions show an association between poor social support and symptomatology. For Gore, stressful life events and low social support have an additive effect on health status.

In light of the breadth of the research enterprise relevant to social support, as well as its ambiguity and conflict, this investigator hesitatingly entered the field. But before being able to worry about the implications of main versus interaction effects, I had to puzzle through a nagging suspicion that social support might not always be unconditionally positive, or even as harmlessly benign, as the literature suggested.

The social support literature provoked the same concern as that elicited by the early stress work in which individuals were assumed to be passive victims of their environments without the capability of withstanding stresses on their own. The social support literature offered a way of understanding how persons might not fall ill in the wake of stressful life events but this is an approach paved by other things or persons and not the stressed individuals themselves. From the social support perspective, one could stay healthy under stress as long as one had other persons to take care of him or her, or sufficient middle-class credentials.

There appeared to be little room or need in this model for individuals' exercise of control, a personal sense of commitment, or an autonomous pursuit of challenge. In fact, those aspects of social support, like the care of concerned others thought to be so helpful, might actually hinder the exercise of hardiness. A student, for example, struggling with the pressures of getting out graduate school applications at a time of exams and deadlines for course papers may be prevented from keeping her life situation engaging, challenging, and under control by an attractive and cohesive student peer group, which encourages her to not worry so much about academic matters and to take some time off to join them for a weekend in the country. A similar threat may be posed by the family of an executive. A husband's encouragement simply to be content with a family that will always love her may deflate the hardiness needed at a time when extra hours have to be put in at work if the company is to get the contract it wants and if the executive is to obtain the promotion and salary increases she wants (see Suls, Chapter 9, this volume, for an extended discussion of potential difficulties posed by social support).

Personality and Social Support Among Lawyers. The results of the previously discussed lawyer study confirmed this investigator's suspicions (Kobasa, 1981). The 157 lawyers were asked simply to list all of those persons with whom they talk over their stressful work experiences (e.g., spouse, close friend, mentor, another lawyer, etc.). This number was entered into a regression analysis along with scores for stressful life events, the personality characteristic of commitment, and two other hypothesized resistance resources (coping techniques and physical exercise) as independent variables. As discussed earlier in this chapter, the dependent variable was strain symptomatology. In line with previous results, stressful life events were found to increase strain, whereas commitment was observed to decrease it. Social support, however, had only a barely significant impact on strain after the effects of stressful life events and personality are taken into account and an impact opposite to that suggested by the social support literature. The more persons lawyers talked with about work stress, the greater their strain. To explain this finding, correlations of the social support measure with other variables were examined. Most revealing was its association with a set of coping techniques that have been dubbed *regressive coping* (cf. Maddi, 1980). The number of persons lawyers talk with is positively correlated with a tendency to handle stressful life events through behaviors like getting angry, drinking and smoking more, feeling apathetic, and physically withdrawing from the stressful situation.

Personality and Social Support Among Executives. The most recent executive data, the analysis of which has not yet been completed, suggest a more positive but also more complex role for social support. In this study, a measure of social support somewhat more refined and psychologically relevant than that used with lawyers was administered. The perceived effect of interactions with others, rather than their mere frequency, was tapped. During the latest monitoring of our executive subjects, designed to cover the period from 1977 to 1980, the Work Environment and Family Environment Scales (Moos, Insel, & Humphrey, 1974) were administered along with the usual stressful life event, illness, and hardiness measures. Most relevant for the social support question were the peer cohesion and staff support work scales and the cohesion and expressiveness family scales. The peer cohesion scale measures the degree to which co-workers are seen as friendly and supportive to each other; staff support indicates the extent to which one's superiors in the company are perceived as supportive; family cohesion refers to the degree to which family members are concerned about and committed to the family, as well as helpful and supportive to each other; and finally, the expressiveness scale assesses the degree to which family members are allowed and encouraged to act openly and to express their feelings directly. All of these perceived social support scales correlate somewhat with hardiness ($r = +.17$, $p < .10$ for combined family scales; $r = +.28$, $p < .05$ for work support), indicating that hardier persons tend to perceive their environments more positively. But these correlations by no means establish identity and allow consideration of the differential impact of hardiness and social support as resistance resources.

Three-way analyses of variance with stressful life events for 1977–1980, each of the environmental perception scales, and personality hardiness as independent variables (with illness for 1977–1980 as dependent) present a much more complicated picture of the function of social support than that suggested in the research literature. Two of these analyses, one involving a composite family environment measure (cohesion plus expressiveness) and the other involving the work staff support scale, are most provocative.

In the three-way analysis with perceived family support, main effects on illness are found for only stressful life events and hardiness and *not* for social support (see Table 1.4). But there are interaction effects. A significant two-way interaction between hardiness and family support establishes that being low in hardiness and at the same time perceiving high cohesiveness and expressiveness in one's family increases an executive's illness score. Further, a significant three-way interaction suggests that executives with high versus low stress be treated as two separate groups. Indeed, the executives who report the most symptomatology are those scoring high on family cohesiveness and expressiveness, high on stressful life events, and low on hardiness. From these results, one is justified in claiming that family support is positively related to health only when one is commenting on persons who are hardy and also under stress. For conditions characterized by low stressful life events and executives who are not committed, in control, and challenged, family support is negatively related to health.

The three-way analysis of variance involving perceived staff support at work presents social support as less dependent on personality for its role in stress

TABLE 1.4
Analysis of Variance on Illness Using Stressful Life Events, Hardiness, and Family Support as Predictors

Classification	*Mean Illness*	n
High Stress Executives		
Low hardiness, low family support	3617.78	27
Low hardiness, high family support	6028.43	14
High hardiness, low family support	2529.07	15
High hardiness, high family support	1028.17	18
Low Stress Executives		
Low hardiness, low family support	1878.14	21
Low hardiness, high family support	2699.25	16
High hardiness, low family support	655.67	18
High hardiness, high family support	1044.28	25
	Main effects	
	Stressful life events	10.92***
	Hardiness	19.22***
	Family support	1.41
	Interactions	
	Stress × Hardiness	2.52*
	Stress × Family Support	.02
	Hardiness × Family Support	4.67**
	Stress × Hardiness × Family	3.30*

*$P < .10$
**$P < .05$
***$P < .001$

resistance, but still only equivocally protective of health. Again, only stressful life events and hardiness have main effects on illness. Social support at work emerges as significant only in a two-way interaction between it and stressful life events. When stressful life events are high for executives, regardless of their hardiness scores, perceiving support from superiors or top management reduces symptomatology.

How does one explain and what can one systematically derive from these different social support findings? Given the preliminary nature of the analyses and the retrospective character of the data they are based on, only speculations can be offered. Family support, but not work support, is associated with a worsening of health status. This may have to do with the specific group under study and the particular nature of its stressful life experience. Throughout this research, at each data collection point, stresses arising in the work place (e.g., gaining a new supervisor, transfer, increase in workload) contributed more to the total stressful life event score than any other kind of stress. To feel alienated, without personal control, and threatened by change in the face of this kind of stress directly and severely limits how successfully one can cope but also to perceive one's family as cohesive and expressive lessens the likelihood that one will even try. If an executive is low on hardiness and finds his family situation unified, warm, and open, then he is more likely to give up the fight with demands of his job situation and simply stay home and let his family take care of him. The executive who is not able to perceive his family as such a safe and compelling refuge is more likely to keep persisting in the confrontation with job stress in an attempt to make this part of his life successful for him. In other words, taking advantage of family support during periods of high work stress stands a chance of making one even more alienated from work, out of control, and unchallenged by work changes than one already is.

The nature of executives' stress experience also clarifies why perceived support at work should have the opposite effect. The public utility under study has recently undergone and continues to face changes that are being orchestrated by the federal government and those at the very top at corporate headquarters on the east coast. Stressful life events reported by executives have been observed to increase in number and seriousness in the wake of some mandate like a job reevaluation program or a change in hiring policy that has been handed down from a source not directly influenced by our individual executive subjects. In times like these, it is crucial for the executive to feel that he is being supported by his immediate superiors. If he cannot agree with an item like "supervisors compliment a subordinate who does something well" or "supervisors really stand up for people," he may, in times of great ambiguity and change in the company, perform actions that only serve to increase his stressful life event score. For example, if an executive receives a vaguely worded order from New York to alter the composition of his work force, but gets no further specification from his boss as to how it should be implemented nor any assurance of support for his eventual decisions, he may engage in the kind of hiring and firing that only provokes additional stresses such as increases in arguments with subordinates and superiors. Regardless of an executive's basic level of hardiness, actions that display control, commitment, and challenge are hard to come by in situations where exactly what the company wants and is willing to give are left unclarified.

These social support results offer some directions for future stress research. Social support is apparently a multidimensional notion. The work with executives demonstrates the importance of distinguishing work from family support for understanding stress resistance. Other populations may require other types of distinctions. In studying how students cope with stressful life events at college, for example, one might want to allow for differential benefit from peer group support, family support, and support from faculty. The specification of what one means by social support also appears worthwhile. In the work reported here, some facilitating of health is related to perceived social support, but none at all to simple frequency of interactions with others. Social psychologists will probably be most interested in distinguishing between those more objective or structural indicators of social support like marital status or income and those of a primarily psychological nature like the enjoyment of an intimate relationship.

Another, and probably the most important, implication of the social support results is the need to be prepared for complexity as one begins to question the role of multiple resistance-resources. Not only is the interpretation of a variety of interactions between variables likely to be required by the data; but also, a struggle with the meaning and implications of even single variables may be called for. The findings presented here, for example, required a much closer look at what exactly was subsumed under the construct of stressful life events, than that originally intended in the research plan. In the introduction to this chapter, the author presented herself as a personality and social psychologist attracted to stressful life events as a way of taking situations seriously. To document a subject's stress score was conceived of as a way of identifying an environment for person variables to interact with. As this research has progressed, and the person variables relevant to stress-resistance have been elaborated, more has also had to be said and explained about situation variables. In raising questions like "Where exactly are the stressful life events that executives confront at work initiated?", these findings have promoted a complex, yet viable, person-in-context research enterprise.

THE MEASUREMENT OF ILLNESS IN HARDINESS STUDIES

A self-report of illness has served as the dependent variable in all of the studies reviewed. There are weaknesses in this approach. One might argue that because of reliance on self-reports, an investigator is only measuring a person's inclination to play the role of a sick person, to enact what Mechanic calls illness behavior. The self-report version of illness may be very different from what one might conclude about a subject's health status by looking at actual physiological or biological indicators like tissue damage or increased white cell count in the blood. This argument is especially provocative when hardiness is paired with health. Is self-report of health merely a reflection of hardiness? Do hardy people tend to not report illness because it conflicts with their self-image as persons who are vigorous and in control of their lives? It could be argued that hardy persons are often not healthy, but they fail to recall or they minimize their illness experiences.

One form of support for the biological or physiological validity of the self-report measure of illness is based on the *kinds* of illnesses that executives and other subjects report. Mild and vague symptoms like indigestion and headache might indeed be overlooked by hardy persons. But it seems unlikely that definite illnesses requiring medical diagnosis and care, such as heart attack, cancer, detached retina, and even hypertension, would be erroneously reported (Mechanic calls these "harder" data). An empirical study of 48 executives supports this claim. The records of medical examinations conducted on these men in the company's medical department on a yearly or more frequent basis were scrutinized. Illnesses reported in the charts were recorded blind and compared with those reported on questionnaires by the executives for the same time period. Complaints of the 12 minor illnesses noted on the self-report instruments (e.g., sore throat) are not typical reasons for a visit to a physician, and could not be validated against medical records. But with regard to the 114 illnesses not amenable to self-diagnosis or treatment (e.g., psoriasis, high blood pressure, peptic ulcer), agreement between self-report and physician's diagnosis ranged from 82% to 93%, with a mean of 89%.

In current work, yet another check on the validity of illness self-reports is being conducted. The medical laboratory results in all of the available medical records on business executives (n = 170) are being used to construct new illness scores. These more objective and specific indicators have been found to correlate with the self-report measures. Most notable are the significant associations between what the executives say about their illness episodes and their laboratory results for white blood cell count, glucose levels, protein bound iodine, red blood cell count, and hemoglobin and hematocrit levels. These and other laboratory tests will be used to construct alternative dependent variables in some future hardiness, stress, and illness studies. Yet other correlational findings show promise for these plans. Stressful life event scores are found to correlate with levels of cholesterol and triglicerides and white blood cell count, as well as laboratory measures not so commonly associated with stress like protein-bound iodine and creatine phosphokinese. The next step in this research is the examination of the extent to which hardiness mediates the new stress and illness associations.

DISCIPLINARY IMPLICATIONS OF STRESS AND HEALTH RESEARCH

The sociologist Richard Sennett, in his book *The Psychology of Society* (1977), took social psychologists to task for not living up to the demands of their subject matter. He accused them of turning away from intellectually and practically important questions about the relationship of the individual to society and of preoccupying themselves with tiny experimental studies and artificial realities like their laboratory small groups. At about the same time, social psychologists (e.g., Elms, 1975; Gergen, 1973; Hendrick, 1976; Schlenker, 1976) were involved in their own self-scrutiny. The status of social psychology as a science, its failure to produce practical knowledge, the ethical problems in its practice, the domination of the field by laboratory and experimental methodology, and the paucity of contemporary theoretical contributions were all held up for review and criticism.

As has been the case with most so-called crises in academic disciplines, responses to the critique of social psychology have been varied. Some social psychologists have treated it as an inevitable, yet transient, growing pain for the field; some have simply ignored it; and yet others appear to have taken it seriously enough to influence the way they conduct research. There are signs that the social psychologists interested in stress, health, and illness (e.g., Taylor, 1978) fall into this third group. It appears to be more than mere coincidence that there was an upsurge of interest among social psychologists in traditionally medical matters soon after the crisis unfolded.

The intellectual objective proposed by many of the major critics appears to have been furthered by the social psychology of health and illness. Among its contributions to a new and more relevant social psychology are the following:

1. An attempt to direct research toward the facilitation of an important human concern (i.e., staying or becoming healthy) (e.g., Cohen, Glass, & Phillips, 1978).
2. An emphasis on field rather than laboratory studies (e.g., Rodin & Langer, 1977).
3. A recognition of individual differences among subjects by virtue of their personal characteristics (e.g., Pennebaker & Skelton, 1978) as well as their social roles (e.g., Snyder & Mentzer, 1978).
4. The rejection of traditional causal methodology and the use of more interactional or process approaches to research (e.g , Lazarus, 1978).
5. Attempts at theoretical elaboration (e.g., Antonovsky, 1979) and interdisciplinary conceptualization (e.g., Adler & Stone, 1979).

The ways in which the author's research may be relevant to real human problems, supportive of a field approach, dependent on formal theorizing as well as data collection, and appreciative of a process or interactional approach to individual and situation variables have been referred to in this chapter. But what should be emphasized here is that as the research has progressed, these "big" questions about its relevance to social psychology as a discipline have loomed larger and larger. One currently ongoing project (Kobasa, 1980a) has demonstrated particularly well the value of Sennett's advice for social psychologists to go beyond the usual boundaries of their disciplines as they seek explanations and to take seriously the realities of the society in which their subjects exist. This project has involved the comparison of personality-based resistance across three professional groups. The finding of discrepancies in how personality functions to keep executives, lawyers, and U.S. Army officers healthy under stress has prevented that easy kind of interpretation that assumes the universality of any single social psychological process. These work-based differences in stress resistance have required the author to examine the diverse occupational and cultural contexts of each of the professional groups for explanations.

The basic procedures and results of the executive and lawyer studies have already been described. The same stress, personality, and illness tests were used with 75 U.S. Army captains and majors (Kobasa, 1980b). Like the other professionals, the officers were all male, and the majority were married, white, college-educated, and Protestant. Officers' total stress and illness reports showed a correlation of .58 ($p < .001$). Although this is an especially strong relationship, hardiness does buffer it. In a stepwise regression analysis, both stressful life events and hardiness emerge as significant predictors of illness. As in the other two studies of professions, stressful life events increase illness, and the commitment and control components of hardiness decrease it. But, distinctively for officers, the challenge component increases symptomatology.

Among the other discrepancies found in the stress, personality, and illness results for the three groups are Army officers' idiosyncratically powerful correlation between stress and illness and lawyers' failure to show any relationship at all between stress and diagnosable illness as indexed by the Wyler et al. (1971) scale. To explain these differences, one requires more than a model that portrays hardiness in interaction with discrete stressful life events. One has to conceive of a more organizationally complex environment that includes the distinctive structures and processes of the professions under study. In other words, one has to go beyond the usual tools of the social psychologist and take advantage of constructs like professional ideology, social climate, and role expectations usually left to other social scientists for explication.

Lawyers' failure to show diagnosable illness following stressful life events, for example, probably has something to do with an ideology, shared by lawyers and the public, that lawyers thrive under stress (cf. Kobasa, 1981). Anecdotes are told about how lawyers never get sick, live very long lives, and perform best in times of great change and when under a lot of pressure (Mayer, 1967). The well-documented traumatic socialization experience of law school (cf. Barry & Connelly, 1978) introduces the strenuous pace that will characterize the rest of the lawyer's professional life. To report illness in the face of stress is simply not expected of lawyers. This ideology may function in several ways to promote stress resistance. It may lead lawyers to postpone labeling their strain symptoms as illness for as long as possible or even to deny that they are suffering from an illness. But it may also serve to help lawyers develop stress-resistance resources like hardiness so that they can live up to the expectations of their profession. Law school, for example, may involve actual training for stress resistance embedded into a radical initiation. To the extent that the profession values this ideology, it may offer the practicing lawyer supports and rewards for this exercise of hardiness. This second line of speculation is supported by lawyers' average level of hardiness, which is higher than that of the other two groups.

Executives and Army officers appear to be in very different ideological contexts. The popular media have spun a new myth about executives, which portrays them as classic stress victims. Magazines carry stories about the up-and-coming executives who suffer heart attacks before the age of 50. The heads of corporations, recognizing the impossibility of reducing stress levels in today's market and economy, are equipping corporate headquarters with cardiac units close to executives' offices. Executives are given surprisingly little encouragement from both the public at large and their own profession to see stress as positive and themselves as capable of handling it. Instead of setting up structures and processes by which executives might develop stress-resistance resources, the gatekeepers of the profession appear to be resigned to the debilitation stress will cause and concerned only to set up mechanisms that will deal with the damage. This lack of ideological commitment to stress resistance within their profession may partially explain why executives show a correlation between stress and diagnosable illness and why lawyers do not.

But as the results presented in this chapter also indicate, the correlation between stress and illness for executives is not that strong, and many executives have developed significant levels of hardiness. The case of the Army officers appears to be more worrisome. Not only do they show extremely large stress and illness correlations, but they also show the lowest hardiness levels of the three professional groups. There is no reason to believe that the Army's distinctiveness is due only to the characteristic of individuals who self-select to join the profession. There are, in fact, things about the current Army's socialization practices, role expectations, and social climate that may hinder the development and practice of hardiness.

For example, since the Vietnam war and with the difficulties of the all volunteer force, the Army has suffered from what organizational theorists would call lack of clarity in professional goals and purpose. That clear sense of and appreciation of one's values and priorities, which have been found to be so crucial for keeping stressful life events in healthy perspective, may be hard to come by in the Army context. Given the still prevalent criticism of the role they play in society and the low recruitment rates to their profession associated with this, Army officers probably find it harder to feel a sense of commitment to self, work, and society than do lawyers and executives.

Even these brief speculations suggest the importance of a socially and culturally elaborated approach to stress resistance. However, looking at how personality interacts with characteristics of professions to keep persons healthy promises to do more than just provide a better understanding of stress and its consequences. It suggests how personality-based stress resistance may be developed in different work contexts. Further, it points out some inroads for intervention attempts by which the exercise of hardiness and, thereby, the enjoyment of health, might be facilitated.

One possible bridge between the conclusions drawn from completed studies and future research stems from intervention attempts derived from existential therapy. The number of practices specializing in therapy for stress management is currently proliferating. Most accept the conclusion that stress leads to illness and teach the patient various techniques of stress avoidance, from relaxation to meditation. Most fail to recognize the psychological, social, and cultural contexts in which stress is occurring. Existential psychotherapy offers an alternative: It seeks to improve persons' perceptions and understanding of themselves and their complex environments—to transform outlooks and actions such that clients become highly aware of, and able to influence, stressful events in their lives. A major goal in this therapy is the recognition of change as inevitable and as an opportunity for the growth of both individuals and societies.

REFERENCES

Adler, N. E., & Stone, G. C. Social science perspectives on the health system. In G. C. Stone, F. Cohen, & N. E. Adler and Associates (Eds.), *Health psychology: A handbook*. San Francisco: Jossey-Bass, 1979.

Alexander, F. Psychoanalytic study of a case of essential hypertension. *Psychosomatic Medicine*, 1939, *1*, 139–152.

Allport, G. W. *Becoming: Basic considerations for a psychology of personality*. New Haven: Yale University Press, 1955.

Altekruse, E. G., & Wilmore, J. H. Changes in blood chemistries following a controlled exercise program. *Journal of Occupational Medicine*, 1973, *15*, 110–113.

Antonovsky, A. Social class and the major cardiovascular diseases. *Journal of Chronic Diseases*, 1968, *21*, 65–106.

Antonovsky, A. *Health, stress, and coping*. San Francisco: Jossey-Bass, 1979.

Antonovsky, A., & Bernstein, J. Social class and infant mortality. *Social Science and Medicine*, 1977, *11*, 453–470.

Averill, J. R. Personal control over adversive stimuli and its relationship to stress. *Psychological Bulletin*, 1973, *80*, 286–303.

Bandura, A. The self system in reciprocal determinism. *American Psychologist*, 1978, *33*, 344–358.

Barry, K. H., & Connelly, P. A. Research on law students: An annotated bibliography. *American Bar Foundation Research Journal*, 1978, *4*, 751–804.

Berlyne, D. E. Novelty. *New Society*, 1964, *87*, 23–24.

Bovard, E. W. The effects of social stimuli on the response to stress. *Psychological Bulletin*, 1959, *66*, 267–277.

Brehm, J. W. *A theory of psychological reactance*. New York: Academic Press, 1966.

Burnet, M. *Genes, dreams, and realities*. New York: Basic Books, 1971.

Caplan, R. D. *Organizational stress and individual strain: A sociopsychological study of risk factors in coronary heart disease among administrators, engineers, and scientists*. Unpublished doctoral dissertation, University of Michigan, 1972.

Cassel, J. The contribution of social environment to host resistance. *American Journal of Epidemiology*, 1976, *104*, 107–123.

Cobb, S. Social support as a moderator of life stress. *Psychosomatic Medicine*, 1976, *38*, 300–314.

Coelho, G. V., Hamburg, D. A., & Adams, J. F. (Eds.). *Coping and adaptation*. New York: Basic Books, 1974.

Cohen, S., Glass, D., & Phillips, S. Environment and health. In H. E. Freeman, S. Levine, & L. G. Reeder (Eds.), *Handbook of medical sociology*. Englewood Cliffs, N.J.: Prentice-Hall, 1978.

Csikszentmihalyi, M. *Beyond boredom and anxiety*. San Francisco: Jossey-Bass, 1975.

Derogatis, L. R., Lipman, R. S., Rickels, K., Uhlenhuth, E. H., & Covi, L. The Hopkins Symptom Checklist (HSCL): A measure of primary symptom dimensions. In P. Pichot (Ed.), Psychological measurements in psychopharmacology. *Modern Problems in Pharmacopsychiatry* 7: 79–110. Basel: Karger, 1974.

Dohrenwend, B. S., Krasnoff, L., Askenasy, A. R., & Dohrenwend, B. P. Exemplification of a method for scaling life events: The PERI Life-Events Scale. *Journal of Health and Social Behavior,* 1978, *19,* 205–229.

Elms, A. The crisis of confidence in social psychology. *American Psychologist,* 1975, *30,* 967–976.

French, J. R. P., Jr. Person role fit. *Occupational Mental Health,* 1973, *3,* 15–20.

Friedman, M., Rosenman, R. H., & Carroll, V. Changes in the serum cholesterol and blood clotting time in men subjected to cyclic variation of occupational stress. *Circulation,* 1958, *17,* 852–861.

Fromm, E. *Man for himself.* New York: Holt, Rinehart, & Winston, 1947.

Gergen, K. J. Social psychology as history. *Journal of Personality and Social Psychology,* 1973, *26,* 309–320.

Glass, D. C., Singer, J. E., & Friedman, L. N. Psychic cost of adaptation to an environmental stressor. *Journal of Personality and Social Psychology,* 1969, *12,* 200–210.

Gore, S. The effect of social support in moderating the health consequences of unemployment. *Journal of Health and Social Behavior,* 1978, *19,* 157–165.

Hahn, M. E. *California Life Goals Evaluation Schedule.* Palo Alto, Cal.: Western Psychological Services, 1966.

Heidegger, M. *Being and time* (J. Macquarrie & E. S. Robinson, trans.). New York: Harper & Row, 1962.

Hendrick, C. Social psychology as history and as traditional science: An appraisal. *Personality and Social Psychology Bulletin,* 1976, *2,* 392–403.

Holmes, T. H., & Masuda, M. Life change and illness susceptibility. In B. S. Dohrenwend & B. P. Dohrenwend (Eds.), *Stressful Life events: Their nature and effects.* New York: Wiley, 1974.

Holmes, T. H., & Rahe, R. H. The Social Readjustment Rating Scale. *Journal of Psychosomatic Research,* 1967, *11,* 213–218.

Hough, R. L., Fairbank, D. T., & Garcia, A. M. Problems in the ratio measurement of life stress. *Journal of Health and Social Behavior,* 1976, *17,* 70–82.

Jackson, D. N. *Personality Research Form Manual.* Goshen, N.Y.: Research Psychologists Press, 1974.

James, W. The energies of men. In H. James, Jr. (Ed.), *Memories and studies.* New York: Longmans, Green, & Company, 1911.

Johnson, J. H., & Sarason, I. G. Life stress, depression and anxiety. Internal–external control as a moderator variable. *Journal of Psychosomatic Research,* 1978, *22,* 205–208.

Kobasa, S. C. Stressful life events, personality and health: An inquiry into hardiness. *Journal of Personality and Social Psychology,* 1979, *37,* 1–11.

Kobasa, S. C. *Personality and stress-resistance across professional groups.* Paper presented at the meeting of the American Psychological Association, Montreal, September 1980. (a)

Kobasa, S. C. *Stress-resistance among Army officers.* Unpublished manuscript, University of Chicago, 1980. (b)

Kobasa, S. C. *Commitment and coping in stress-resistance among lawyers. Journal of Personality and Social Psychology,* 1982, *42,* 707–717.

Kobasa, S. C., & Hill, L. *Women and stress-resistance.* Unpublished manuscrpit, University of Chicago, 1981.

Kobasa, S. C., & Maddi, S. R. Existential personality theory. In R. Corsini (Ed.), *Current personality theories.* Itasca, Ill.: T. F. Peacock, 1977.

Kobasa, S. C., Maddi, S. R., & Courington, S. *Personality and constitution as mediators in the stress-illness relationship. Journal of Health and Social Behavior,* 1981, *22,* 368–378.

Kobasa, S. C., Maddi, S. R., & Kahn, S. *Hardiness and health: A prospective study. Journal of Personality and Social Psychology,* 1982, *42,* 168–177.

Lazarus, R. S. A strategy for research on psychological and social factors in hypertension. *Journal of Human Stress,* 1978, *4,* 35–40.
Lazarus, R. S., & Cohen, J. B. Environmental stress. In J. Altman & J. F. Wohlwill (Eds.), *Human behavior and the environment: Current theory and research.* New York: Plenum Press, 1977.
Lefcourt, H. M. *Locus of control: Current trends in theory and research.* Hillsdale, N.J.: Lawrence Erlbaum Associates, 1978.
Lowenthal, M. F., & Haven, C. Interaction and adaptation: Intimacy as a critical variable. *American Sociological Review,* 1968, *33,* 20–30.
Luborsky, L., Todd, T. C., & Katchen, A. H. A self-administered social assets scale for predicting physical and psychological illness and health. *Journal of Psychosomatic Research,* 1973, *17,* 109–120.
Maddi, S. R. The existential neurosis. *Journal of Abnormal Psychology,* 1967, *72,* 311–325.
Maddi, S. R. The search for meaning. In M. Page (Ed.), *Nebraska Symposium on Motivation* (Vol. 18). Lincoln: University of Nebraska Press, 1970.
Maddi, S. R. *Personality as a resource in stress resistance.* Paper presented at the meeting of the American Psychological Association, Montreal, September 1980.
Maddi, S. R., Kobasa, S. C., & Hoover, M. An alienation test. *Journal of Humanistic Psychology,* 1979, *19,* 73–76.
Mayer, M. *The lawyers.* New York: Harper & Row, 1967.
Mechanic, D., & Volkart, E. Stress, illness behavior, and sick role. *American Sociological Review,* 1961, *26,* 51–58.
Mischel, W. *Personality and assessment.* New York: Wiley, 1968.
Mischel, W. Toward a cognitive social learning reconceptualization of personality. *Psychological Review,* 1973, *80,* 252–283.
Moos, R. H., Insel, P. M., & Humphrey, B. *Family, work and group environment scales manual.* Palo Alto, Cal.: Consulting Psychologists Press, 1974.
Moss, G. E. *Illness, immunity, and social interaction.* New York: Wiley, 1973.
Mullen, B., & Suls, J. "Know thyself": Stressful life changes and the ameliorative effect of private self-consciousness. *Journal of Experimental Social Psychology,* 1982, *18,* 43-55.
Myers, J., Lindenthal, J. J., & Pepper, M. P. Life events, social integration and psychiatric symptomatology. *Journal of Health and Social Behavior,* 1975, *16,* 121–127.
Nuckolls, K. B., Cassel, J., & Kaplan, B. H. Psychological assets, life crisis and the prognosis of pregnancy. *American Journal of Epidemiology,* 1972, *95,* 431–441.
Pelletier, K. R. *Mind as healer, mind as slayer.* New York: Delta, 1977.
Pennebaker, J. W., & Skelton, J. A. Psychological parameters of physical symptoms. *Personality and Social Psychology Bulletin,* 1978, *4,* 524–530.
Rabkin, J. G., & Struening, E. L. Life events, stress and illness. *Science,* 1976, *194,* 1013–1020.
Rahe, R. H. Life-change measurement as a predictor of illness. *Proceedings of the Royal Society of Medicine,* 1968, *61,* 1124–1126.
Rahe, R. H. The pathway between subjects' recent life changes and their near-future illness reports: Representative results and methodological issues. In B. S. Dohrenwend & B. P. Dohrenwend (Eds.), *Stressful life events: Their nature and effects.* New York: Wiley, 1974.
Rodin, J., & Langer, E. J. The effects of choice and enhanced personal responsibility for the aged: A field experiment in an institutional setting. *Journal of Personality and Social Psychology,* 1977, *34,* 191–198.
Rotter, J. B., Seeman, M., & Liverant, S. Internal vs. external locus of control of reinforcement: A major variable in behavior theory. In N. F. Washburne (Ed.), *Decisions, values, and groups.* London: Pergamon, 1962.
Sartre, J. P. *Being and nothingness* (H. Barnes, trans.). New York: Philosophical Library, 1956.
Schlenker, B. R. Social psychology as science: Another look. *Personality and Social Psychology Bulletin,* 1976, *2,* 418–420.

Seligman, M. E. P. *Helplessness*. San Francisco: Freeman, 1975.

Selye, H. *The stress of life*. New York: McGraw-Hill, 1956.

Sennett, R. (Ed.). *The psychology of society*. New York: Random House, 1977.

Smith, R. E., Johnson, J. H., & Sarason, I. G. Life change, the sensation seeking motive, and psychological distress. *Journal of Consulting and Clinical Psychology*, 1978, *46*, 348–349.

Snyder, M. L., & Mentzer, S. Social psychological perspectives on the physician's feelings and behavior. *Personality and Social Psychology Bulletin*, 1978, *4*, 541–547.

Taylor, S. E. A developing role for social psychology in medicine and medical practice. *Personality and Social Psychology Bulletin*, 1978, *4*, 515–523.

Weiner, H. *Psychobiology and human disease*. New York: Elsevier, 1977.

Weiss, J. M. Effects of coping behavior in different warning signal conditions on stress pathology in rats. *Journal of Comparative and Physiological Psychology*, 1971, *77*, 1–13.

White, R. W. Motivation reconsidered: The concept of competence. *Psychological Review*, 1959, *66*, 297–333.

Wolfe, S. W. Avoid sickness—How life changes affect your health. *Family Circle*, May 1972, pp. 30; 166–170.

Wyler, A. R., Masuda, M., & Holmes, T. H. Magnitude of life events and seriousness of illness. *Psychosomatic Medicine*, 1971, *33*, 115–122.

Zyzanski, S. J., Jenkins, C. D., Ryan, T. J., Flessas, A., & Everist, M. Psychological correlates of coronary angiographic findings. *Archives of Internal Medicine*, 1976, *136*, 1234–1237.

2 Social Psychology of the Type A Coronary-Prone Behavior Pattern

Charles S. Carver
Charlene Humphries
University of Miami

Coronary heart disease (CHD) is a leading cause of death in the United States. Attempts to understand and control this disease have traditionally focused on the relationship between CHD and risk factors such as advancing age, gender, elevated levels of blood cholesterol and fats, hypertension, cigarette smoking, diabetes mellitus, family history of heart disease, obesity, and physical inactivity (e.g., Brand, Rosenman, Scholtz, & Friedman, 1976; Dawber & Kannel, 1961). Each of these factors contributes to enhanced risk. However, even the best combination of these risk factors fails to identify most new cases of CHD before they occur (Jenkins, 1971). As a part of the broadening search for antecedents of CHD, researchers have begun to focus on a psychological/behavioral variable: the so-called Type A behavior pattern.

Pattern A has been described as an "action-emotion complex" that is characterized by a competitive achievement orientation, a sense of time urgency, and excessive hostility (Friedman, 1969; Rosenman, 1974). Early on, research established that these behavioral characteristics are overrepresented among coronary patients. Indeed, one subsequent study found that Type A's have twice the incidence of CHD as do Type B's, who are defined by the absence of the Type A pattern (Rosenman, Brand, Jenkins, Friedman, Straus, & Wurm, 1975). This difference in CHD risk has been demonstrated in numerous retrospective and prospective studies (see e.g., Blumenthal, Williams, Kong, Schlanberg, & Thompson, 1978; Jenkins, Rosenman, & Zyzanski, 1974; Rosenman, Friedman, Straus, Wurm, Jenkins, & Messinger, 1966; Rosenman et al., 1975). Most of this research has focused on men, but there is also evidence of an association of Pattern A with CHD among women (e.g., Bengtsson, 1973). Pattern A behavior is only one risk factor contributing to cardiovascular pathology, of course, but it is a risk factor that is clearly behavioral in nature. Thus, it has been of considerable interest to psychologists as well as medical practitioners.

MECHANISMS OF ASSOCIATION

The association of Pattern A with CHD is partially mediated by traditional risk factors. That is, Type A's have been found to have higher levels of blood cholesterol than do Type B's (Friedman & Rosenman, 1959; Rosenman & Friedman, 1974). Type A's also show more lability in blood pressure than do Type B's (e.g., Dembroski, MacDougall, Shields, Petitto, & Lushene, 1978; Manuck, Craft, & Gold, 1978), although Pattern A apparently is not related to chronic hypertension (e.g., Shekelle, Schoenberger, & Stamler, 1976). Nevertheless, even when statistical controls were introduced to partial out the effects of several traditional risk factors, at least one study still found a significant association between Pattern A and CHD (Rosenman et al., 1975). Thus the behavior pattern appears to constitute an independent risk factor.

How, then, does Pattern A increase the risk of CHD? As is discussed later in this chapter, there is now considerable evidence that Type A's respond to the social and psychological stresses of day-to-day life with stronger physiological reactions than do Type B's. By reacting vigorously and often to stress-inducing stimuli in their environments, Type A's thus may experience more frequent and more extended periods of high levels of sympathetic arousal. Repeated arousal of this "defense reaction"—a pattern of physiological changes that serves to mobilize the organism for action—has been found to be associated with cardiovascular and biochemical changes harmful to the heart and blood vessels (e.g., Charvat, Dell, & Folkow, 1964; Eliot, 1974; Herd, 1978; Obrist, 1976).

The release of catecholamines by nerve terminals and the adrenal medulla is a component of this stress response which has been directly related to heart disease. It is significant in this regard that Type A's have been shown to exhibit higher serum levels of the catecholamine norepinephrine than Type B's (Friedman, St. George, Byers, & Rosenman, 1960). They also have been found to excrete more epinephrine in response to competitive challenge (Friedman, Byers, Diamant, & Rosenman, 1975) and in response to competitive challenge combined with harassment (Glass, Krakoff, Contrada, Hilton, Kehoe, Mannucci, Collins, Snow, & Elting, 1980). Catecholamine secretion may potentiate CHD by facilitating atherosclerosis and by increasing the chances of acute clinical events in other ways. Accordingly, these processes are beginning to be investigated in more detail with regard to Pattern A.

Atherosclerosis

Atherosclerosis is the depositing of lipids in the lining of the coronary arteries that supply blood to the heart. Eventually this process results in arterial damage and occlusion. A number of studies have reported a positive relationship between

Type A behavior and severity of artery occlusion (Blumenthal et al., 1978; Frank, Heller, Kornfeld, Sporn, & Weiss, 1978), although some of these studies have not been successfully replicated (see Dimsdale, Hackett, Catanzano, & White, 1979; Dimsdale, Hackett, Hutter, Block, Catanzano, & White, 1978).

Moreover, Pattern A has also been associated in at least one study with the *progression* of atherosclerosis (Krantz, Sanmarco, Selvester, & Matthews, 1979). In this research, male coronary outpatients underwent repeated examinations for coronary occlusions over a 17-month period. Type A's were more likely than Type B's to show progression of the disease over this period. The authors cautioned, however, that the results might have been subject to biases (i.e., factors such as volunteering for the study) because the research was conducted with subjects already identified as diseased. Thus, it is desirable that these results be replicated in additional samples.

Underlying Mechanisms. Researchers have gone further than merely noting the relationship between Type A and atherosclerosis. They have also attempted to understand and explore some of the underlying mechanisms through which the behavior pattern results in arterial damage. Possible links between Pattern A, catecholamine release, and subsequent artery damage have received the most attention thus far.

The atherosclerosis process is currently believed to occur in the following way. A slight injury first occurs in the internal lining of the coronary artery. The body responds to injury with a buildup of smooth muscle cells and blood platelets in the area. Lipids then accumulate here, forming plaques. Eventually this tissue breaks down, perhaps closing the artery, and releasing thrombi composed of plaque material.

There is evidence that catecholamines aggravate almost all of these processes. Excitement of the heart through sympathetic nervous system input may increase the speed, force, and turbulence of blood flow, thereby contributing to an initial injury. Catecholamines may also break down fats in the body, contributing to higher levels of lipids, lipoproteins, and fats in the blood. Carlson, Levi, and Oro (1968) have found that this process occurs during periods of stress. High levels of circulating cholesterol have also been implicated as a cause of artery tissue damage (Ross & Harker, 1976). It is of some interest in this regard that Type A's have been found to exceed B's in the levels of both lipoproteins and cholesterol in their blood (Friedman & Rosenman, 1959). Elevated levels of serum cholesterol have even been found in Type A's as young as college age (Glass, 1977).

Blood clotting mechanisms that may play a role in atherosclerosis are also affected by catecholamines. Norepinephrine has been found to enhance the platelet-aggregation process (Davies & Reinert, 1965; Davis, 1974). It is therefore of some interest that Type A's have been shown to exhibit less of a decrease in platelet aggregation than Type B's after treadmill exercise (Simpson, Olewine, Jenkins, Ramsey, Zyzanski, Thomas, & Hames, 1974) and to experience more rapid blood clotting under stress (Rosenman & Friedman, 1974).

In addition to these physiological pathways to the development of CHD, there are also A-type behavioral characteristics that might influence the incidence or severity of CHD in other ways. Speculations regarding this possibility are presented in later sections of the chapter in which those behavioral characteristics are described in considerable detail.

ASSESSMENT

We have reviewed the evidence of an association between Pattern A and risk of CHD and some of the speculations regarding possible mechanisms by which this link is created. Let us now examine the behavior pattern itself. A very basic question is this: How are people categorized as Type A's or Type B's for purposes of research? The technique that was developed first, and which is still widely regarded as most valid, is referred to as the *structured interview*. This is a one-on-one interview—designed to be stressful—in which the subject is asked questions concerning his or her ambition, competitiveness, feelings of hostility, and time urgency (Friedman, 1969; Jenkins, Rosenman, & Friedman, 1968). In making classifications based on this interview, more weight is placed on the manner and tone of the response than on its actual content. Rapid, loud speech and explosive vocal intonations are some of the dimensions that distinguish Type A's from Type B's (Schucker & Jacobs, 1977). On the basis of this interview, individuals may be classified as fully developed A's, incompletely developed A's, incompletely developed B's, and fully developed B's. For the purposes of most epidemiological research, however, a simple A–B dichotomy is typically used.

The A–B classification deriving from the interview does not distinguish among the various Pattern A attributes. However, a factor analysis of interview data (Matthews, Glass, Rosenman, & Bortner, 1977) has revealed several relatively discrete factors including competitive drive, past achievement, nonjob achievement, impatience, and speed. These factors are consistent with the typical conception of the Type A style, except that hostility did not form a separate factor. Data pertaining to hostility loaded primarily on impatience or competitive drive.

A second method of assessment is the Jenkins Activity Survey for Health Prediction (JAS), a self-report questionnaire based on the questions used in the interview. Subjects are asked to judge to what extent they feel they exhibit certain A-type qualities and to judge how others perceive their behavior in that regard. The JAS yields a continuous distribution of scores. Research subjects are usually dichotomized by division at the median or by selection from the top and bottom portions of the distribution. Factor analyses of the JAS have yielded a "hard-driving and competitive" factor as well as a factor of "speed and impatience" (see Glass, 1977, Appendix A; Zyzanski & Jenkins, 1970). Hostility has failed to emerge from these analyses as a separate component, just as was the case in factor analyses of the interview (Matthews et al., 1977).

Interestingly, the JAS and the structured interview do not always show high levels of agreement in distinguishing Type A's from Type B's. The JAS is less accurate than the interview in classifying individuals who are not extreme Type A's or B's. Presumably this is because the stress-inducing character of the interview "pulls" Type-A behavior from susceptible individuals, thus distinguishing them more clearly from Type B's. The interview is also a better predictor of CHD morbidity and mortality than is the JAS. However, the JAS *does* predict mortality reliably. For this reason, and because it is much easier and cheaper to administer than is the interview, the JAS has been used extensively in research on Pattern A.

Other methods are occasionally used for assessing Pattern A, besides the two already discussed. These include the Gough Adjective Checklist, (Gough 1952), the Thurstone Temperament Schedule, (Thurstone, 1949) and Bortner's Short Rating Scale as a Potential Measure of Pattern A behavior (Bortner, 1969). However, as there has been little validation research done using these measures, they are less frequently used in research than the interview or the JAS.

BEHAVIORAL MANIFESTATIONS OF PATTERN A

Pattern A, as assessed by both the structured interview and the JAS, has repeatedly been found to be associated with risk of CHD. Until relatively recently, however, little more than anecdotal evidence had been gathered concerning whether people designated as Type A actually did behave in the ways ascribed to them. That is, are Type A's really more prone to aggression? Do they tend to be more competitively oriented than Type B's? Do they have a sense of time urgency? Indeed, are there other behavioral characteristics not part of the original conceptualization that distinguish Type A's from Type B's? A good deal of research has been aimed at answering these questions, beginning with the work of Glass and his associates (see Glass, 1977).

Hostility and Aggressiveness

Hostility and aggressiveness have been an integral part of Pattern A since its formulation. Indirect evidence of this type of behavior was obtained in a study in which Type A's became more irritable than Type B's when frustrated or blocked in an attempt to achieve a goal (Glass, Snyder, & Hollis, 1974, Experiment 3). In later research, Carver and Glass (1978) assessed the hostility component more directly. In this study, subjects were informed that their task was to teach another subject (actually a confederate of the experimenter) in a concept-formation task.

More specifically, the subject was to punish the other person for incorrect responses by administering shocks and to reward him for correct responses. The confederate actually received no shocks, but instead monitored the intensity chosen by the subject on each trial. The mean shock intensity chosen by the subject over trials served as the measure of aggression.

Prior to the bogus learning session, some participants were provoked by the confederate, who belittled their efforts to complete a task, which was actually insoluble within the time provided. Other participants in a control condition were not provoked. Provocation resulted in significant increases in aggression among Type A's but not among Type B's (Carver & Glass, 1978, Experiment 1). Further research (Carver & Glass, 1978, Experiment 2) revealed that overt provocation was not necessary to produce heightened aggressiveness among Type A's. The frustration generated by the insoluble task was sufficient by itself to produce a significant increase in aggression among Type A's. Type B's, in contrast, were quite indifferent to frustration.

It is important to note that in this research Type A's were not more aggressive than Type B's independent of experimental treatment. No A–B difference was found in the control condition in either experiment. This is one instance of a recurring finding in the validation research—that environmental circumstances, and specifically threats to the Type A's mastery of a situation, are instrumental in eliciting Pattern A behavior. In the absence of such circumstances, the Type A behaves no differently than does the Type B.

Time Urgency

Another component of Pattern A is a strong sense of time urgency. Type A's have been found to estimate that a time interval of 1 minute has elapsed sooner than do Type B's (Bortner & Rosenman, 1967; Burnam, Pennebaker, & Glass, 1975). Gastorf (1980) has reported a related finding. Type A's and Type B's were asked to appear for an experiment at a given time and place. Type A's appeared significantly earlier for their scheduled appointments than did Type B's.

This strong concern with time, and the characteristic impatience of the Type A, may indirectly influence other types of behavior. For example, Type A's perform more poorly than Type B's on tasks that require delayed responses (so-called DRL tasks). DRL tasks require the subject to wait a specified interval before responding to a stimulus. Reward is based on the ability to tolerate delay, because a premature response resets a timer and prevents reinforcement. In a study that made use of such a task (Glass et al., 1974), Type A's were found to receive fewer reinforcements than Type B's because they were unable to delay their responses to the stimulus. Consistent with this picture, during their sessions nearly 50% of the A's but only 12% of the B's displayed tense and hyperactive movements while waiting to respond.

Competitive Achievement Striving

The third component of the Type A pattern as originally defined is an exaggerated competitive achievement orientation. This component of Pattern A is often viewed as underlying the others. That is, the Type A's sense of time urgency may be seen as stemming from an attempt to accomplish more and more in less time, and the A's hostility appears to arise when an accomplishment has been thwarted.

Evidence for this achievement orientation among Type A's comes from a number of sources. In one study college students were asked to complete a series of arithmetic problems and were given either an explicit deadline or no deadline (Burnam et al., 1975). Type A's attempted more problems than did B's when there was no explicit deadline. The mention of a deadline, however, caused A's and B's to perform at the same high level. This finding suggests that Type A's do not need a salient deadline in order to work at their maximum capacity.

The relationship between Pattern A and traditional measures of achievement motivation has also been examined. Weak though significant relationships have been found between JAS scores and scores on the Edwards (1957) measure of achievement motivation (r's = .14 and .17 in two samples, see Glass, 1977). Another study found no significant relationship between Pattern A and TAT measures of need for achievement (Matthews & Saal, 1978). However, subjects in the latter study who were very high in achievement motivation but who had little fear of failure also were found to have very extreme Type A scores on the JAS.

It might be expected that having a psychological orientation toward achievement might result in greater *actual* achievements. There is, in fact, some evidence of this. Glass (1977) reported that Type A college students earned more honors than their Type B counterparts and that more A's than B's planned to attend graduate and professional schools. Moreover, a small but reliable relationship is typically found between Pattern A and educational attainment and occupational and socioeconomic status (Mettlin, 1976; Shekelle et al., 1976; Waldron, 1978; Waldron, Zyzanski, Shekelle, Jenkins, & Tannenbaum, 1977). More direct evidence of achievement comes from a study by Matthews, Helmreich, Beane, and Lucker (1980). These researchers found that Type A social scientists were cited more frequently in professional publications than their Type B counterparts. This presumably reflects either a greater output of work within a given period of time by Type A's or the production of work that is of particularly high quality.

In another study that bears on this issue, the A-type characteristics of incoming freshmen were related to their actual performance in their first semester of college (Ovcharchyn, Johnson, & Petzel, 1980). Pattern A was found to be significantly and positively related to grade point averages. Current credit hours taken and amount of responsibility outside of school were also significantly greater among Type A's than Type B's. Interestingly, although Type A's were more likely to increase their workload both in and out of school over the semester, they did not report feeling any more pressured in their schoolwork than did B's.

Although a good deal of research has established that Type A's are achievement oriented, less attention has been paid to the competitive aspect of that orientation. At least one study has examined this question, however, by pairing subjects in a mixed-motive zero-sum game (Van Egeren, 1979). Type A pairs were found to emit reliably more competitive responses in this situation than either Type B pairs or mixed pairs. Subjects in the study also had the opportunity to communicate with their partners. Type A pairs were found to send more competitive and antisocial messages and fewer cooperative or conciliatory messages than either Type B or mixed pairs.

The achievement orientation of Type A's also has implications for the strategies that they prefer to use in achieving their goals. Type A's have been found to prefer working alone on a stressful task (Dembroski & MacDougall, 1978) apparently because working alone provides the greatest control over the finished product. Prior to beginning the task, however, A's preferred to wait with other people rather than waiting alone. Presumably this was because waiting with others provides an opportunity to gain task-relevant information through social comparison.

This tendency to engage in social comparison can have other influences on behavior as well. In particular, consider the phenomenon known as social facilitation. It is widely known that the presence of another person often improves one's performances on simple tasks but impairs performances on complex tasks (see, e.g., Zajonc, 1965). It has been found that having either the motive or the opportunity to engage in social comparison with a coactor during task performance results in such effects (cf. Sanders, Baron, & Moore, 1978). If Type A's are particularly likely to engage in the social comparison process, they should also be especially susceptible to the facilitation effect.

This, indeed, seems to be the case. Gastorf, Suls, and Sanders (1980) have reported that when working on a simple task with a coactor who was either similar or superior to themselves, Type A's displayed enhanced performances, whereas B's did not. When the task was complex, the performances of Type A's (but not Type B's) were impaired by the presence of the coactor.

It is worthy of some additional note that Type A's were affected by the presence of coactors whether those coactors were portrayed as being similar to themselves or as superior. This appears to be yet another reflection of the Type A's competitive achievement orientation.

Research concerning the achievement orientation of Pattern A has been particularly prolific. And it has been particularly fruitful in the sense that the investigation has broadened to include phenomena that are only indirectly related to achievement per se. These phenomena themselves are quite interesting, however, and these studies have led to an awareness of a facet of Pattern A behavior that has important implications in its own right.

Symptom Suppression

One might expect the hard-driving achievement orientation of the Type A to be associated with the tendency to ignore or attempt to suppress subjective states that would tend to threaten one's performance. Fatigue, for example, is a condition that makes effective performance difficult and therefore threatens task mastery. The reasoning that Type A's might suppress their awareness of such states was investigated by Carver, Coleman, and Glass (1976). This study approached the question quite directly: Would Type A's suppress their fatigue in order to persist at a tiring but challenging treadmill-walking task? Each subject walked on a motorized treadmill at increasingly sharp angles of incline (cf. Balke, 1954; Balke, Grillo, Konecci, & Luft, 1954). The subject rated his fatigue every 2 minutes according to a labeled 11-point scale. Each subject walked until he felt he wished to go no farther. The maximum aerobic capacity of each subject (i.e., maximum rate of oxygen absorption) was later assessed by a running test. This allowed each subject's walking performance to be scored as a percentage of his maximum capacity.

Type A's and Type B's were not found to differ in physical characteristics such as percentage of body fat. However, Type A's expressed having significantly less fatigue than Type B's on each of the last four ratings before termination of walking. At the same time, the A's had pushed themselves to 91.4% of their aerobic capacity, whereas the B's had averaged only 82.8% of their capacities. Thus, Type A's reported less fatigue than B's but actually worked closer to the limits of their endurance.

Similar reasoning was examined in a field study of college football players (Carver, DeGregorio, & Gillis, 1981). In this study, coaches were asked to rate their players according to the degree to which they felt the players exerted themselves to their limits in practice and in actual games. No difference was found between Type A's and Type B's, except among those players who faced the greatest degree of challenge—playing while injured. Head coaches and assistant coaches alike reported that injured Type A players exerted themselves closer to their limits than injured Type B players.

Weidner and Matthews (1978) have extended this line of inquiry to a different kind of subjective experience. Subjects in their research were exposed to a series of noise bursts while attempting to perform a task. They were then asked to rate any physical symptoms they were experiencing in response to the noise. Some subjects were told that the task was finished. No difference between A's and B's was found in this condition. However, among subjects who believed that the task was not yet completed, Type A's reported fewer symptoms than did Type B's. Type A's thus apparently suppressed or ignored their symptoms in order to complete the task at hand. But when the task was perceived as completed, there was no longer a need to suppress the symptoms.

These various findings regarding symptom suppression have very straightforward implications for the link between Pattern A and CHD. If A's are less aware than B's of fatigue and other symptoms, perhaps Type A's are more likely than Type B's to drive themselves past normal points of exhaustion and thus to severely deplete their physical resources with greater consistency. Further, fatigue is the most common and earliest symptom of an impending heart attack (Greene, Moss, & Goldstein, 1974). By ignoring such symptoms, Type A's may wait longer to get help, leading to clinical events of greater severity than might otherwise be the case.

Attentional Style: Cognitive Implications. One important question regarding these various findings is whether Type A's are really less aware of intrusive, task-irrelevant stimuli or are simply denying their impact for purposes of public display. Matthews and Brunson (1979) have presented evidence in support of the position that Type A's actively suppress their attention to intrusive, task-irrelevant stimuli such as physical symptoms and are therefore actually less aware of them. More specifically, their findings (using research paradigms from cognitive psychology) indicate that when Type A's are engaged in a task that has been designated to be of central importance, they focus their attention on that task to the exclusion of peripheral stimuli or events. Thus, pain, fatigue, or other tasks or events perceived as being less important than the central task may be so excluded.

The difference between Type A's and Type B's in allocation of attention also has implications for other cognitive processes such as the formation and use of categories. As a person begins to form a mental representation of a category, the attributes that appear most frequently in category-relevant stimuli may be regarded as being central to the definition of that category. If (as is implied by the findings of Matthews & Brunson) Type A's restrict their attention to centrally important information, they may focus on the emerging central tendencies in an evolving category and correspondingly ignore less frequently occurring attributes. This means that the categories formed by Type A's should be characterized by relatively restrictive definitions. Type B's, who are less likely to ignore peripheral attributes, should form categories that have broader definitions, encompassing both frequent and infrequent attributes.

When asked to judge whether new stimuli fit the category, A's should then be expected to differ from B's in the following way: A's should be more confident than B's of the category membership of stimuli incorporating high-frequency attributes, and should be more confident of the *non*membership of stimuli incorporating lower-frequency attributes. This reasoning has been given support in research conducted recently by Humphries, Carver, and Neumann (in press). In addition, as is true of many studies of Pattern A behavior, the emergence of the A–B difference in this research was highly dependent on the presence of situational challenge. When subjects were simply informed that the study concerned people's responses to visual stimuli, there was no difference between groups. Reliable differences emerged only when the procedure was portrayed as part of a challenging intelligence test.

PATTERN A AND CONTROL

At several points in the preceding discussion we have noted the importance of situational challenge in eliciting Type A characteristics. We now take up this point more explicitly. The fact that some sort of situational challenge appears to be required in order for A-type behavior to emerge has led Glass (1977) to characterize Pattern A as being a response style that is aimed at gaining and maintaining control over important aspects of the environment. Type A's appear to desire to exercise personal control over the outcomes of their actions, and Pattern A behavior emerges when situational elements begin to threaten that control. The loss of time, for example, may be seen as a threat to control, resulting in a sense of time urgency. Frustration creates a threat to control, leading to aggression. But recent studies in several domains have provided even more direct support for the notion that control is very important to the Type A.

Much of his research stems from a line of reasoning developed to explain why persons who are exposed to uncontrollable outcomes sometimes attempt to reassert control and other times give up. Wortman and Brehm (1975) have argued that exposure to uncontrollable events threatens one's sense of control. If the threat is not strong enough to eliminate the perception of (potential) control, it induces a state of reactance (Brehm, 1966; Wicklund, 1974). The result is an attempt to reassert control, thereby removing the threat. If, however, the threat is so strong that the person believes control of the situation is truly lost, the result is a giving-up response, sometimes termed learned helplessness (cf. Seligman, 1975). Often the difference between these two states is determined by the length of the exposure to cues signifying lack of control. Short exposures constitute threat; longer exposures suggest that control has been lost.

Explaining these phenomena in terms of threats to one's sense of control has some interesting implications for Pattern A. If Type A's have greater interest in control than Type B's, they might therefore be expected to respond more strongly to the threat posed by an uncontrollable outcome. This has led Glass (1977; see also Glass & Carver, 1980) to propose that both reassertion and helplessness might be particularly strong among Type A's under the appropriate circumstances. Several studies have supported this reasoning.

Reassertion of Control

Three studies have examined reassertion of control among Type A's and Type B's after limited exposure to cues denoting the loss of control. Krantz and Glass (in Glass, 1977) exposed subjects to a pretreatment consisting of 12 bursts of

100-db noise. For some subjects this treatment could be escaped by pressing a lever, but other subjects could not escape the noise. All subjects were then asked to complete a reaction-time task, which included long intertrial intervals. Type A's typically perform quite poorly on this type of task, as they become impatient and inattentive between trials and respond more slowly once the stimulus appears. It was reasoned, however, that when motivated by exposure to an uncontrollable stressor, Type A's might take the opportunity to reassert their mastery of the situation by performing particularly well on a subsequent task. In this case, A's were expected to try to overcome their characteristic impatience, thus producing better performances on the reaction-time task. This reasoning was confirmed. Type A's exposed to the uncontrollable stressor (inescapable noise) exhibited shorter reaction times than did Type B's in the same condition. Type A's in the escapable noise condition displayed the usual pattern of longer reaction times than Type B's.

These findings were conceptually replicated in a second study (see Glass, 1977). In the first phase of this experiment, subjects were asked to solve two cognitive problems (taken from Hiroto & Seligman, 1975). In the control condition, veridical feedback was given to the subjects in their attempts to solve the problems. Other subjects received random feedback during the problem-solving session, which was intended to heighten their feelings of lack of control. The second phase of the study involved a DRL procedure on which, as mentioned earlier, Type A's tend to do more poorly than Type B's. Type A subjects exposed to veridical feedback did perform more poorly than comparable Type B's. However, exposure to uncontrollable feedback caused Type A's to exhibit superior performances. In contrast, the same manipulation led to performance decrements among Type B's.

Finally, Fazio, Cooper, Dayson, and Johnson (1981) gave subjects a proofreading task. This was the only task for half the subjects, but other subjects also worked on two additional tasks simultaneously. The extra demands imposed on the latter groups were expected to threaten their feelings of control of the situation. This, in turn, should have led to a reassertion response on the part of the Type A's. No A–B difference in accuracy on the proofreading task was found in either condition. Differences did occur, however, in speed of performance. When faced with multiple demands, Type A's corrected more lines than did Type B's in the same amount of time, a relationship that was reversed when only a single task was presented. The authors attributed the superior performance of the Type A's under multiple-demand conditions to an attempt to reassert control when threatened with its loss.

Reactance. If the eagerness of Type A's to reassert control when threatened with its loss truly represents a reactance phenomenon, then it would not be surprising if Type A's demonstrated strong reactance effects in more traditional reactance paradigms as well. One such paradigm is based on the notion that people resist attempts at coercive persuasion. The behavior of Type A's in such circumstances has been examined in at least two research projects (Carver, 1980; Snyder & Frankel, 1980). Although the patterns of results in these projects were not identical, both found that Type A's showed more resistance than did Type B's to the attempts of an external agent to change their opinions, consistent with the assumptions of reactance theory.

Helplessness

The results of all these studies underscore the importance that Type A's ascribe to control over significant aspects of the environment. They will try, if possible, to reassert control when it is threatened. But maintaining control is not always possible. If a stressor is truly uncontrollable, at some point the realization must come that control has been lost. One result of the perception that control has been irretrievably lost is a decrease in effort, known as helplessness. Based on the foregoing characterization of Pattern A, it might be expected that the realization of loss of control would affect Type A's more strongly than Type B's, leading to stronger helplessness effects. Several studies have investigated this possibility.

Krantz, Glass, and Snyder (1974) manipulated feelings of control by exposing subjects to either escapable or inescapable noise. This pretreatment is similar to one used in a study discussed earlier investigating reassertion. However, the study discussed earlier was intended merely to *threaten* the subject's control. The Krantz et al. (1974) procedure was intended to induce the perception that control was completely lost. To accomplish this, subjects were exposed to 35 bursts of noise, rather than the 12 used in the other study. Intensity of the noise was also varied in this experiment, with some subjects receiving a loud noise (105 db) and others hearing only moderately loud noise (78 db). Subjects were then asked to perform a different task in which it was now possible for all subjects to escape from or even completely avoid the noise bursts by emitting an appropriate response. A criterion of three consecutive escape/avoidance responses constituted the dependent measure. Greater helplessness would be indicated by a greater number of trials to criterion.

The results were somewhat more complex than expected. When the noise stressor was intense, Type A's in the inescapable noise condition did show greater helplessness effects than B's, taking longer to reach criterion than their counterparts in the escapable noise condition. When the noise stressor was less intense, however, Type A's did not display helplessness.[1]

---

[1]Our presentation of the findings of this and subsequent studies concerning helplessness is somewhat restricted by virtue of our focus on the behavior of Type A's. Type B's also displayed a response impairment in this study, but under conditions of *low* salience. Subsequent research by Brunson and Matthews (1981), discussed later in this section, provides grounds for viewing this effect as reflecting what Miller and Norman (1979) termed "pseudo-helplessness." See Brunson and Matthews (1981) for further elaboration of this point.

The finding that noise intensity influenced helplessness indicates the presence of a mediating factor. One possibility is that the uncontrollable stimuli in the two noise-intensity conditions varied in their salience. Glass (1977) has argued that when cues signifying loss of control are low in salience (e.g., the moderate noise condition) Type A's might be able to ignore suggestions that they are no longer in control. But, when such cues are high in salience (e.g., a highly intense stressor) it may no longer be possible to ignore the cues. The result, then, is helplessness. This explanation is wholly consistent with findings reviewed earlier that Type A's tend to suppress subjective symptom states (Carver et al., 1976; Weidner & Matthews, 1978) and to selectively ignore stimuli under certain conditions (Humphries et al., in press; Matthews & Brunson, 1979).

Armed with this reasoning, Glass undertook a second helplessness study that took the salience factor into account (Hollis & Glass, in Glass, 1977). In this study subjects were exposed to a pretreatment consisting of either random or veridical feedback on cognitive problems. Four such problems were used to induce perceptions that control was lost rather than just threatened. Salience of the control cues was varied by requiring subjects in the high salience condition to keep detailed records of their performance on the cognitive tasks. Subjects in the low salience condition kept no such records. The dependent measure in this study was subsequent performance on an anagram task (taken from Hiroto & Seligman, 1975).

Results supported the salience hypothesis. When cues signifying loss of control were highly salient, Type A's showed greater helplessness after an uncontrollable pretreatment than did Type B's, as reflected by taking more trials to reach the performance criterion. Under low salience conditions, however, Type A's did not display the helplessness pattern.

Additional research by Brunson and Matthews (1981) has provided information regarding the cognitive and affective events that underlie such responses to loss of control. In their study, Type A and Type B undergraduates were presented with four soluble discrimination problems, followed by four insoluble discrimination problems. Subjects' affect and attributions were monitored by having the subjects verbalize their thoughts continuously while attempting to solve all eight problems. The researchers also monitored the type of problem-solving strategies employed by the subjects, particularly noting any changes that occurred after the shift from soluble to insoluble tasks. Salience of failure was manipulated by requiring subjects in the high salience condition to keep a written record of feedback received on their task performances. At the end of the study, subjects filled out questionnaires indicating their attributions for success and failure.

Performances were analyzed in terms of sophistication of the problem-solving strategies used by subjects. The performances of Type A's in the high salience condition (but not in the moderate salience condition) deteriorated markedly over failure trials. These Type A's turned to inefficient strategies and included statements outlining inefficient strategies in their verbalizations. They were annoyed with their "stupidity" and were not optimistic about future performance. They attributed responsibility for failure more to lack of ability than to task difficulty. Although Type B's were unhappy with their failure, they remained relatively optimistic, attributing the failure more to external explanations such as task difficulty. These self-report patterns are consistent with the notion that A's have an enhanced susceptibility to the helplessness experience, relative to B's.

In contrast to the consistent picture presented by the three studies just described, however, an investigation by Lovallo and Pishkin (1980) has failed to find that Type A's respond to loss of control with helplessness. The greatest threat to control in this study consisted of failures on two pretreatment tasks, while being exposed to random bursts of noise. This procedure is quite different from those employed in the Krantz et al. and the Hollis and Glass studies, most notably in the use of random noise bursts as a secondary manipulation of loss of control. Inasmuch as evidence reviewed earlier indicates that Type A's suppress attention to task-irrelevant stimuli, it is difficult to know whether that manipulation exerted its intended influence. Nevertheless, it is clear from the data that Type A's in the Lovallo and Pishkin study showed no evidence of greater helplessness than did Type B's. Thus, the reliability of the relationship between the two variables should probably be regarded with some caution.

At this point it seems appropriate to reexamine the reasons underlying the interest in the possibility of a link between Pattern A and susceptibility to helplessness. As was indicated earlier, research examining this relationship was undertaken with a specific theoretical goal in mind. That is, such a relationship is predicted by the conceptualization of Pattern A as an orientation to life experiences in which gaining and maintaining control is of paramount importance (Glass, 1977). But there is a second basis for interest in this possibility, as well. Specifically, it suggests another way in which Pattern A may be associated with CHD.

A number of writers have suggested that the sense of helplessness and uncontrollability that can be induced by negative life events may potentiate the onset of a variety of diseases (e.g., Engel, 1968; Paykel, 1974; Schmale, 1972). Consistent with this reasoning is the finding that sudden death is uncommonly frequent among men who have had a period of depression immediately preceding their deaths (Greene, Goldstein, & Moss, 1972). If Type A's are especially prone to respond to a very salient loss of control in laboratory settings with a helplessness or giving-up response, it may be that Type A's are also susceptible to such effects when they occur in their daily lives. This giving-up response, then, may have adverse health implications.

Consistent with this reasoning, Glass (1977) found in a retrospective study that coronary patients reported an unusually high incidence of uncontrollable events in their lives during the year prior to their hospitalization. In subsequent research Suls, Gastorf, and Witenberg (1979) found that Type A's differed from

Type B's in what kinds of life events were perceived as most distressing. It was events perceived to be undesirable, unexpected, and of uncertain controllability that produced the most distress among Type A's. Among Type B's, in contrast, the more uncontrollable the event was perceived to be, the less was the distress that accompanied it. These findings are consistent with the notion that A's are more likely than B's to be bothered by uncertainty concerning the controllability of events, and thus perhaps more likely to respond eventually with helplessness.

PHYSIOLOGICAL REACTIVITY UNDER STRESS

Up to this point, we have stressed the behavioral manifestations of Pattern A as they occur under conditions of implicit or explicit stress. We should point out, however, that people respond to stressors in a multitude of physiological as well as behavioral ways. A number of researchers have thus begun to ask whether the *behavioral* hyperresponsivity of the Type A is paralleled by *physiological* hyperresponsivity.

Research in this area has focused on assessing physiological responses in situations that have been found to elicit A–B differences in behavior. In one early study of this sort, heart rate, blood pressure, and galvanic skin potential were examined in college students who had been JAS-classified as Type A or Type B (Dembroski, MacDougall, & Shields, 1977). Measures were taken during performance of a choice reaction-time task, in which the importance of speed and accuracy had been emphasized to subjects. Type A's showed greater changes in both heart rate and blood pressure from base line to task period than did Type B's.

In a similar study, Manuck, Craft, and Gold (1978) found that Type A males (but not females) exhibited greater elevations of systolic blood pressure than Type B's in response to a difficult cognitive task. In yet another study (Manuck & Garland, 1979), Type A's were found to exhibit larger systolic blood pressure responses than Type B's to a cognitive task, although no difference was found between the groups in either heart rate or diastolic blood pressure.

Dembroski et al. (1978) monitored Type As' and Type Bs' physiological reactions while they performed three difficult tasks involving perceptual-motor and cognitive skills, thus establishing a situational challenge. The need for rapid and accurate responding was stressed to the subjects. Interview-defined fully developed Type A's showed the largest systolic blood pressure and heart rate changes during the task (averaged across trials), followed by incomplete Type A's. Type B's showed the least amount of change in systolic blood pressure and heart rate. When subjects were divided at the median JAS score, a significant A–B difference in diastolic blood pressure was also found.

These differences in physiological responding have also been found in coronary patients (Dembroski, MacDougall, & Lushene, 1979). These patients and a group of hospitalized controls completed the structured interview and a challenging American history quiz while the researchers monitored their blood pressure and heart rate. Type A coronary cases and Type A controls exhibited greater increases in systolic blood pressure than Type B's in both the interview and quiz periods. Interestingly, both A and B coronary patients responded with increased systolic blood pressure during the quiz as compared to the preceding interview. This occurred in spite of the fact that many patients were on medication that tends to inhibit such changes. Diastolic blood pressure differences were found between Type A's and Type B's, but only during the latter part of the interview.

The foregoing studies indicate that distinctive physiological reactions are associated with the Type A behavioral style and that such reactions occur under the same conditions that elicit A-type behavioral characteristics. But none of these studies systematically investigated the role of challenge in producing these physiological responses, despite the fact that challenge was obviously implicit in many of the experimental procedures. Further investigation of the role of situational challenge has been one of the aims of more recent research.

One project examined this question by varying instructions given to male college students before cold-pressor and reaction-time tasks (Dembroski, MacDougall, Herd, & Shields, 1979). Some subjects were informed that the task was routine and easily completed. Other subjects heard instructions that emphasized the difficulty of the task and the need for much "willpower" (for the cold-pressor test) or aggressiveness (for the reaction-time task) to complete the task successfully. Type A's exhibited significantly greater heart rate and systolic blood pressure changes from resting levels (as compared with Type B's) on both tasks. This was particularly so in the high-challenge conditions, although the interaction between type and condition was not significant. Under low-challenge conditions, those Type A's who also exhibited high levels of hostility were found to differ from both Type B's and other A's in the amount of heart rate and blood pressure changes they exhibited. When this group was separated from the others, however, no significant A–B difference remained in the low-challenge condition.

Challenging situations also tend to be stressful in nature. Could it be that the role of challenge in eliciting Pattern A has been confounded with the presence of stress? At least two studies have investigated this possibility. Pittner and Houston (1980) found that Type A's displayed increases in heart rate and blood pressure when a cognitive task (memory span for digits) was presented as challenging and important. But subjects who attempted the same task under conditions involving physical threat (potential receipt of painful shocks) as a motivator displayed no A–B difference in cardiovascular response. The authors concluded that Type A's respond physiologically to psychological threats but not to physical threats.

Goldband (1980) has examined this question using somewhat different procedures. Two groups attempted a reaction-time task, some of them with an instructional set emphasizing speed, competitiveness, and time urgency. Other subjects were asked to blow up balloons until they popped, a task that Goldband considered stressful but not competitively challenging. All subjects were monitored for heart rate and pulse transit time, an analog of blood pressure considered to be an indicator of sympathetic activation. The data showed that excessive physiological responsiveness occurred among Type A's only when the challenging instructional set was presented in the reaction-time task. No A–B difference emerged either in the nonchallenging condition, or when A's were exposed to the mastery-irrelevant stressor.

A study by Holmes, Solomon, and Spreier (1979) has determined that the kind of stress associated with physical exercise is also unrelated to A–B differences in physiological reactivity. Subjects in this study completed a challenging IQ test and a rigorous exercise task. Type A males (but not females) exhibited heart rate acceleration while taking the IQ test, but no physiological difference was found during the physical exercise. The authors concluded that the Type A's greater reactivity to challenge represents a psychologically mediated reaction to a specific stimulus—challenge—and is not reflective of a physical makeup that simply overreacts to any demands placed on it.

At least one other study has been conducted examining physiological reactions of Type A's to challenge. Glass et al. (1980) monitored the blood pressure, heart rate, and catecholamine levels of Type A's and Type B's who were engaged in a competitive electronic game with a confederate. Half the subjects were harassed and insulted by the confederate while completing this procedure; the other subjects were not. The results showed that competitive challenge alone produced increases in systolic blood pressure and heart rate among both Type A's and Type B's, with no significant difference between the groups. With harassment, however, Type A's (but not Type B's) exhibited additional physiological changes, including a pronounced increase in plasma epinephrine.

Component Analyses

A question that is present in all research on coronary-prone behavior—but one that we have not addressed until now—is the following: Is the Type A behavior *pattern* associated with increased risk of CHD (or indeed any of the behavioral effects discussed in this chapter), or is some *component* of the pattern responsible for the effects? It is unknown, in fact, to what degree these various A-type characteristics actually do comprise a coherent cluster in people. Although this problem is present in all aspects of research in the area, it has been confronted most directly by some of the researchers who study physiological responsiveness among Type A's. That is, these investigators have attempted to determine whether different aspects of the Type A pattern differentially predict cardiovascular responsiveness under conditions of stress, a technique referred to as *component analysis*.

The findings of this research have been intriguing. Dembroski et al. (1978), for example, have found that the hostility component of Pattern A was highly predictive of physiological change under stress. Among Type A subjects in this study there was a reliable correlation between hostility, as measured by the structured interview, and the amount of change in systolic blood pressure experienced under stress. Hostility has also been found to be an effective predictor of physiological changes during the interview itself and during a challenging history quiz (Dembroski, MacDougall, & Lushene, 1979). In fact, Type A's who possess especially high potentials for hostility appear to experience cardiovascular hyperreactivity even when challenge is minimal. High-hostility Type A's show as much physiological reactivity (in response to cold-pressor and reaction-time tasks) after low-challenge instructions as do all A's after high-challenge instructions (Dembroski, MacDougall, Herd, & Shields, 1979). These findings imply that in their reactions to only mildly challenging events highly hostile Type A's may experience more frequent periods of physiological activation than other persons. As was discussed earlier, it is often argued that such overly frequent activation is a root cause of atherosclerosis and eventual CHD.

Indeed, the link between hostility and exaggerated physiological responsiveness is especially interesting in view of the finding that hostility appears to be the best predictor of CHD out of all the elements of Pattern A (Matthews et al., 1977). It thus seems not unreasonable to speculate that hostility and its resulting physiological reactivity may be one path linking Pattern A to CHD.

The suggestion that a specific component of the Type A pattern relates to cardiovascular reactivity also comes from another study (Scherwitz, Berton, & Leventhal, 1978) in which the physiological reactions of Type A's and Type B's were measured during a series of tasks including cold pressor, mental arithmetic, and generation of emotion. No overall A–B difference emerged on these tasks. However, when the researchers separated out Type A's who exhibited greater "self-involvement" (indicated by the number of personal pronouns verbalized during the interview and emotion sessions) from those who exhibited less self-involvement, marked differences were found between the two groups. Highly self-involved A's showed reliable blood pressure increases and heart rate decreases under stress, which were not found among less self-involved A's.

Future Directions. The aspects of Pattern A that have been found to be related to cardiovascular reactivity are only a small subset of the characteristics that have been ascribed to Type A's. Future research is likely to be aimed at ascertaining whether this set of findings is reliable and exhaustive, or whether any of the other aspects of Pattern A are associated with exaggerated cardiovascular reactivity in response to situational challenge. The nature of the environmental factors that elicit physiological changes must also be clarified. For instance, harassment in the presence of competition has been shown to produce elevated physiological responses among Type A's (Glass et al., 1980). But it is unclear whether harassment alone was responsible for the effect, or whether it was the combination of harrassment plus competition.

Finally, more investigation is necessary to determine the exact nature of the responses elicited by stress. Thus far, researchers have concentrated on studying heart rate and blood pressure changes as a response to challenge. Attention is now shifting to the underlying processes that may contribute to the changes observed in those indices. It is unclear whether the Type A's physiological hyperreactivity represents: (1) a tendency toward greater sympathetic arousal in general (cf. Obrist, 1976); (2) a tendency toward exaggeration of either of two global physiological response patterns (cf. Williams, 1978); or (3) a tendency to react to certain stimuli with a specific emotion such as anger. These represent quite different conceptualizations, and they may have quite different implications. Which is most accurate can only be determined by further research.

PATTERN A AND SOCIAL RELATIONS

Let us return now to the domain of overt behavior and consider a separate question that is beginning to attract research attention. Most of the Type A's behavioral characteristics are instrumental, in the sense that they are aimed at attaining performance goals. Earlier in the chapter, we detailed support for the assertion that Pattern A is characterized by aggressiveness when thwarted, a sense of time urgency, an orientation toward competition and achievement, and a tendency to suppress the awareness of stimuli or events that have not been defined as centrally important. This may, in fact, be a very effective work style (although even this point is arguable, as is shown later). At a minimum, the Type A style ensures that things get done when necessary and that responsibilities are taken seriously. But there is some question as to whether this pattern of behavior constitutes a very adaptive way of life outside the work arena.

There are at least two studies that have direct implications in this regard. DeGregorio and Carver (1980) have investigated the psychological adjustment of A's and B's as a function of sex and sex-role orientation. Based on the assumption that A-type characteristics are adaptive only in masculine domains, it was predicted that Type A's who did not have a substantial masculine component in their sex-role identities would be more poorly adjusted than other groups, in terms of low social self-esteem, social anxiety, and depression. Furthermore, because our culture expects women to be more socially adept than men, these effects were expected to be more pronounced among Type A low-masculine women than comparable men. These predictions found considerable support in the data. Pattern A apparently is less functional in strictly interpersonal domains than in task applications.

Although the DeGregorio and Carver study collected no data on this point, it seems reasonable to suggest some further implications of their findings, keeping in mind that these suggestions remain speculative. One potential implication stems from the fact that anxiety and depression have physiological concomitants. To the degree that Type A's (or at least a subset of Type A's) experience these emotions frequently in their social encounters, it may contribute to the more general pattern of physiological overreactivity that was described earlier in the chapter. A second implication is based on the fact that low self-esteem often creates a "vicious cycle" (cf. Brockner & Hulton, 1978). That is, it lowers expectations for future success, leading to diminished efforts in the relevant behavioral domain, leading in turn to the anticipated unsuccessful outcomes. If a subset of Type A's tend to have poor interpersonal adjustment, the result may be further withdrawal from social relations among those A's and, perhaps, a corresponding further immersion in work activities.

A related but separate set of inferences can be drawn from data reported by Burke, Weir, and DuWors (1979). Their study proceeded from the assumption that the clash between the Pattern A style and the demands of social interaction does not exert its influence solely on the person who has that behavior pattern. It may also have an impact on the *family* of the Type A. Burke et al. (1979) found a significant association between Type A behavior among male civil service employees and decreased marital satisfaction and emotional well-being among their wives. Wives of Type A men reported having relatively few friends and social contacts and not feeling a part of surrounding social networks. They also reported more feelings of depression, worthlessness, anxiety, tension, guilt, and isolation than wives of Type B men.

Once again, it seems reasonable to suggest secondary inferences from these data, although the inferences remain to be substantiated by further research. Specifically, it seems likely that there is a reciprocal influence between the marital dissatisfaction of the wives of Type A's and the behavioral manifestations of Pattern A among the husbands. That is, depression, tension, and isolation among the wives represent frustrating and uncontrollable situations for the husbands, situations that they are ill-equipped to deal with successfully. The result may be increases in manifest hostility on the husband's part and/or a tendency to bury himself further in his work environment, isolating himself from the difficulties at home, and perhaps denying the existence of those difficulties (cf. Pittner & Houston, 1980). This, in turn, should further exacerbate the sense of guilt, depression, and isolation among the wives. The result should be a continuing spiral of stress, with all of the pathogenic influences associated with stress.

Indeed, this line of reasoning also raises questions as to whether Pattern A ultimately is truly effective as a work style. Friedman and Rosenman (1974) have suggested that Type A's—though productive—may tend to produce stereotyped products by virtue of the driven, time-urgent nature of their efforts. Further, if their performances are in any way hampered by the presence of co-workers or collaborators (a possibility that is suggested by the findings of Gastorf et al., 1980), Type A's may be especially likely to choose to work in relative isolation (cf. Dembroski & MacDougall, 1978). If this were so, it would effectively remove the Type A even further from social influences that might potentially prevent or diminish such stereotyped activity.

The more general tendency to withdraw from social interaction—implicit in both lines of speculation just presented—may well have health-relevant consequences in and of itself. That is, there is evidence that networks of "social support" provide some degree of protection against a wide variety of pathological states (see, e.g., Cobb, 1976). By withdrawing from the social network, both within and outside of the work arena, the Type A may be forsaking those potential benefits, thereby contributing to increased risk of disease.

INTERVENTION

With the role of Pattern A behavior as a risk factor for CHD firmly established (though mechanisms by which it exerts its influence somewhat more speculative), researchers have begun to explore ways to modify Type A behavior, thereby reducing CHD risk (e.g., Rosenman & Friedman, 1977; Roskies, Spevack, Surkis, Cohen, & Gilman, 1978; Suinn & Bloom, 1978). These approaches have been based for the most part on findings that Type A's respond to environmental stressors with cardiovascular hyperresponsivity (e.g., Dembroski et al., 1977; Dembroski et al., 1978; Manuck et al., 1978) and the assumption that it is this heightened responsiveness over long periods of time that leads to deterioration of the cardiovascular system and thus potentiates CHD. Intervention strategies based on this reasoning attempt (through a variety of methods) to reduce the Type A's tendency toward heightened physiological arousal. This may be accomplished either by changing subjects' perceptions of the stressors that they commonly confront or by reducing their physiological reactions to the stressors (Roskies, 1980).

The relatively few studies that have been conducted in this area thus far have all been the subject of some degree of criticism. Roskies et al. (1978) examined the relative influences on Type A characteristics of a behavioral therapy technique (which included progressive muscle relaxation and deep breathing exercises) and a psychoanalytically oriented therapy. Significant pre- to posttreatment reductions in mean systolic blood pressure, serum cholesterol, self-reported time pressures, and a number of self-reported psychological symptoms were found for both groups after the 14-week treatment period. The authors concluded from these findings that Type A behavior and resulting CHD risk may indeed be amenable to change. But the study did not allow a conclusion as to which approach was preferable.

Suinn and Bloom (1978) trained Type A's in a program similar to Roskies et al.'s behavioral therapy. This Anxiety Management Training program included deep muscle relaxation and the use of imagery to modify subjects' reactions to environmental stressors. A 3-week training period resulted in lower scores on the hard-driving and speed-impatience subscales of the JAS (compared to controls). The treatment group also reported less trait and state anxiety (by questionnaire) after treatment. However, significant reductions in lipid levels and blood pressure, expected on the basis of prior studies using a similar treatment (Suinn, 1975a, 1975b), did not occur.

Other projects have taken more eclectic approaches to intervention. Friedman and Rosenman (1974) have viewed the acquisition and maintenance of Pattern A characteristics as stemming from the belief that such behaviors are essential for socioeconomic success (see also Rosenman & Friedman, 1977). Their intervention strategy incorporated an attempt to reorient subjects away from this belief and also from the belief in the paramount importance of career success. Subsequent elaborations of their program have included behavioral drills and environmental management strategies to eliminate Type A habits, practice in deceleration of motor activities, use of progressive muscle relaxation, and development of skills to cope with challenging situations (Rosenman & Friedman, 1977). Type A's have also been encouraged to develop soothing avocational interests unrelated to their careers and to remove from their immediate environments stimuli that would unnecessarily elicit A-type behavior. Although conceptually reasonable, such an approach would seem to be difficult to implement over the long run in a culture that emphasizes an achievement-oriented work ethic, as is the case in the United States.

Roskies has expanded her behavioral treatment plan to encompass a multimodal approach similar to that of Rosenman and Friedman. In a study of this approach (Roskies & Avard, in press), four separate types of therapy were offered to the participants. These included progressive muscle relaxation to help Type A's deal with their physical reactions to stress, rational-emotive therapy, training in problem-solving skills, and stress inoculation to help modify subjects' perceptions of and cognitive responses to stress. Physiological measures and subjective reports are used to assess the treatment. Although the physiological data are not yet in, subjects have reported success in feelings of enhanced well-being, in controlling emotional outbursts, and so on.

Criticisms of Intervention Studies

These attempts at intervention research have not been without criticism, as noted earlier. Indeed, some of the projects can hardly be called "research" at all (except in an exploratory or pilot sense), in that they have been conducted with very small samples, have confounded several treatment procedures with each other, and have typically lacked necessary control groups. However, many problems confront even the best attempts to intervene in the Type A pattern.

Criterion Measures. Perhaps the most basic problem is defining "improvement" in an acceptable fashion. The ultimate criterion for improvement in this syndrome is a reduction in CHD morbidity and mortality. But the expense, difficulty, and length of time necessary for assessment in this regard have resulted in the substitution of alternative criteria. Most studies have used either: (1) changes in subjects' responses on self-report or interview measures of Pattern A; or (2) changes in physiological indices that are believed to be relevant to pathogenesis of CHD. It is not at all clear whether either of these is ultimately predictive of reduced risk of CHD. Moreover, both of these approaches have additional problems.

Use of the structured interview or the JAS to measure change in Type A characteristics has been criticized on the grounds that these instruments were designed as initial assessment techniques, and not as improvement criteria for intervention. For example, the JAS contains items that pertain to the individual's past history, which cannot be influenced by intervention (Chesney, 1978). On the other hand, although the interview is effective in initial identification of Type A's and Type B's, it is somewhat less sensitive to variation within these categories and may not detect changes in a Type A that are less than a full scale conversion to a Type B (Roskies, 1980).

The use of physiological measures (including blood pressure, heart rate, and lipid levels) is also fraught with difficulty. Much care is needed to make accurate measurements, and such measures are often quite expensive to carry out on a large scale (Roskies, 1980). Moreover, the relationship between even these measures and CHD is still uncertain. Perhaps the worst problem with use of physiological criteria, however, is that Pattern A behavior has been shown to convey CHD risk *independently* of these physiological factors. It may very well be possible, then, to demonstrate changes in various physiological risk factors without ultimately lowering Type A related risk (Chesney, 1978).

Pattern or Components? A second major problem in intervention research is the problem (as we noted earlier in the chapter) that is confronted by *all* research on coronary-prone behavior. Specifically, it is not at all clear whether the statistical relationship between Pattern A and CHD is based on the entire behavior pattern or whether a single component of that pattern *uniquely* increases risk. It may be that many components of the Type A pattern are not related to CHD at all. If so, interventions that attempt to change all aspects of Type A behavior may entail a great deal of wasted effort. It has also been pointed out that the broader effects of such grand-scale reengineering of the Type A's life style are unknown and that it is entirely possible that such programs may adversely influence Type

As' productivity, career advancement, and views of themselves. Researchers in this area are thus beginning to question the wisdom of massive intervention until it is clearer where an intervention should be focused (Chesney, 1978; Gentry & Suinn, 1978; Roskies, 1980).

Cost Effectiveness. A related problem with intervention efforts is this: Although there is a statistically reliable association between the presence of Type A characteristics and eventual CHD, the fact remains that few Type A's ever have a heart attack or any other clinical manifestation of CHD (Scherwitz, Leventhal, Cleary, & Laman, 1978). Should behavioral interventions be conducted on large numbers of people who will derive no benefit in order to benefit the one individual who would have developed heart disease through Type A behavior? This is a very real issue—an issue that has important implications for public policy decisions.

Choice of Target Populations. Another important question is whether to focus on persons who are at risk for CHD, but who have not yet developed clinical symptoms, or to focus instead on persons who have already had a heart attack. It would seem desirable to be able to *prevent* disease rather than simply react to it. However, the person with no clinical manifestations of CHD is often less interested in changing his or her behavior patterns than is the patient who has just had a heart attack. The danger of heart disease probably seems quite remote to the former, although it is obviously not remote to the latter. The result may be differences in involvement in the intervention program, differences in compliance with the demands of the program, and differences in long-term maintenance of the desired changes. This again raises the issue of cost effectiveness.

Recidivism. One final problem must be faced by all programs that attempt to induce voluntary changes in behavior. Even if behavior is effectively altered, there is a great deal of backsliding (i.e., of returning to former habits). This problem has been graphically illustrated in areas of behavioral change such as diet and smoking (Bernstein & McAllister, 1976; Stunkard, 1977). Given the importance of A-type characteristics in the Type A's overall life style, one might expect a high degree of relapse after treatment. Encouragingly, Pattern A has been found in at least one study to be amenable to long-term influences from intervention (Roskies, Kearney, Spevack, Surkis, Cohen, & Gilman, 1979), and a number of suggestions have been advanced for ways to facilitate this long-term influence. For example, participants might keep detailed records of their progress or report back for periodic "booster" sessions (Chesney, 1978; Roskies, 1980). It has also been suggested that Type A's could be "inoculated" for relapse so that temptations or actual incidents of relapse could be dealt with constructively (Marlatt & Gordon, 1980; Roskies, 1980).

SUMMARY

The Type A behavior pattern has been found to be a source of risk for coronary heart disease, independent of traditional risk factors. There are several possible mechanisms by which Pattern A might contribute to CHD risk. One line of research and theory implicates Type A characteristics in long-term increases in atherosclerosis and other pathological physiological states. Moreover, the nature of the behavioral and cognitive characteristics of this behavior pattern suggest additional ways in which CHD may be potentiated or aggravated.

Pattern A has been validated in behavioral research as an action-emotion complex consisting of competitive achievement striving, a sense of time urgency, and aggressiveness in response to frustration of goal attainment. This pattern is also associated with an attention-allocation bias, such that centrally important activities are focused on closely and attention is actively inhibited to peripheral or secondarily important stimuli. This results in suppression of awareness of fatigue and other physical symptoms during attempts to meet behavioral challenges.

Pattern A behavior has been characterized as being aimed at maintaining control over significant aspects of one's environment. Consistent with this characterization, threats to the Type A's control have been found to lead to reassertion attempts and reactance responses. Moreover, very salient loss of control has led to pronounced helplessness responses among Type A's. In addition to these behavioral responses to environmental challenges, Type A's have also been found to be hyperresponsive physiologically to personally challenging situations. The latter findings are consistant with the argument that repeated arousal, leading eventually to atherosclerosis, provides an important mechanism by which Pattern A contributes to CHD risk.

Pattern A also has implications for social adjustment and satisfaction, both among Type A's and among their immediate families. Type A's who lacked a masculine component in their sex-role identities have been found to have a reduced sense of social self-esteem. And the wives of Type A's have been found to feel depressed, isolated, and set apart from social networks. This mutual dissatisfaction may result in a further-widening gap between the Type A and other persons who normally represent important sources of support.

Several studies have been conducted to examine ways of altering Type A characteristics. But these studies appear to have raised as many questions as they have answered. The questions include the appropriateness of various assessment criteria in assessing meaningful change, the cost effectiveness of large-scale intervention strategies, the issue of what aspect of Pattern A should be the target of any intervention attempt, and the problem of recidivism.

Throughout these areas of research, from the defining of CHD risk to the planning of intervention, an important question that has often been neglected is this: Exactly what is it about the Type A behavior pattern that constitutes "coronary-prone behavior?" Future research will attempt to provide an answer to this question, because it is a question with profound implications for our understanding of the effects of behavior on cardiovascular health.

REFERENCES

Balke, B. Optimale koerperliche leistunsfaehigkeisihre messung und veraenderung infrolage arbeitsermuedung. *Arbeitsphysiologie,* 1954, *15,* 311–323.

Balke, B., Grillo, G. P., Konecci, E. B., & Luft, U. C. Work capacity after blood donation. *Journal of Applied Physiology,* 1954, *7,* 231–238.

Bengtsson, C. Ischaemic heart disease in women. *Acta Medica Scandinavia,* 1973, *549,* 1–28.

Bernstein, D. A., & McAllister, A. L. The modification of smoking behavior: Progress, and problems. *Addictive Behavior,* 1976, *1,* 89–102.

Blumenthal, J. A., Williams, R. B., Kong, Y., Schlanberg, S. M., & Thompson, L. W. Type A behavior pattern and coronary atherosclerosis. *Circulation,* 1978, *58,* 634–639.

Bortner, R. W. A short rating scale as a potential measure of Pattern A behavior. *Journal of Chronic Diseases,* 1969, *23,* 87–91.

Bortner, R. W., & Rosenman, R. H. The measurement of Pattern A behavior. *Journal of Chronic Diseases,* 1967, *20,* 525–533.

Brand, R. J., Rosenman, R. H., Sholtz, R. I., & Friedman, M. Multivariate prediction of coronary heart disease in the Western Collaborative Group Study compared to the findings of the Framingham Study. *Circulation,* 1976, *53,* 348–355.

Brehm, J. W. *A theory of psychological reactance.* New York: Academic Press, 1966.

Brockner, J., & Hulton, A. J. B. How to reverse the vicious cycle of low self-esteem: The importance of attentional focus. *Journal of Experimental Social Psychology,* 1978, *14,* 564–578.

Brunson, B., & Matthews, K. A. The Type A coronary-prone behavior pattern and reactions to uncontrollable stress: An analysis of performance strategies, affect, and attributions during failure. *Journal of Personality and Social Psychology,* 1981, *40,* 906–918.

Burke, R. J., Weir, T., & DuWors, R. E. Type A behavior of administrators and wives' reports of marital satisfaction and well-being. *Journal of Applied Psychology,* 1979, *64,* 57–65.

Burnam, M. A., Pennebaker, J. W., & Glass, D. C. Time consciousness, achievement striving, and the Type A coronary-prone behavior pattern. *Journal of Abnormal Psychology,* 1975, *84,* 76–79.

Carlson, L. A., Levi, L., & Oro, L. Plasma lipids and urinary excretion of catecholamines in man during experimentally induced emotional stress, and their modification of nicotinic acid. *Journal of Clinical Investigation,* 1968, *47,* 1795–1805.

Carver, C. S. Perceived coercion, resistance to persuasion, and the Type A behavior pattern. *Journal of Research in Personality,* 1980, *14,* 467–481.

Carver, C. S., Coleman, A. E., & Glass, D. C. The coronary-prone behavior pattern and the suppression of fatigue on a treadmill test. *Journal of Personality and Social Psychology,* 1976, *33,* 460–466.

Carver, C. S., DeGregorio, E., & Gillis, R. Challenge and Type A behavior among intercollegiate football players. *Journal of Sport Psychology,* 1981, *3,* 140–148.

Carver, C. S., & Glass, D. C. Coronary-prone behavior pattern and interpersonal aggression. *Journal of Personality and Social Psychology,* 1978, *36,* 361–366.

Charvat, J., Dell, P., & Folkow, B. Mental factors and cardiovascular diseases. *Cardiologia,* 1964, *44,* 124–141.

Chesney, M. *Coronary-prone behavior and heart disease: Intervention strategies.* Paper presented at the annual meeting of the American Psychological Association, Toronto, 1978.

Cobb, S. Social support as a moderation of life stress. *Psychosomatic Medicine,* 1976, *38,* 300–313.

Davies, R. F., & Reinert, H. Arteriosclerosis in the young dog. *Journal of Atherosclerosis Research,* 1965, *5,* 181–188.

Davis, R. Stress and hemostatic mechanisms. In R. S. Eliot (Ed.), *Stress and the heart.* Mt. Kisco, N.Y.: Futura, 1974.

Dawber, T. R., & Kannel, W. B. Susceptibility to coronary heart disease. *Modern Concepts in Cardiovascular Disease,* 1961, *30,* 671–676.

DeGregorio, E., & Carver, C. S. Type A behavior pattern, sex role orientation, and psychological adjustment. *Journal of Personality and Social Psychology,* 1980, *39,* 286–293.

Dembroski, T., & MacDougall, J. M. Stress effects on affiliation preferences among subjects possessing the Type A coronary-prone behavior pattern. *Journal of Personality and Social Psychology,* 1978, *36,* 23–33.

Dembroski, T., MacDougall, J. M., Herd, J. A., & Shields, J. L. Effects of level of challenge on pressor and heart rate responses in Type A and B subjects. *Journal of Applied Social Psychology,* 1979, *9,* 209–228.

Dembroski, T. M., MacDougall, J. M., & Lushene, R. Interpersonal interaction and cardiovascular response in Type A subjects and coronary patients. *Journal of Human Stress,* 1979, *5,* 28–36.

Dembroski, T. M., MacDougall, J. M., & Shields, J. L. Physiologic reactions to social challenge in persons evidencing the Type A coronary-prone behavior pattern. *Journal of Human Stress,* 1977, *3,* 2–10.

Dembroski, T. M., MacDougall, J. M., Shields, J. L., Petitto, R., & Lushene, R. Components of the Type A coronary-prone behavior pattern and cardiovascular responses to psychomotor performance challenge. *Journal of Behavioral Medicine,* 1978, *1,* 159–176.

Dimsdale, J. E., Hackett, T. P., Catanzano, D. M., & White, P. J. The relationship between diverse measures for Type A personality and coronary angiographic findings. *Journal of Psychosomatic Research,* 1979, *23,* 289–293.

Dimsdale, J. E., Hackett, T. P., Hutter, A. M., Block, P., Catanzano, D., & White. P. Type A personality and extent of coronary atherosclerosis. *American Journal of Cardiology,* 1978, *42,* 583–586.

Edwards, A. L. *Manual for the Edwards Personal Preference Schedule* (rev. ed.). New York: Psychological Corporation, 1957.

Eliot, R. S. (Ed.). *Stress and the heart.* Mt. Kisco, N.Y.: Futura, 1974.

Engel, G. L. A life setting conducive to illness: The giving-up complex. *Annals of Internal Medicine,* 1968, *69,* 293–300.

Fazio, R. H., Cooper, M., Dayson, K., & Johnson, M. Control and the coronary-prone behavior pattern: Responses to multiple situational demands. *Personality and Social Psychology Bulletin,* 1981, *7,* 97–102.

Frank, K. A., Heller, S. S., Kornfeld, D. S., Sporn, A., & Weiss, M. Type A behavior and coronary angiographic findings. *Journal of the American Medical Association,* 1978, *240,* 761–763.

Friedman, M. *Pathogenesis of coronary artery disease.* New York: McGraw-Hill, 1969.

Friedman, M., Byers, S. O., Diamant, J., & Rosenman, R. H. Plasma catecholamine response of coronary-prone subjects (Type A) to a specific challenge. *Metabolism,* 1975, *4,* 205–210.

Friedman, M., & Rosenman, R. H. Association of a specific overt behavior pattern with increases in blood cholesterol, blood clotting time, incidence of arcus senilis and clinical coronary artery disease. *Journal of the American Medical Association,* 1959, *169,* 1286–1296.

Friedman, M., & Rosenman, R. H. *Type A behavior and your heart.* Greenwich, Conn.: Fawcett, 1974.

Friedman, M., St. George, S., Byers, S. O., & Rosenman, R. H. Excretion of catecholamines, 17-ketosteroids, 17-hydroxycorticoids, and 5-hydroxyindole in men exhibiting a particular behavior pattern (A) associated with high incidence of clinical coronary artery disease. *Journal of Clinical Investigation,* 1960, *39,* 758–764.

Gastorf, J. W. Time urgency of the Type A behavior pattern. *Journal of Consulting and Clinical Psychology,* 1980, *48,* 299.

Gastorf, J. W., Suls, J., & Sanders, G. S. The Type A coronary-prone behavior pattern and social facilitation. *Journal of Personality and Social Psychology,* 1980, *38,* 773–780.

Gentry, W. D., & Suinn, R. M. Section summary: Behavioral intervention. In T. M. Dembroski, S. M. Weiss, J. L. Shields, S. G. Haynes, & M. Feinleib (Eds.), *Coronary-prone behavior.* New York: Springer-Verlag, 1978.

Glass, D. C. *Behavior patterns, stress and coronary disease.* Hillsdale, N.J.: Lawrence Erlbaum Associates, 1977.

Glass, D. C., & Carver, C. S. Helplessness and the coronary-prone personality. In J. Garber & M. E. P. Seligman (Eds.), *Human helplessness: Theory and application.* New York: Academic Press, 1980.

Glass, D. C., Krakoff, L. R., Contrada, R., Hilton, W. F., Kehoe, K., Mannucci, E. G., Collins, C., Snow, B., & Elting, E. Effects of harassment and competition upon cardiovascular and plasma catecholamines responses in Type A and Type B individuals. *Psychophysiology,* 1980, *17,* 453–463.

Glass, D. C., Snyder, M. L., & Hollis, J. F. Time urgency and the Type A coronary-prone behavior pattern. *Journal of Applied Social Psychology,* 1974, *4,* 125–140.

Goldband, S. Stimulus specificity of physiological response to stress and the Type A coronary-prone behavior pattern. *Journal of Personality and Social Psychology,* 1980, *39,* 670–679.

Gough, H. G. *The Adjective Check List.* Berkeley, California: University of California Press, 1952.

Greene, W. A., Goldstein, S., & Moss, A. J. Psychosocial aspects of sudden death: A preliminary report. *Archives of Internal Medicine,* 1972, *129,* 725–731.

Greene, W. A., Moss, A. J., & Goldstein, S. Delay, denial, and death in coronary heart disease. In R. S. Eliot (Ed.), *Stress and the heart.* Mt. Kisco, N.Y.: Futura, 1974.

Herd, J. A. Physiological correlates of coronary prone behavior. In T. M. Dembroski, S. M. Weiss, J. L. Shields, S. G. Haynes, M. Feinleib (Eds.), *Coronary-prone behavior.* New York: Springer-Verlag, 1978.

Hiroto, D. S., & Seligman, M. E. P. Generality of learned helplessness in man. *Journal of Personality and Social Psychology,* 1975, *31,* 311–327.

Holmes, D. S., Solomon, S., & Spreier, B. J. *Cardiac and subjective response to cognitive challenge and to controlled physical exercise by male and female coronary prone (Type A) and non-coronary prone persons.* Unpublished manuscript, University of Kansas, Psychology Department 1979.

Humphries, C., Carver, C. S., & Neumann, P. G. Cognitive characteristics of the coronary-prone behavior pattern. *Journal of Personality and Social Psychology,* in press.

Jenkins, C. D. Psychologic and social precursors of coronary disease. *New England Journal of Medicine,* 1971, *284,* 244–255.

Jenkins, C. D., Rosenman, R. H., & Friedman, M. Replicability of rating the coronary-prone behavior pattern. *British Journal of Preventive and Social Medicine,* 1968, *22,* 16–22.

Jenkins, C. D., Rosenman, R. H., & Zyzanski, S. J. Prediction of clinical heart disease by a test for the coronary-prone behavior pattern. *New England Journal of Medicine,* 1974, *290,* 1271–1275.

Krantz, D. S., Glass, D. C., & Snyder, M. L. Helplessness, stress level and the coronary-prone behavior pattern. *Journal of Experimental Social Psychology,* 1974, *10,* 284–300.

Krantz, D. S., Sanmarco, M. E., Selvester, R. H., & Matthews, K. A. Psychological correlates of progression of atherosclerosis in men: A preliminary report. *Psychosomatic Medicine,* 1979, *41,* 467–475.

Lovallo, W. R., & Pishkin, V. Performance of Type A (coronary-prone) men during and after exposure to uncontrollable noise and task failure. *Journal of Personality and Social Psychology,* 1980, *38,* 963–971.

Manuck, S. B., Craft, S. A., & Gold, K. J. Coronary-prone behavior pattern and cardiovascular response. *Psychophysiology,* 1978, *15,* 403–411.

Manuck, S. B., & Garland, F. N. Coronary-prone behavior pattern, task incentive and cardiovascular response. *Psychophysiology,* 1979, *16,* 136–147.

Marlatt, G., & Gordon, J. Determinants of relapse: Implications for the maintenance of behavior change. In P. O. Davidson, & S. M. Davidson (Eds.), *Behavioral medicine: Changing health lifestyles.* New York: Brunner/Mazel, 1980.

Matthews, K. A., & Brunson, B. I. The attentional style of Type A coronary-prone individuals: Implications for symptom reporting. *Journal of Personality and Social Psychology,* 1979, *37,* 2081–2090.

Matthews, K. A., Glass, D. C., Rosenman, R. H., & Bortner, R. W. Competitive drive, Pattern A, and coronary heart disease: A further analysis of some data from the Western Collaborative Group Study. *Journal of Chronic Diseases,* 1977, *30,* 489–498.

Matthews, K. A., Helmreich, R. L. , Beane, W. E., & Lucker, G. W. Pattern A, achievement-striving, and scientific excellence: Does Pattern A help or hinder? *Journal of Personality and Social Psychology,* 1980, *39,* 962–967.

Matthews, K. A., & Saal, F. E. The relationship of the Type A coronary-prone behavior pattern to achievement, power, and affiliation motives. *Psychosomatic Medicine,* 1978, *40,* 631–636.

Mettlin, C. Occupational careers and the prevention of coronary-prone behavior. *Social Science and Medicine,* 1976, *10,* 367–372.

Miller, I. W., & Norman, W. H. Learned helplessness in humans: A review and attribution-theory model. *Psychological Bulletin,* 1979, *86,* 93–118.

Obrist, P. A. The cardiovascular-behavioral interaction—as it appears today. *Psychophysiology,* 1976, *13,* 95–107.

Ovcharchyn, C. A., Johnson, H. H., & Petzel, T. P. *Type A behavior, academic aspirations, and academic success.* Unpublished manuscript, 1980.

Paykel, E. S. Life stress and psychiatric disorder: Applications of the clinical approach. In B. S. Dohrenwend & B. P. Dohrenwend (Eds.), *Stressful life events: Their nature and effects.* New York: Wiley, 1974.

Pittner, M. S., & Houston, B. K. Response to stress, cognitive coping strategies and the Type A behavior pattern. *Journal of Personality and Social Psychology,* 1980, *39,* 147–157.

Rosenman, R. H. The role of behavior patterns and neurogenic factors in the pathogenesis of coronary heart disease. In R. S. Eliot (Ed.), *Stress and the heart.* Mt. Kisco, N.Y.: Futura, 1974.

Rosenman, R. H., Brand, R. J., Jenkins, C. D., Friedman, M., Straus, R., & Wurm, M. Coronary heart disease in the Western Collaborative Group Study: Final follow-up experience of 8½ years. *Journal of the American Medical Association,* 1975, *233,* 872–877.

Rosenman, R. H., & Friedman, M. Neurogenic factors in pathogenesis of coronary heart disease. *Medical Clinics of North America,* 1974, *58,* 269–279.

Rosenman, R. H., & Friedman, M. Modifying the Type A behavior pattern. *Journal of Psychosomatic Research,* 1977, *21,* 323–333.

Rosenman, R. H., Friedman, M., Straus, R., Wurm, M., Jenkins, C. D., & Messinger, H. Coronary heart disease in the Western Collaborative Group Study: A follow-up experience of two years. *Journal of the American Medical Association,* 1966, *195,* 130–136.

Roskies, E. Considerations in developing a treatment program for the coronary-prone (Type A) behavior pattern. In P. O. Davidson, & S. M. Davidson (Eds.), *Behavioral medicine: Changing health lifestyles.* New York: Brunner/Mazel, 1980.

Roskies, E., & Avard, J. Teaching healthy managers to control their coronary-prone (Type A) behavior. In K. Blankstein, & J. Polivy (Eds.), *Self control and self modification of emotional behaviors.* New York: Plenum, in press.

Roskies, E., Kearney, H., Spevack, M., Surkis, A., Cohen, C., & Gilman, S. Generalizability and durability of treatment effects in an intervention program for coronary-prone (Type A) managers. *Journal of Behavioral Medicine,* 1979, *2,* 195–207.

Roskies, E., Spevack, M., Surkis, A., Cohen, C., & Gilman, S. Changing the coronary-prone (Type A) behavior pattern in a non-clinical population. *Journal of Behavioral Medicine,* 1978, *1,* 201–217.

Ross, R., & Harker, L. Hyperlipidemia and atherosclerosis. *Science,* 1976, *193,* 1094–1100.

Sanders, G. S., Baron, R. S., & Moore, D. L. Distraction and social comparison as mediators of social facilitation effects. *Journal of Experimental Social Psychology,* 1978, *14,* 291–303.

Schmale, A. H. Giving up as a final common pathway to changes in health. *Advances in Psychosomatic Medicine,* 1972, *8,* 18–38.

Scherwitz, L., Berton, K., & Leventhal, H. Type A behavior, self-involvement and cardiovascular response. *Psychosomatic Medicine,* 1978, *40,* 593–609.

Scherwitz, L., Leventhal, H., Cleary, P., & Laman, C. Type A behavior: Consideration for risk modification. *Health Values: Achieving High Level Wellness,* 1978, *2,* 291–296.

Schucker, B., & Jacobs, D. R., Jr. Assessment of behavioral risk for coronary disease by voice characteristics. *Psychosomatic Medicine,* 1977, *39,* 219–228.

Seligman, M. E. P. *Helplessness: On depression, development, and death.* San Francisco: Freeman, 1975.

Shekelle, R. B., Schoenberger, J. A., & Stamler, J. Correlates of the JAS Type A behavior pattern score. *Journal of Chronic Diseases,* 1976, *29,* 381–394.

Simpson, M. T., Olewine, D. A., Jenkins, C. D., Ramsey, F. H., Zyzanski, S. J., Thomas, G., & Hames, C. G. Exercise induced catecholamines and platelet aggregation in the coronary-prone behavior pattern. *Psychosomatic Medicine,* 1974, *36,* 476–487.

Snyder, M. L., & Frankel, A. *Reactance and the Type A.* Unpublished manuscript, Dartmouth College, Department of Psychology, 1980.

Stunkard, A. Behavioral treatment of obesity: Failure to maintain weight loss. In R. B. Stuart (Ed.), *Behavioral self-management: Strategies, techniques and outcome.* New York: Brunner/Mazel, 1977.

Suinn, R. Anxiety management training for general anxiety. In R. Suinn, & R. Weigel (Eds.), *The innovative psychological therapies: Critical and creative contributions.* New York: Harper, 1975. (a)

Suinn, R. The cardiac stress management program for Type A patients. *Cardiac Rehabilitation,* 1975, *5,* 13–15. (b)

Suinn, R., & Bloom, L. Anxiety management training for Pattern A behavior. *Journal of Behavioral Medicine,* 1978, *1,* 25–35.

Suls, J., Gastorf, J. W., Witenberg, S. H. Life events, psychological distress and the Type A coronary-prone behavior pattern. *Journal of Psychosomatic Research,* 1979, *23,* 315–319.

Thurstone, L. L. *The Thurstone Temperament Schedule: Examiners Manual.* Chicago: Science Research Associates, 1949.

Van Egeren, L. F. Cardiovascular changes during social competition in mixed motive game. *Journal of Personality and Social Psychology,* 1979, *37,* 858–864.

Waldron, I. Sex differences in the coronary-prone behavior pattern. In T. M. Dembroski, S. M. Weiss, J. L. Shields, S. G. Haynes, & M. Feinleib (Eds.), *Coronary-prone behavior.* New York: Springer-Verlag, 1978.

Waldron, I., Zyzanski, S. J., Shekelle, R. B., Jenkins, C. D., & Tannenbaum, S. The coronary-prone behavior pattern in employed men and women. *Journal of Human Stress,* 1977, *3,* 2–19.

Weidner, G., & Matthews, K. A. Reported physical symptoms elicited by unpredictable events and the Type A coronary-prone behavior pattern. *Journal of Personality and Social Psychology,* 1978, *36,* 213–220.

Wicklund, R. A. *Freedom and reactance.* Hillsdale, N.J.: Lawrence Erlbaum Associates, 1974.

Williams, R. B. Psychophysiological processes, the coronary-prone behavior pattern, and coronary heart disease. In T. M. Dembroski, S. M. Weiss, J. L. Shields, S. G. Haynes, & M. Feinleib (Eds.), *Coronary-prone behavior*. New York: Springer-Verlag, 1978.

Wortman, C. B., & Brehm, J. W. Responses to uncontrollable outcomes: An integration of reactance theory and the learned helplessness model. In L. Berkowitz (Ed.), *Advances in experimental social psychology*. New York: Academic Press, 1975.

Zajonc, R. B. Social facilitation. *Science*, 1965, *149*, 269–274.

Zyzanski, S. J., & Jenkins, C. D. Basic dimensions within the coronary-prone behavior pattern. *Journal of Chronic Diseases*, 1970, *22*, 781–795.

3 Who Is Responsible for Your Health? The Construct of Health Locus of Control

Kenneth A. Wallston
School of Nursing
Vanderbilt University

Barbara Strudler Wallston
George Peabody College
Vanderbilt University

In the summer of 1964, Norman Cousins, the former editor of the *Saturday Review*, was diagnosed as having ankylosing spondylitis, a collogen disease leading to disintegration of the connective tissue in the spine. Upon being told by his doctor that a leading specialist gave him "one chance in five hundred" of recovering, Cousins (1979) decided it was about time he took an active interest in his own case: "All this gave me a great deal to think about. Up to that time I had been more or less disposed to let the doctors worry about my condition. But now I felt a compulsion to get into the act. It seemed clear to me that if I was to be that one in five hundred I had better be something more than a passive observer [p. 35]." Cousins (1979) details how he developed his own treatment regimen, formed a partnership with his physician, and ultimately was freed from this crippling, degenerative disease.

The issue of who is responsible for an individual's degree of health or illness is one for which there are no definitive answers but plenty of opinions. Many patients and most physicians behave as if doctors are primarily responsible; when a health problem arises it is the doctor's job to set things right. Other people strongly believe that the ultimate responsibility for one's health either lies squarely with the individual or ought to lie there. As Ginzberg (1977) writes: "No improvement in the health care system will be efficacious unless the citizen assumes responsibility for his own well-being [p. 239]." This exemplifies the viewpoint that if we as a society are to do anything about the rising cost of health care in the United States today, people must begin to take charge of their own health and not leave such an important matter up to the so-called experts. Still others believe that nobody is ultimately responsible for health or illness; if you are healthy, you are lucky or have been rewarded by God; if you are sick, you are ill-fated or have been punished by God.

The example of Cousins' actions in the face of ankylosing spondylitis shows that responsibility for recovering from an illness need not rest solely on the patient or on the doctor. A partnership can be struck between doctor and patient in which responsibility is jointly held and shared. Cousins did not merely give up and accept his fate, nor did he dismiss his doctor and carry on exclusively on his own. Instead, he gathered as much information as he could, formulated an unorthodox treatment plan, consulted with his physician, garnered the support of family and friends, and proceeded to take charge of his own life.

THE THEORETICAL FRAMEWORK

A social psychologist familiar with Cousins' story might speculate that Cousins' behavior exemplifies a person with an ''internal locus of control'' belief orientation. Social learning theory (Rotter, 1954) posits that: ''the potential for a behavior to occur in any specific psychological situation is a function of the expectancy that the behavior will lead to a particular reinforcement in that situation and the value of that reinforcement [Rotter, 1975, p. 57].'' Cousins, who highly valued being a healthy, vigorous, alive human being, confronted overwhelming odds and professional pessimism with direct health-enhancing action because he truly believed that his actions would make a difference. The generalized expectancy that one's outcomes (or reinforcements) are directly the result of one's behavior or relatively enduring characteristics is termed an *internal* locus of control orientation (Rotter, 1966). This is opposed to believing that one's outcomes (reinforcements) are under the control of powerful other people or are randomly determined by forces such as fate, luck, or chance—beliefs that are indicative of an *external* locus of control orientation.

According to Rotter's theory, peoples' behavior can be predicted from a knowledge of how they view the situation, their expectancies about their behavior, and how they value the outcomes that might occur as a result of their behavior in that situation. According to Strickland (1978): ''If a situation is novel or ambiguous, then an individual will depend on generalized expectancies that have served him/her in the past. More specific expectancies are used when the aspects of the situation are straightforward or routine [p. 1193].'' Locus of control beliefs have been treated as both generalized and situation-specific expectancies; likewise, individual differences in these beliefs have been considered as either relatively stable personality factors or as transitory social cognitions influenced by a host of situational cues and changes.

Much research has tested various aspects of Rotter's social learning theory (see Rotter, Chance, & Phares, 1972), but the construct that has received the greatest amount of attention has been locus of control. There have been well over 1000 published papers dealing with individual differences in locus of control beliefs, not to mention the myriad of unpublished theses, dissertations, and studies that have investigated this construct (Rotter, 1979). Although there has been quite a diversity of findings and conclusions, it has generally been the case that—compared to those persons espousing external locus of control expectancies—internals are more potent, competent, effective persons, likely to take responsibility for their actions and to take steps to change aversive life situations.[1]

An increasing number of health researchers have measured locus of control beliefs and have attempted to relate these expectancies to a host of health-related behaviors and statuses.[2] Some of these investigations have utilized measures of locus of control that include no mention of health or illness (e.g., Rotter's I–E Scale, Rotter, 1966; Levenson's I, P, & C Scales, Levenson, 1973, 1981); more recently, health-specific measures of this construct have been developed and have been adopted by investigators in the health fields (Wallston & Wallston, 1981). The linkage between assuming responsibility for one's own health and endorsing internal locus of control beliefs has a certain compelling logic to it. Also, Strickland (1978) reports that early "results of research conducted with various [I–E] instruments suggest that beliefs about internal versus external control are related in significant and even dramatic ways to health-related behaviors [p. 1192]." Thus, from both a theoretical and empirical perspective, the exploration of locus of control and health-related phenomena seems warranted.

This chapter summarizes current knowledge regarding the relationship between the health locus of control beliefs of adults[3] and: (1) measurements of other psychological constructs; (2) health information and preventive measures; (3) reactions to physical conditions; (4) responses to health-related interventions; and (5) interactions with health care settings.[4] It begins with a brief description

---

[1]For reviews of this research, see Joe (1971) Lefcourt (1966, 1976, 1981) Phares (1973, 1976), Rotter (1966, 1975).

[2]See Strickland (1978) and Wallston and Wallston (1978) for reviews of some of the earlier work in this field.

[3]A health locus of control scale specifically developed for use with school-age children has been published by Parcel and Meyers (1978). The Children's Health Locus of Control Scale has been used in a number of studies, but work with this scale or other studies involving children is not reviewed in this chapter.

[4]The organization of this chapter, partially modeled after Strickland (1978) is radically different from another recent chapter written by the authors (Wallston & Wallston, 1981). The present chapter includes some studies completed after the other chapter was written and less detail, in general, about specific studies.

of the health related locus of control scales, followed by a suggested typology based on multidimensional patterns of belief.

THE HEALTH LOCUS OF CONTROL SCALES

The degree to which individuals believe that their health is controlled by internal versus external factors (i.e., whether the locus of control is or is not within the individual) is typically assessed by the extent to which individuals agree or disagree with a series of belief statements such as: ''I am directly responsible for my health''; ''Other people play a big part in whether I stay healthy or become sick''; ''When I stay healthy I'm just lucky,'' presented via questionnaire or verbal interview. A belief scale score is the sum of responses to a number of such statements. The more the responses on a given scale intercorrelate with one another, the more internally consistent the scale is, and thus, the greater is the likelihood that the scale is reliably measuring the underlying belief system (Selltiz, Wrightsman, & Cook, 1976).

The first published version of a locus of control measure specific to the domain of physical health/illness was the work of Kirscht and his colleagues (Dabbs & Kirscht, 1971; Kirscht, 1972). In their early attempts, there was some confounding of expectancy and motivational statements. (An example of the latter was, ''I really work at it to stay in good health.'') Only a few items assessing expectancies tapped the construct of health locus of control. The measure developed by Kirscht has had minimal impact on the field and is not dealt with further in this chapter.

The first health-related locus of control measure developed by the authors, the Health Locus of Control (HLC) Scale (Wallston, Wallston, Kaplan, & Maides, 1976), consisted of 11 items with a 6-point, Likert response format (i.e., *strongly agree, moderately agree, slightly agree, slightly disagree,* etc.). High scores on the HLC Scale indicate agreement with the six externally worded statements and disagreement with the five internally worded items. Individuals with scores above the median are sometimes labeled ''health-externals''; those with scores below the median are ''health-internals.''

Two years later, multidimensional versions of the HLC scale were published (Wallston, Wallston, & DeVellis, 1978). Modeled after Levenson's I, P, & C Scales (Levenson, 1973, 1981), the Multidimensional Health Locus of Control (MHLC) Scales consist of three 6-item scales, again using a 6-point, Likert response format. The major contribution of Levenson's multidimensional approach was in splitting externality into two distinct components. The PHLC Scale assesses beliefs that one's health is determined by powerful other people (e.g., doctors, nurses, family, or friends), and the CHLC Scale measures the extent to which one believes that health/illness is a matter of fate, luck, or chance. The two external scales—PHLC and CHLC—are treated as separate measures of health locus of control beliefs; they have not been combined with one another to form an overall measure of health externality. The IHLC Scale measures health internality, or the extent to which individuals believe that internal factors are responsible for their health/illness. Low scores on the IHLC Scale do not mean that individuals believe that external factors determine their health; all that can be said about low IHLC scores is that they are not indicative of internal beliefs. The three dimensions tapped by the MHLC Scales are more or less statistically independent (i.e., scores on the three scales do not substantially intercorrelate).

The MHLC Scales are superior to the unidimensional HLC Scale in at least two ways. Psychometrically, the individual MHLC Scales are more internally consistent (thus, more reliable) than the HLC Scale, which is comprised of both internally and externally worded items. Conceptually, the HLC Scale only contains a single powerful-others item ("I can only do what my doctor tells me to do."), whereas the MHLC has an entire scale (PHLC) devoted to this important construct. As the remainder of this chapter illustrates, some of the most interesting findings regarding locus of control and health-related phenomena come from the PHLC Scale.[5]

A HEALTH LOCUS OF CONTROL TYPOLOGY

Conceptualizing locus of control as a multidimensional rather than a unidimensional contruct makes it much more difficult to think and talk about types of individuals or situations. With two external dimensions—chance and powerful others—what does it mean to label a person as an *external* or to describe a situation as one that induces externality? Also, if the separate dimensions are statistically independent of one another, it is quite possible that a given person can simultaneously score high on two or even three dimensions. Do such patterns of scores make sense conceptually, and is it worthwhile to make separate predictions for persons exhibiting such patterns? Are there types of situations that are more or less favorable to persons exhibiting different patterns of health locus of control beliefs? In this section, we propose a typology of persons based upon possible patterns of scores on the MHLC Scales. This typology is highly speculative because no research has yet been done confirming its existence or demonstrating its validity. In proposing such a typology, there is no intention on our part to suggest that these are personality types (i.e., relatively enduring characteristics of individuals); rather, we take the position that at any one point in time a person's belief pattern may be heuristically described using this typology.

[5]Information relevant to the development of the health locus of control scales and the actual scale items can be found in Wallston, Wallston, Kaplan, and Maides (1976, the HLC Scale) and Wallston, Wallston, and DeVellis (1978, the MHLC Scales). Information about the scales' reliability and validity and normative data can be found in Wallston and Wallston (1981).

Figure 3.1 presents eight different patterns of health locus of control expectancies based on whether an individual is relatively high or low on each of the three dimensions: IHLC, PHLC, and CHLC. The first three patterns are "pure" types; each consists of an endorsement of only one of the three dimensions. The second three types consist of high scores on two of the dimensions, low scores on the other. Type IV might be termed a "double health-external" because both

Type I
"Pure" Internal

	IHLC	*PHLC*	*CHLC*
High	X		
Low		X	X

Type II
"Pure" Powerful Others External

	IHLC	*PHLC*	*CHLC*
High		X	
Low	X		X

Type III
"Pure" Chance External

	IHLC	*PHLC*	*CHLC*
High			X
Low	X	X	

Type IV
Double External

	IHLC	*PHLC*	*CHLC*
High		X	X
Low	X		

Type V
Believer in Control

	IHLC	*PHLC*	*CHLC*
High	X	X	
Low			X

Type VI

	IHLC	*PHLC*	*CHLC*
High	X		X
Low		X	

Type VII
"Yea-Sayer"

	IHLC	*PHLC*	*CHLC*
High	X	X	X
Low			

Type VIII
"Nay-Sayer"

	IHLC	*PHLC*	*CHLC*
High			
Low	X	X	X

FIG. 3.1. A multidimensional health locus of control typology.

external belief dimensions are endorsed, but the individaul does not agree with the internal statements. Type V is possibly the most adaptive of all. By scoring high on both IHLC and PHLC and low on CHLC, individuals express the belief that their health is controllable, either by themselves or other people, and not a matter of fate, luck, or chance. This constellation of beliefs could be particularly beneficial to a person who has to cope with a chronic illness (e.g., diabetes or hypertension) where much of the responsibility for successfully treating the condition lies with the patient carrying out the treatment regimen prescribed by the physician. In an earlier paper (Wallston & Wallston, 1973), we referred to such an individual as a "responsible internal." Norman Cousins is probably such a person.

Type VI—high on IHLC and CHLC, low on PHLC—is probably nonexistent or extremely rare. Inasmuch as the IHLC and CHLC Scales are only slightly negatively correlated, this pattern is mathematically possible but conceptually difficult to understand. One possible explanation is that individuals have learned that there are certain aspects about their health that they can control and other aspects that are totally unpredicatable. In responding to the MHLC belief statements, the Type VI person is merely expressing this dualism.

The last two patterns (i.e., all three dimensions simultaneously high or low) can arise because they validly reflect HLC beliefs or because of response biases (see Couch & Keniston, 1960). "Yea-sayers"—persons who indiscriminately agree with a statement regardless of content—would be Type VII; "nay-sayers" would be Type VIII. If these patterns are not simply the result of response biases, then the same explanation proferred earlier for Type VI would hold for Type VII; individuals have also learned that certain aspects of their health are controlled by powerful others. Such an individual might even be better off than a Type V because the endorsement of CHLC beliefs might provide a convenient rationalization for those instances where one's best shot and the best efforts of others have all come to naught. Being a Type VIII might be indicative of a very selective "nay-sayer"; such persons might just be expressing the opinion that the sample of items contained in the MHLC scales does not reflect their own particular health locus of control expectancies. For example, someone who strongly believes that God controls health and illness might be Type VIII. No claim has been made that all possible HLC beliefs are tapped by the three MHLC dimensions (Wallston & Wallston, in press).

MEASUREMENT OF OTHER PSYCHOLOGICAL CONSTRUCTS

Aside from correlating health locus of control beliefs with other measures of locus of control expectancies, several studies have related HLC or MHLC scores to other constructs, some of which were themselves health-specific measures. Dishman, Ickes, and Morgan (1980) found a modest but significant relationship between HLC scores and their own measure of self-motivation. Those individuals scoring in the internal direction on the HLC expressed a higher degree of self-motivation. This correlation would probably be stronger with the individual MHLC scales, but they have not been correlated to date. Those scoring high on the PHLC might be high or low on self-motivation depending on what their IHLC and CHLC beliefs are.

Strickland (1978) suggested a relationship between Type A behavior characteristics (see Carver & Humphries, Chapter 2, this volume) and holding internal locus of control beliefs. Macri (1980) correlated the MHLC scales with the Type A subscale of the Jenkins Activity Survey (JAS) (Jenkins, Zyzanski, & Rosenman, 1979) but found no significant relationships. Her sample, consisting of men hospitalized for chest pain, was quite small ($n = 14$), so it is still possible that persons exhibiting Type A behavior might differ in their health locus of control beliefs from those who are not Type A.

Tolor (1978), studying a diverse group of graduate students and community volunteers, found no significant relationships between HLC scores and death anxiety or adjustment. Brown, Perman, and Dobbs (1981) studied a sample of geriatric patients all of whom recently had pacemakers implanted and found that HLC internality was correlated significantly with life satisfaction and the will-to-live. Hatz (1978) found high positive correlations between IHLC scores and past and expected future life satisfaction in a sample of chronic hemodialysis patients.

DeVellis, DeVellis, Wallston, and Wallston (1980a, 1980b) administered a depression scale (CES-D) (Radloff, 1975) along with the MHLC Scale in a survey of persons with epilepsy. CES-D scores were significantly correlated with CHLC and, to a lesser extent, PHLC beliefs. Similarly, in a sample of cancer patients receiving chemotherapy on an outpatient basis at Vanderbilt Hospital, we are also finding CHLC to be highly correlated with depression as assessed by the Zung Depression Scale (Zung, 1965). Nice (1980a) found that CHLC was significantly correlated with situational depressive affect (Ryman, Biersner, & LaRocco, 1974) among navy wives whose husbands were at sea, but correlations with IHLC and PHLC were not significant. Nice (1980a) reports: "This differential relationship between the chance and powerful other subscales of the MHLC on the criterion measure of depressive affect may provide a valuable extension of the work relating both learned helplessness and external locus of control to depression [p. 11]."

Krantz, Baum, and Wideman (1980) reported only modest correlations in one sample and no correlation in a second sample between HLC scores and the two subscales of the Krantz Health Opinion Survey (KHOS). One subscale (I) purportedly measures preferences for health-related information; the other (B) assesses desire for behavioral involvement (i.e., self-care and active participation) in medical care. In a recent study (Smith, Wallston, & Wallston 1981), we administered the KHOS along with the MHLC Scales to a sample of community volunteers and found highly significant interrelationships among the two KHOS subscales and the three MHLC Scales, with Krantz's B scale and the PHLC strongly negatively correlated. This suggests that these two scales are essentially tapping the same construct. The modest correlations found by Krantz et al. (1980) between the KHOS and HLC Scale were due to the fact that the HLC Scale does not measure PHLC beliefs. Further evidence for this assertion comes from Dunn (1980) who found a significant negative correlation between PHLC and attitude toward self-care (see Linn & Lewis, 1979), a construct similar to Krantz's measure of behavioral involvement.

In the Smith et al. (1981) study referred to earlier, we found IHLC scores to be uncorrelated with a general (nonhealth-specific) measure of desire for control (Burger & Cooper, 1979). Surprisingly, IHLC was also uncorrelated with a measure of expectancy for control in a specific health-related situation (as a patient in the hospital dying of a terminal illness), but it was positively correlated with desire for control in that same setting. CHLC and PHLC scores were also independent of the situation-specific expectancy measure, but both were negatively correlated with the measures of general and situation-specific desire for control. It is unclear why the health locus of control scales, which are measures of expectancies of control, demonstrate stronger correlations with measures of desire for control than with expectations for control in a particular health care setting; this latter measure, however, deals with control over the health care delivery process, whereas the MHLC Scales assess beliefs about control over outcomes (i.e., health and illness).

We are not aware of any studies correlating PHLC scores to measures of authoritarianism [e.g., Adorno, Frenkel-Brunswik, Levinson, & Sanford, 1950] or interpersonal trust (e.g., Rotter, 1967), two psychological constructs that in theory ought to correlate with beliefs that one's health is controlled by powerful other persons. As doctors and nurses are aften perceived by patients as authority figures, and as they usually act accordingly, it is logical to assume that people endorsing PHLC beliefs would also espouse authoritarian attitudes.

Individuals high in interpersonal trust, especially trust of health professionals, who also believed that powerful others controlled their health would not experience much dissonance (see Festinger, 1957). However, a person with high PHLC beliefs who did not trust other people would indeed be in a conflict state. Such an individual might be what Hochreich and others have termed a "defensive external" (see Phares, 1979), a person who answers a locus of control scale in an external direction but behaves like someone who actually holds internal beliefs. Hochreich (1974) has operationalized the defensive external as a person who scores high on the I–E Scale (Rotter, 1966) and low on the Interpersonal Trust Scale (Rotter, 1967). To date there have been no attempts to identify those persons who are defensive externals in regard to their health locus of control beliefs. If there are persons who distort their health locus of control beliefs, presumably to avoid blame if their health actions do not bring about desired results, this could explain why certain studies have not confirmed the hypothesized relationships between health locus of control beliefs and health behaviors.

Most of the findings reported in this section attest to the construct validity of the HLC scales. The most consistent relationship is between depressive affect and the belief that one's health is unpredictable (i.e., CHLC).

HEALTH INFORMATION AND PREVENTIVE MEASURES

One means by which individuals assume responsibility for their own health is to behave in a health-enhancing manner, thus maximizing the possibility of maintaining a satisfactory level of physical and mental well-being and helping to avoid illness or accidents. Some widely accepted ''healthy'' behaviors are: getting sufficient rest and exercise, eating and drinking in moderation, avoiding smoking (and others who are smoking), brushing and flossing the teeth regularly, wearing seat belts, and—although a matter of continuing controversy—receiving periodic physical examinations. Another aspect of behaving responsibly is to be informed and knowledgeable about all aspects of health and illness, including the health care system.

Strickland (1978) summarized the research relating measures of locus of control to health knowledge and precautionary measures by saying:

> With some exceptions, the bulk of the reported research on I–E and precautionary health practices lends credence to the expected theoretical assumptions that individuals who hold internal as opposed to external expectancies are more likely to assume responsibility for their health. Internals appear to attempt to maintain their physical well-being and guard against accidents and disease to a greater extent than individuals who hold external expectancies [p. 1194].

At the time Strickland did her review, there were only two published studies using the health locus of control scale (Wallston, Maides, & Wallston, 1976; Wallston, Wallston, Kaplan, & Maides, 1976). How does Strickland's conclusion stand up now, after a number of additional studies have been conducted using the health-specific locus of control measures?

Health Information Seeking

The initial studies investigating health locus of control beliefs and health-related information seeking (Wallston, Maides, & Wallston, 1976) established that persons who highly valued health[6] and who were classified as ''internals'' using the

[6]In these studies, high health value was operationalized as rank ordering health—among 10 terminal values—above the group's median ranking of health.

HLC Scale indicated a willingness to read more hypertension-related information than high health value HLC externals. The subjects for these studies were college students who were asked to pretend (i.e., to role play) that they had just been diagnosed as being hypertensive. DeVito, Reznikoff, and Bogdanowicz (1979) partially replicated this finding, but their attempt to extend the results to an actual measure of information seeking was not successful, nor was our attempt to generalize the finding to information seeking about obesity (see Wallston & Wallston, 1981).

Three studies have been done using the foregoing paradigm with the MHLC scales, and results are mixed (see Wallston & Wallston, 1981). One study of hypertension information seeking (again using college students who played the role of a newly diagnosed patient) failed to replicate the earlier findings. A second study, however, provided significant results. This latter study also included an actual information-seeking measure—whether or not the subject asked a question about the disease when given the opportunity to do so. Splitting subjects at the median on their MHLC scores and looking only at those who highly valued health, high IHLC, low CHLC, and high PHLC subjects asked more questions about hypertension than did their counterparts (i.e., low IHLC, high CHLC, low PHLC subjects). The measure of number of hypertension-related pamphlets the subjects said they would read was greater for high PHLC and low CHLC high health value subjects than their counterparts. High IHLC subjects did not choose more pamphlets than did low IHLC subjects. These MHLC results suggest that the Wallston, Maides, and Wallston (1976) findings with the HLC scale were due to the fact that those classified as HLC internals were actually low "chance externals" and not especially high in the belief that their own behavior influenced their health.

A third study attempting to generalize these findings to a different medical condition (herpes simplex virus) did not show the expected pattern of findings. Thus, for college students role playing hypertensive patients and indicating that they valued health highly, health locus of control beliefs are related to hypertension information seeking. But it is not necessarily the health internality dimension that is responsible for these findings. Significantly, in the one MHLC study that produced results (described earlier), high PHLC scorers sought more information than low PHLC scorers. This provides some further justification for separating the two external MHLC dimensions. Why these studies only "work" for hypertension and not for other medical conditions remains a puzzle.

There is some evidence that the hypertension information-seeking results might generalize beyond college students. Toner and Manuck (1979) had persons participating in a public health screening fill out the HLC Scale. After their blood pressure was measured, the subjects were allowed to choose from among 23 hypertension-related informational pamphlets. Within the older half of their subjects (mean age = 57.3 years), HLC internals chose significantly more pamphlets than HLC externals; no such difference was found for the younger half of the sample (mean age = 25.2). This latter null finding could, perhaps, be explained by the fact that Toner and Manuck did not assess health value. Inasmuch as health value is highly dependent on age—the older the person, the higher the value placed on health—Toner and Manuck's older sample probably contained mostly health-oriented persons, whereas the younger sample was mixed, thus washing out the HLC results.

In another study, Sproles (1977) administered the HLC Scale to renal dialysis patients and found that HLC internals knew more about their condition, desired to know even more, and were more willing to attend patient education classes than were HLC externals. We can only speculate about what results Sproles would have obtained if she had used the MHLC Scales, but it would be consistent with other findings to expect that Sproles' results would have been different for those espousing PHLC beliefs than for those high on CHLC.

Krantz et al. (1980) reported a nonsignificant correlation between college students' HLC scores and the number of questions asked of a clinic nurse during a visit for minor complaints. A three-way split of HLC scores appeared to suggest that those persons with moderate HLC beliefs asked the fewest number of questions. In a study of persons visiting a dental hygienist for regular checkups, we failed to find any relationship between MHLC scores and the hygienist's ratings of whether the person was an above average, below average, or average asker of questions compared to the typical patient in that situation. This result could have been due to the lack of validity of the hygienist's ratings, just as Krantz et al.'s (1980) findings may have been due to some invalidity in the clinic nurse's behavioral reports. Nevertheless, neither of those two studies provide much support for the relationship of health locus of control beliefs to the direct asking of questions to health professionals. Although Roter (1977) was able to train an experimental group to be more internal and ask more questions during physician visits than a control group, HLC scores did not correlate with questions asked. The power of her intervention may have wiped out the effect of individual differences, or the intervention may have been differentially effective, depending on initial health locus of control beliefs, but these analyses were not conducted. Further discussion of this study is provided in the section on "Responses to Health Care Interventions."

In a nationwide survey of persons with epilepsy (DeVellis et al., 1980b), we included a measure of epilepsy-relevant information seeking. The best single predictor of the subjects' expressed willingness to expose themselves to information about epilepsy was their PHLC scores, with high PHLC beliefs correlating significantly with high information seeking. Thus, here is a second piece of evidence that one does not have to hold exclusively internal health locus of control beliefs in order to seek health-relevant information. No studies, however, have shown that persons who are high in CHLC beliefs engage in health-related information seeking. One study, in fact, has found CHLC scores to be negatively correlated to medical self-care knowledge (Dunn, 1980). Therefore, a belief that one's health is controllable either by oneself or other persons (Types I, II, or V) may lead to information seeking, but a belief that one's health is unpredictable (i.e., Type III—high CHLC beliefs) does not dispose individuals to learn more about their health.

Preventive Health Behaviors

With the exception of three studies on smoking reduction, research correlating health locus of control beliefs with measures of behaviors carried out to maintain or enhance health has produced few significant relationships. Six separate surveys, each looking at a different sample of individuals—clerical workers (Baughman, 1978), health maintenance organization clients (Lauver, 1978), pregnant women (Lowenstein, 1979), health-fair attendees (Wallston & Wallston, 1978), and two nationwide surveys (Stuart, 1979)—have failed to find meaningful correlations between health locus of control beliefs and a wide range of health behaviors. In contrast to these mostly null results, Bronson (personal communication, 1981) studied adults undergoing comprehensive health examinations and found that those scoring above the mean on the IHLC Scale scored significantly higher on measures of health behavior, knowledge about health problems, and health plans than those scoring below the mean on IHLC. In a study of Welsh wives of skilled manual workers, Pill (1981) reported a negative relationship between PHLC scores and an interview-derived measure of salience of life style as a contributor to health. In other words, those Welsh women who rejected the notion that powerful others controlled their health were more likely to spontaneously mention life-style factors (e.g., diet, exercise) as causing or preventing illness. In those studies that have looked at specific (as opposed to broadly based) health behaviors, the findings have also been mixed. For example, Olbrisch (1975) reported no differences between HLC internal and HLC external gonorrhea patients in plans to take future precautions against the disease, and McCusker and Morrow (1979) found no relationship between HLC scores and preventive cancer behaviors.

Although not quite statistically significant, Fischberg (1979) found women who value their health highly and who were also high on IHLC were slightly more likely to practice breast self-examination than those low on IHLC. Grady (personal communication, 1981) found that scores on a shortened version of the MHLC Scales contributed 4% of the variance in the number of breast self-examination records returned. This was due predominantly to high CHLC women and high PHLC women returning less records (i.e., conducting fewer examinations) than low CHLC or low PHLC women.

Dishman et al. (1980) found that persons who stayed with a physical activity program had more internal HLC scores than persons who dropped out of the program. Kaplan (1974) however, did not find similar differences in dropouts from a weight management program. Saltzer (1979) also could not distinguish completers of a weight management program from noncompleters using the MHLC scores, but she did find that the completers were more internal on a weight-specific locus of control scale of her own design.

Grady (personal communication, 1981) found that persons who agreed to participate in her breast self-examination study had higher PHLC and IHLC scores than those who refused to participate but who were interviewed over the telephone. Perhaps holding beliefs that health can be controlled (Type V in our suggested typology) predisposes a person to cooperate with health education programs.

Carnahan (1979) failed to predict college students' scores on a dental plaque index from either their MHLC scores or a multidimensional dental health locus of control scale that she constructed. We were equally unsuccessful in correlating MHLC scores to self-reports of brushing and flossing or hygienists' ratings of teeth and gums in a study of adult patients receiving regular prophylactic care.

Three studies of mothers' preventive health behavior vis-á-vis their children failed to find any relationship with MHLC beliefs. The behaviors examined were immunization levels (Berger, 1980), vitamin supplementation (Gossler, 1980), and car seat usage (Guske, 1980).

In the area of smoking reduction, Kaplan and Cowles (1978) found that high health value, HLC internals reduced their cigarette consumption and maintained the reduction to a greater extent than other subjects. Wildman, Rosenbaum, Framer, Keane, and Johnson (1979) reported similar findings, although they did not measure health value. HLC internals cut back more during treatment and maintained more of the reduction than did HLC externals. Shipley (1980), using the MHLC scales, found results similar to those of Wildman et al. but only for the IHLC and CHLC scales; scores on the PHLC were unrelated to the ability to stop smoking.

Given Strickland's (1978) summary of the early research in this area, it is indeed disappointing that health locus of control beliefs are not more strongly related to measures of preventive health behaviors because these behaviors are what most people think about when they think of assuming responsibility for their health. One explanation for this almost total lack of expected findings is that preventive health behaviors are multidetermined, and it is simplistic to believe that any single construct such as locus of control will predict much of the variance in individual health behaviors (Rotter, 1975; Wallston & Wallston, 1981). This may even be the case for those studies that have included a measure of health value and have attempted to predict health behavior from the interaction of health locus of control beliefs and the importance placed on health as an outcome. Although in theory this bivariate predictor approach appears superior, it is undoubtedly the case that still other variables, such as specific beliefs about the behavior(s) in question, carry most of the weight in predicting behavior. Moreover, it has been argued that attitude-behavior prediction can be improved by broadening the scope of behavioral measures and multiple observations (Ajzen & Fishbein, 1977; Epstein, 1979; Weigel & Newman, 1976). Although health behaviors are frequently uncorrelated (e.g., Steele & McBroom, 1972), indices summing over a variety of health behaviors would take into account different behavioral expressions of the same attitude or expectancy. Thus, locus of control beliefs may make better predictions of such behavioral indices than any specific health behavior.

It is also quite likely that many people believe one thing but behave quite differently when it comes to protecting their health. Nurses, for example, have one of the highest smoking rates of any profession (cf. National Clearinghouse for Smoking & Health, 1977), yet they are fully cognizant of the health risks involved and would strongly oppose the behavior in their patients. Engaging in preventive health behavior is often quite costly either because the behavior itself involves some effort (e.g., flossing one's teeth, exercising regularly, practicing birth control) or because something very reinforcing has to be reduced or eliminated altogether (e.g., desserts, cigarettes). Even people who highly value their health and who believe their behavior influences their health will, on occasion, behave contradictorily to their beliefs and values. At those moments, there are other outcomes the individual values even more than good health.

Inasmuch as Strickland (1978) reviewed mostly studies using general rather than health-specific measures of locus of control and reached such optimistic conclusions about the relationship between locus of control beliefs and preventive health behaviors, it is puzzling why the studies cited in this chapter, which utilized the health locus of control scales, for the most part failed to demonstrate significant relationships. It would be wrong to infer that general locus of control beliefs are related to engaging in preventive health behaviors, whereas health-specific locus of control beliefs are not; no study has yet shown this to be the case. Rather, as with many other areas in social psychology, as more studies are done in a particular "promising" area using refined methodologies, we learn that the world is not as simple as we would have it be.

REACTIONS TO PHYSICAL CONDITIONS

Because expectancies with respect to locus of control are learned, health and illness status as well as experiences with the health care system should influence these beliefs. Moreover, health locus of control beliefs (in conjunction with health value and aspects of the situation) should influence one's responses to symptoms and to chronic illness. In this section, literature is reviewed on the health locus of control beliefs of persons with a variety of physical conditions, the relation between such beliefs and responses to symptoms, and the adherence with medical regimens of persons whose beliefs vary.

Responses to Disability

Strickland (1978) noted:

> Any impending or disabling disorder, whether chronic or temporary, has a varying degree of influence on the responses of the persons faced with the handicap. The severity of the disorder, the time of the onset, the current status of the patient, the support that he/she receives, and so on, all interact with what is probably a complex set of cognitions about the disorder. When an individual is more helpless than he/she once was, or is handicapped in relation to others, beliefs about locus of control would be expected to be, and apparently are, related to reactions to the disorder [p. 1198].

Reviewing the literature on generalized locus of control beliefs conducted primarily with chronically handicapped children (e.g., Eggland, 1973; Goldstein, 1976), Strickland concluded that such individuals tend to be more external than their healthy counterparts. Studies of adult health locus of control beliefs appear to confirm these early findings (see Wallston & Wallston, 1981).

In particular, across a variety of chronic patient samples, beliefs in chance and in powerful others as the locus of control for one's health are relatively high, whereas beliefs in internal health locus of control are similar to those of healty adults. Such findings are relatively consistent across diverse conditions, including cancer, diabetes, epilepsy, and respiratory disease (Wallston & Wallston, 1981). However, as these data are not longitudinal, one can only hypothesize that such beliefs arise out of experience with illness. Persons with a history of illness (and therefore in frequent interaction with the health care system) may develop complex and differentiated beliefs in relation to the locus of causality of health and illness. While maintaining beliefs in IHLC, chronically ill persons may recognize that they did not bring about their illness, and thus an increased belief in CHLC may develop. Moreover, persons with chronic conditions are more reliant on family members or health professionals for care, and thus high PHLC beliefs are likely to develop. This is a case where Type VII (yea-sayers) may reflect a reasonable belief structure rather than response scale bias.

Some additional evidence that health locus of control beliefs develop in relation to illness experiences comes from our national survey of persons with epilepsy (DeVellis et al., 1980a). A modest but significant proportion of the variance in beliefs in chance, internal, and powerful others health locus of control was predicted from seizure history variables (e.g., having an aura, whether a seizure can be avoided, seizure severity, age of first seizure, and number of years with seizures). Interestingly, the best prediction was to PHLC beliefs. As these data are correlational and also cross-sectional rather than longitudinal, one could argue that reports of history were influenced by respondents' beliefs. However, the concrete nature of some of the history variables (e.g., number of years with seizures) suggests that history with epilepsy has influenced these beliefs. Tolor (1978) similarly found, for women but not for men, that those with severe and frequent childhood accidents and illness held more HLC external beliefs. Longitudinal investigations are needed to further our understanding of responses to disability.

Symptoms

There is some indication that women with internal HLC beliefs report fewer menstrual symptoms (deHaas & vanReken, 1979). Also, Nice (1980b) found CHLC scores correlated with number of physical symptoms reported by naval wives separated from their husbands away at sea. In a stepwise regression, CHLC was the best predictor of physical symptoms. For his total sample, including navy wives whose husbands were not at sea, Nice (personal communication, 1981) found that CHLC correlated positively and IHLC correlated negatively with reported number of symptoms. Inasmuch as Nice's data are prospective, they suggest that endorsement of CHLC beliefs may result in heightened sensitivity to symptoms. However, chance locus of control beliefs may develop as a response to increased symptomatology. Nice's longitudinal data provide a means of differentiating among these hypotheses, although such analyses have not yet been done.

Adherence to Medical Regimens

Although Strickland (1978) noted that: "internal adults . . . attempt to influence health care to a greater extent than externals [p. 1198]," Wallston and Wallston (1978) concluded that: "the relation between compliance with medical regimen and locus of control is unclear [p. 112]." Research using the HLC and MHLC Scales continues to provide conflicting data.

Although research using only the I–E distinction provides some evidence that internality is related to judged dietary compliance among male hypertensives (Wallston & McLeod, 1979) and self-reported medication compliance for hypertensives who also perceived a high level of assistance in following their regimen (Lewis, Morisky, & Flynn, 1978), contrary data also exist. Key (1975) found better adherence by HLC externals in terms of medication taking (indexed by urinary drug levels) and diet among the predominantly black, female hypertensive patients investigated. Two studies (Key, 1975; Wallston & McLeod, 1978) found no relationship between HLC and appointment keeping or self-reported medication taking.

The distinction between chance and powerful-others health locus of control seems particularly important in understanding adherence behavior, and multidimensional studies provide somewhat more consistent data. There is no indication that beliefs in CHLC are predictive of adherence (e.g., Goldstein, 1980; Hatz, 1978; Levin & Schulz, 1980). However, some studies indicate that internality is the best predictor of adherence, whereas others suggest the importance of a powerful-others orientation. Levin and Schulz (1980) found that renal dialysis patients scoring high on IHLC adhered more closely to their diet and restricted weight gain more than did low scorers, whereas PHLC scores were unrelated to these adherence measures. McGrath (1980) similarly found that those mothers she classified as internal more regularly administered anticonvulsants to their epileptic children than those mothers with the strongest beliefs in powerful others; however, her comparison of each person's IHLC, PHLC, and CHLC scores failed to take into account normative differences among the scales.[7] Goldstein (1980) found that beliefs in internality and in powerful others were positively related to a diabetic management index among adult insulin-dependent diabetics. Hatz (1978) found that beliefs in powerful others but not internality was related to less weight gain between treatments, a reasonable proxy measure of adherence by dialysis patients. However, Nagy (personal communication, 1981) found no relation between MHLC scores and clinic visits, medication taking, or other adherence behaviors among the diabetic, hypertensive, and pulmonary patients she studied.

DeVellis et al. (1980b) found that MHLC variables explained a significant amount of variance in an index of self-reported health-related behaviors of persons with epilepsy. The adherence behaviors investigated were medication taking, refraining from driving, and refraining from drinking alcohol. The best three predictors of the behavioral index were PHLC, IHLC multiplied by health value, and IHLC alone. This latter factor correlated negatively with the index, reflecting that—without regard to the value placed on health—internals with epilepsy were more likely to admit driving, drinking, and failing to take their medication. Those internals with high health value, however, were more likely to report adherence. For persons with mild epilepsy, driving and drinking in moderation might be viewed as adaptive behaviors, even though persons with epilepsy are told not to engage in either.

Thus, beliefs in internality and in powerful others health locus of control may be conducive to adherence. More work is needed distinguishing between types of adherence and investigating typologies of beliefs in this area. We have noted that a partnership with health professionals may entail both IHLC and PHLC beliefs

---

[7]Because within the American culture beliefs in IHLC are typically stronger than beliefs in CHLC and PHLC, comparisons among scores should be made only after standardizing within each scale. Most persons score above the theoretical mean on IHLC and below the theoretical mean on CHLC. Drawing comparisons between raw scores for an individual without taking this general tendency into account is inappropriate.

(i.e., Type V) and that such a partnership is particularly important for patients with chronic diseases.

RESPONSES TO HEALTH CARE INTERVENTIONS

Health locus of control expectancies can contribute to understanding responses to health care interventions in two ways. As we have previously noted (Wallston & Wallston, 1978), many interventions, particularly health education programs, emphasize patient responsibility and internal beliefs. One indicator of the success of such programs would be changes in expectancies regarding health locus of control, utilizing such beliefs as a dependent measure. Alternatively, health locus of control beliefs may be considered an independent variable, and programs may prove differentially effective for persons with differing beliefs. We have previously argued for the potential value of tailoring programs to individuals' expectancies (Wallston & Wallston, 1978). Strickland (1978) has similarly concluded: "Congruence between locus of control expectancies and the structure of the therapeutic endeavor appears to lead to the most pervasive changes [p. 1203]." For example, Cromwell, Butterfield, Brayfield, and Curry (1977) found that among cardiac patients, only those in incongruent conditions (externals with high participation or internals with low participation in self-treatment) either returned to the hospital or died within 12 weeks following their hospital stay. Research utilizing health-specific measures of these expectancies can now be reviewed, considering such expectancies as dependent and independent variables.

Health Locus of Control as a Dependent Variable

Several studies of health education programs have failed to find changes in locus of control beliefs consistent with program intent (Davis, 1979; Nagelberg, 1979; Schiller, Stekler, Dawson, & Heyman, 1979). Whether these findings are suggestive of problems with the programs or the scales is not clear. Moreover, all of these programs involved healthy participants with relatively high beliefs in internality at the outset. Thus, a ceiling effect may have been involved or the programs may have been aimed at the wrong audience. Moreover, Davis (1979) and Schiller et al. (1979) report relatively high program attrition. There is some indication in the Schiller et al. (1979) study that completers had stronger internal beliefs than those who did not attend class regularly (see Wallston & Wallston, 1981, for a more detailed discussion). Davis (1979) presented no pretest data on program dropouts. Special intervention may be necessary to maintain the health education class participation of healthy individuals with low beliefs in internality.

Roter's (1977) health education intervention, designed to increase question asking during a medical visit, successfully increased scores on internal health locus of control beliefs for experimental group patients in comparison to placebo group patients. As this sample was predominantly black, female, elderly, and chronically ill, it is impossible to gauge whether the nature of the intervention or the subject population accounted for the success of this study in contrast to those reported earlier.

Two studies with cancer patients provide some evidence for intervention effectiveness in influencing HLC beliefs. Mastectomy patients who received a special counseling intervention were significantly less external than the standard care comparison group 2 months after surgery (Bloom, 1979). There was some indication of increased externality among control group cancer patients after 3 months in comparison to the experimental group receiving a psychosocial rehabilitation intervention (Diller, Gordon, Friedenbergs, Ruckdeschel-Hibbard, Levine, Wolf, Ezrachi, Lipkins, Lucido, & Francis, 1979; see also, Wallston & Wallston, 1981). But significant changes over time were not reported in another report of the study (Gordon, Friedenbergs, Diller, Hibbard, Wolf, Levine, Lipkins, Ezrachi, & Lucido, 1980). However, control group dropouts at 6 months were more external, whereas intervention group dropouts did not differ on this variable. Gordon et al. (1980) conclude:

> The cluster of variables associated with attrition [in the control group] (older, less educated, high external locus of control, etc.) may be viewed as potential barriers to rehabilitation, since they are factors that work against a patient's maintaining contact with components of the health care system. . . . In contrast, intervention appeared to militate against these sources of attrition, since systematic intervention had the benefit of maintaining contact with those who might have been lost at follow-up [p. 757].

Each study discussed in this section has utilized a different intervention with a different sample. Further work is clearly needed on the nature of appropriate interventions if changes in health locus of control expectancies are desired. Such changes would be appropriate were there sufficient evidence that particular belief structures are related to health behaviors. For example, if we knew for certain that Type I individuals (pure internals) were the ones most likely to live a healthy life style, we might want to increase the number of Type I persons in the population. Additional research investigating belief-behavior relationships is necessary before interventions to change beliefs are recommended.

Moreover, interventions must be designed with the nature of the clients in mind. Somewhat more success has been evident in interventions with chronically ill samples than with healthy samples. This may be because healthy persons who volunteer for health education interventions are the ones whose expectancies are already in line with the intervention. For example, participants at a YMCA health fair had higher internal and lower chance health locus of control beliefs compared with typical adult samples (Wallston & Wallston, 1978). More research is needed on attracting and maintaining contact with persons who most need health education intervention.

Health Locus of Control as an Independent Variable

Although there is still reason to believe that tailoring treatments to locus of control beliefs has great promise, the limited evidence to date is not yet encouraging. Two studies of self-medication classes for psychiatric patients preparing for discharge (Battle & Halliburton, 1979; Witt, 1978) failed to impact on medication adherence for internals and externals. However, at the time of discharge, external low health value patients were the least adherent in one of these studies (Battle & Halliburton, 1979) as would be expected theoretically. Saltzer (1979, 1980) found no differences in effectiveness or completion of a medical weight reduction program in relation to generalized health locus of control beliefs. However, her own weight locus of control scale was predictive of behavior. Program completers were more internal with respect to expectancies regarding weight loss, and weight locus of control internals who valued health or physical appearance were more likely to translate their behavioral intentions to lose weight into successful weight loss.[8]

In the one study clearly designed to test the notion of tailoring treatments, the findings were mixed (Wallston, Wallston, Kaplan, & Maides, 1976). Although HLC internals expressed greater satisfaction with a self-directed weight management program and HLC externals (PHLC and CHLC combined) were more satisfied with the therapist-directed program, weight loss data were in the expected direction but not statistically significant.

Inasmuch as three of the four reported studies did not utilize interventions specifically tailored to locus of control expectancies, the lack of differerential effects is not surprising. Further work on tailoring treatments to HLC expectancies is clearly needed.

INTERACTION WITH HEALTH CARE SETTINGS

Little work has been done on differential responses to health care settings in relation to health locus of control expectancies. In a theoretical analysis, Taylor (1979) has characterized the hospital environment as one in which people have

[8]The findings regarding physical appearance suggest the importance of measuring the value of the appropriate reinforcer. Behaviors we classify as health-relevant may have other reinforcing properties.

little control. This should be particularly problematic for persons who expect and desire control. Research on differential utilization of health systems and responses to such systems can now be reviewed.

Health System Utilization

Differential utilization of health systems has been found by persons differing in health locus of control beliefs. Krantz et al. (1980) found that HLC internal college students reported fewer clinic visits, perhaps indicative of self-reliance. A second sample of HLC internals was more likely to use self-diagnosis. However, Krantz's own Health Opinion Survey was a better predictor of these behaviors than the HLC Scale.

The importance of the distinction between chance and powerful-others health locus of control is evident from Nice's data on navy wives' visits to physicians (personal communication, 1981). The women with higher beliefs in PHLC had some tendency to visit physicians more frequently, whereas beliefs in CHLC and IHLC were unrelated to this behavior. However, when data were analyzed separately for navy wives separated from their husbands who were at sea, none of the MHLC scales correlated with the number of physician visits. The separated wives visited physicians more frequently than control group wives (Nice, 1980b). Symptoms were the major predictor of physician visits for the separated wives, and as already discussed, CHLC is positively correlated with reporting of symptoms. Thus, beliefs in CHLC have an indirect, rather than a direct, influence on doctor visits because they moderate perception or reporting of symptoms.

Macri (1980) found that PHLC was negatively correlated with total delay in seeking treatment among males hospitalized with chest pain. Neither IHLC nor CHLC beliefs were related to total delay. Using Safer, Tharps, Jackson, and Leventhal's (1979) distinctions between appraisal delay (deciding one is ill), illness delay (deciding that medical care is needed), and utilization delay (time between illness delay and seeking care), it appears that the correlation with total delay is due to the relationship between PHLC beliefs and illness delay. It is theoretically consistent that recognition of the need for medical care would come more quickly for those with strong PHLC beliefs. No MHLC belief dimension predicted utilization delay, but appraisal delay was significantly related to CHLC beliefs. As 93% of this sample ranked health value high, linear relations with health locus of control beliefs are to be expected. Although the small sample size of this study makes one wary of generalization, the data are consistent theoretically and provide further indication of the importance of the multidimensional distinctions.

Butler (1980) studied first-time clients of chiropractors, nutrition counselors, and medical doctors. Clients of alternative practitioners had lower CHLC beliefs than medical-doctor clients. Clients of medical doctors reported the highest

PHLC beliefs, whereas clients of nutrition counselors evidenced the lowest PHLC beliefs. Although nutrition-counselor clients were the most internal and medical-doctor clients the least internal, the IHLC dimension did not discriminate between groups because this highly educated, predominantly white sample evidenced high IHLC beliefs relative to adult normative data. Inasmuch as long symptom duration was the best discriminator between clients of alternative practitioners and those of medical doctors, low PHLC beliefs may reflect the lack of positive response by the medical system to clients' health problems. In addition to long-standing health problems, these clients of alternative practitioners had seen more health practitioners within the last year and expressed more negative attitudes regarding the professional competence of medical doctors. Butler's findings are particularly important because they account for more variance than most of the studies in the utilization research literature (see Mechanic, 1979, for a review); they also emphasize the importance of the multivariate health locus of control distinctions.

Responses to Health Systems

Krantz et al. (1980) found that internal college students who visited the clinic were more likely to assert themselves by requesting specific medications than moderate scorers or those with more external health locus of control beliefs.

Roter (personal communication, 1981) analyzed verbal content and filtered speech of patients interacting with physicians. Among internals, verbal content showed high scorers to be less anxious, more satisfied, and more assertive than low scorers. High internal scorers' filtered speech also showed less anxiety, and they were judged as more likely to return to the clinic. For externals, no relationships were found on verbal content analyses. For filtered speech, high external scorers evidenced more anxiety and were judged less likely to return to the clinic than low external scorers.

Although Binik and Devins (1979) found no differences in HLC beliefs among renal dialysis patients on staff-assisted hospital dialysis, patient-managed hospital dialysis, and home dialysis patients, Levin and Schulz (1980) found some distinctions. Hospital hemodialysis patients evidenced stronger PHLC beliefs than did self-care patients, although the groups did not differ in CHLC or IHLC beliefs.

In a recent study (Smith et al., 1981), we have found that participants wishing to die in a hospital had higher PHLC scores than those expressing a preference for dying at home or in a hospice facility. These groups did not differ in CHLC or IHLC beliefs.

Nicholson (1980) found that mothers involved in prepared childbirth expressed decreased IHLC beliefs and increased CHLC beliefs following delivery. Experiences during hospitalization (e.g., being bullied by the doctor) could account for these changes.

Although data on responses to health systems are limited, they support the importance of differentiating internal, chance, and powerful-others HLC beliefs. Work investigating and manipulating control in health care settings in relation to people's expectancies is an important direction for future research.

THE TYPOLOGY REVISITED

The bulk of the research reviewed in this chapter has concentrated on individual differences in beliefs and behaviors and has typically ignored situational factors. Too little attention in this research has been paid to the situation and the actual contingencies that are present. Many people, including ourselves, have often taken the naive position that it is important to strengthen internal beliefs and create "internals" or Type I's (cf. Wallston & Wallston, 1973), but there may be instances when this is unwarranted. Wortman and Dunkel-Schetter (1979) noted that internal beliefs may be maladaptive for some persons with cancer if, indeed, there is nothing that they themselves can do about their condition. High IHLC (Type I) cancer patients might expend valuable energy and resources in futile attempts to alter the course of their condition positively (e.g., flying to a foreign country to obtain Laetril or some other highly touted "cure" not available locally), or they might refuse to take advantage of some possibly effective treatment (e.g., chemotherapy or radiation), the availability of which is mediated by powerful others.

Another drawback to being a strong Type I individual is that espousing such beliefs may alienate potential helpers who, when alienated, might be all too willing to let the patient assume total responsibility and then turn around and blame the patient if and when things go wrong. The movement toward getting persons to assume more of the responsibility for their own health can be viewed as an abrogation of responsibility on the part of the health care system. We may see a great deal of "blaming the victim" (cf. Ryan, 1971) when patients' efforts in contributing to their own health come to naught. This is not to suggest that strong beliefs in IHLC are not adaptive under some conditions.

Patients with chronic diseases are often heavily reliant on health professionals or other people such as family or friends. In these instances, strong PHLC beliefs reflect actual situational contingencies and are probably adaptive, but only if other people are willing and able to be of assistance. The person who believes exclusively in control by powerful others (Type II in our suggested typology) would be totally helpless if others were not there to give help and direction.

Although Bulman and Wortman (1977) found that taking responsibility for an accident related to positive coping by spinal cord injury patients, CHLC beliefs can be a positive response to the question "Why me?," which frequently is the initial reaction to illness onset or accidental injury. Strickland (1978) noted: "It may be that a defensive stance is helpful when a person who is accustomed to considerable personal control is suddenly faced with events beyond his or her influence [p. 1198].'' It might be better to believe that you were singled out for misfortune on a strictly random basis than to feel that you brought your troubles on yourself or that someone else was out to get you.

Thus, in the early stages of trying to come to grips with ill health—especially if you are in the hands of competent health professionals—there might be definite advantages to being Type III or IV. The linkage between CHLC and depressive affect and the reporting of physical symptoms, however, suggests that Type III beliefs may not be generally adaptive; that is, only when no real control is possible is it likely that perception of lack of control is highly adaptive. In fact, Langer (1975, 1977) has argued for the adaptiveness of perceiving more control than may be present, and research on depression (cf. Arnkoff & Mahoney, 1979; Golin, Terrell, & Johnson, 1977) suggests that persons who are depressed more accurately perceive situational contingencies. The value of Type III (chance external) beliefs is an open question.

Earlier in this chapter we discussed the Type V belief pattern (high IHLC, high PHLC, low CHLC) as conducive to forming a partnership between health care consumer and provider. At that time we were only referring to the consumer's beliefs. Obviously, however, it takes two to form a partnership. Nothing is known about the health locus of control beliefs of health care providers, particularly about which beliefs they would want their patients to hold. We can speculate that the ideal partnership between provider and consumer is one in which they mutually believe that each has something to bring to the partnership and that only by working together will they optimize the outcomes. The relationship between Norman Cousins and his personal physician exemplifies this.

In order for such partnerships to form and work, however, a revolutionary change needs to take place in the socialization of health professionals, especially physicians who often develop a self-perception of omnipotence and omniscience (Kane & Kane, 1969). According to one leader of this revolution (Mendelsohn, 1979), in the new medicine: ''Health neither begins nor ends with the doctor. The doctor's role is somewhere in the middle [p. 171].'' This medical ''heretic'' goes on to say: ''The doctor–patient relationship is democratic in the sense that both doctor and patient share information equally [p. 173].'' Getting doctors to inform patients fully of relevant facts is a revolutionary concept and one that will entail great behavioral changes on the part of many providers. The Type V patient, however, will be eager and ready to have that information.

As currently organized, the health care system in general is oriented toward removing control from patients and placing it in the hands of health care professionals. This is particularly true within hospitals (Taylor, 1979). However, the system and individuals in the system give patients mixed messages. On the one hand, hospitals are total institutions (cf. Goffman, 1961) filled with dehumanization and loss of control for patients. On the other hand, as patients leave the hospital, particularly those with chronic conditions, they are told to take care of themselves and assume responsibility for their health. Little preparation for such responsibility is provided to patients, and they are blamed when they do not follow doctors' orders and engage in health and sick role behaviors. Yet even the term *compliance* suggests a hierarchical rather than partnership relationship between patients and physicians (see Leventhal & Hirschman, Chapter 7, this volume). "Good patients" are those who obey orders and do not question the doctor's authority (Taylor, 1979).

What are the implications of these ideas for research on control and health care delivery? It is clear that a personological approach is too narrow. Person and situation (Lewin, 1951) must be considered. Research must take into account actual situational potential for control, patients' perceptions and expectancies regarding control, and the expectancies of health care providers. Only by studying the complex interaction of these factors will we be able to predict health behavior and thus intervene effectively to enhance health.

ACKNOWLEDGMENTS

Work on this chapter has been facilitated by Grant #HS 04096 from the National Center for Health Services Research. The chapter was written while the second author was on leave at the Department of Medical Psychology, Uniformed Services University of the Health Sciences, Bethesda, Md. and the Department of Psychology, University of Maryland, College Park. The authors wish to thank Patricia Williamson for her assistance in preparing this manuscript.

REFERENCES

Adorno, T., Frenkel-Brunswik, E., Levinson, D., & Sanford, N. *The authoritarian personality.* New York: Harper, 1950.

Ajzen, I., & Fishbein, M. Attitude-behavior relations: A theoretical analysis and review of empirical research. *Psychological Bulletin,* 1977, *84,* 888–918.

Arnkoff, D. B., & Mahoney, M. J. The role of perceived control in psychopathology. In L. C. Perlmuter & R. A. Monty (Eds.), *Choice and perceived control.* Hillsdale, N.J.: Lawrence Erlbaum Associates, 1979.

Battle, E. H., & Halliburton, A. *Self-medication among psychiatric inpatients and adherence after discharge.* Unpublished manuscipt, Veterans Administration Medical Center, Murfreesboro, Tenn., 1979.

Baughman, M. K. *The relationship of locus of control and value beliefs to health status and behavior among clerical workers.* Unpublished doctoral dissertation, University of Cincinnati, 1978.

Berger, D. M. *The relationship between health locus of control and health values of the mother and immunization levels of her children.* Unpublished master's thesis, Virginia Commonwealth University, Richmond, 1980.

Binik, Y. M., & Devins, G. *Personal control in end-stage renal disease.* Paper presented at the annual meeting of the American Psychological Association, New York, 1979.

Bloom, J. R. Psychosocial measurement and specific hypotheses: A research note. *Journal of Consulting and Clinical Psychology*, 1979, *47*, 637–639.

Brown, J. S., Perman, B. S., & Dobbs, J. L. The will to live. *Research on Aging*, 1981, *3*(2), 182–201.

Bulman, R. J., & Wortman, C. B. Attributions of blame and coping in the "real world": Severe accident victims react to their lot. *Journal of Personality and Social Psychology*, 1977, *35*, 351–363.

Burger, J. M., & Cooper, H. M. The desirability of control. *Motivation and Emotion*, 1979, *3*, 381–393.

Butler, J. *The utilization of alternative health services*. Unpublished doctoral dissertation, George Peabody College for Teachers of Vanderbilt University, 1980.

Carnahan, T. M. *The development and validation of the multidimensional dental locus of control scales*. Unpublished doctoral dissertation, State University of New York, Buffalo, 1979.

Couch, A., & Keniston, K. Yeasayers and naysayers: Agreeing response set as a personality variable. *Journal of Abnormal and Social Psychology*, 1960, *60*, 151–174.

Cousins, N. *Antomy of an illness as perceived by the patient*. New York: Norton, 1979.

Cromwell, R. L., Butterfield, D. C., Brayfield, F. M., & Curry, J. J. *Acute myocardial infarction: Reaction and recovery*. St. Louis: Mosby, 1977.

Dabbs, J. M., & Kirscht, J. P. Internal control and the taking of influenza shots. *Psychological Reports*, 1971, *28*, 959–962.

Davis, P. T. *Effect of exposure to the health hazard appraisal on the scores obtained on the multidimensional health locus of control scales*. Unpublished master's thesis, Virginia Commonwealth University, 1979.

deHaas, P. A., & vanReken, M. K. *Menstrual cycle symptoms as a function of health locus of control*. Paper presented at the Association for Women in Psychology Conference, Dallas, Tex., 1979.

DeVellis, R. F., DeVellis, B. M., Wallston, B. S., & Wallston, K. A. Epilepsy and learned helplessness. *Basic and Applied Social Psychology*, 1980, *1*, 241–253. (a)

DeVellis, R. F., DeVellis, B. M., Wallston, K. A., & Wallston, B. S. *Epilepsy as an analogue of learned helplessness*. Paper presented at the annual meeting of the American Psychological Association, Montreal, 1980. (b)

DeVito, A. J., Reznikoff, M., & Bogdanowicz, J. *Actual and intended health-related information seeking and health locus of control*. Paper presented at the annual meeting of the American Psychological Association, New York, 1979.

Diller, L., Gordon, W. A., Friedenbergs, I., Ruckdeschel-Hibbard, M., Levine, L. R., Wolf, C., Ezrachi, O., Lipkins, R., Lucido, D., & Francis, A. *Demonstration of benefits of early identification of psychosocial problems and early intervention toward rehabilitation of cancer patients* (National Cancer Institute Contract #N01–CN–55188, Final Report). New York University Medical Center, 1979.

Dishman, R. K., Ickes, W., & Morgan, W. P. Self-motivation and adherence to habitual physical activity. *Journal of Applied Social Psychology*, 1980, *10*, 115–132.

Dunn, D. A. *The relationship of health locus of control and health value to medical self-care knowledge and attitudes of undergraduate and graduate health education majors in Oregon*. Unpublished doctoral dissertation, University of Oregon, Portland, 1980.

Eggland, E. T. Locus of control and children with cerebral palsy. *Nursing Research*, 1973, *22*, 267–270.

Epstein, S. The stability of behavior: I. On predicting most of the people much of the time. *Journal of Personality and Social Psychology*, 1979, *37*, 1097–1126.

Festinger, L. *A theory of cognitive dissonance*. Stanford, Cal.: Stanford University Press, 1957.

Fischberg, E. B. *Frequency of breast self-examination and health locus of control in women who do and do not participate in consciousness raising*. Unpublished master's thesis, Pace University, 1979.

Ginzberg, E. The sacred cows of health manpower. *Man and Medicine*, 1977, *2*, 235–242.

Goffman, E. *Asylums*. Garden City, N.Y.: Doubleday Anchor, 1961.

Goldstein, A. M. Denial and external locus of control as mechanisms of adjustment in chronic medical illness. *Essence*, 1976, *1*, 5–22.

Goldstein. L. *Relationship of health locus of control and individual diabetic management*. Unpublished master's thesis, Pace University, 1980.

Golin, S., Terrell, F., & Johnson, B. Depression and the delusion of control. *Journal of Abnormal Psychology*, 1977, *86*, 440–442.

Gordon, W. A., Friedenbergs, I., Diller, L., Hibbard, M., Wolf, C., Levine, L., Lipkins, R., Ezrachi, O., & Lucido, D. Efficacy of psychosocial intervention with cancer patients. *Journal of Consulting and Clinical Psychology*, 1980, *48*, 743–759.

Gossler, J. L. *The study of the non prescription vitamin giving behaviors of mothers of preschool and schoolaged children*. Unpublished master's thesis, University of Oregon, Portland, 1980.

Guske, S. J. *Factors determining the usage of infant car seats by mothers in the Kaiser Permanente medical program*. Unpublished master's thesis, University of Oregon, Portland, 1980.

Hatz, P. S. *The relationship of life satisfaction and locus of control in patients undergoing chronic hemodialysis*. Unpublished master's thesis, University of Illinois, 1978.

Hochreich, D. Defensive externality and attribution of responsibility. *Journal of Personality*, 1974, *42*, 543–557.

Jenkins, C. O., Zyzanski, S. J., & Rosenman, R. H. Progress toward validation of a computer scored test for the Type A coronary-prone behavior pattern. *Psychosomatic Medicine*, 1979, *33*, 193–202.

Joe, V. C. Review of the internal–external control construct as a personality variable. *Psychological Reports*, 1971, *28*, 619–640.

Kane, R. L., & Kane, R. A. Physicians' attitudes of omnipotence in a university hospital. *Journal of Medical Education*, 1969, *44*, 684–690.

Kaplan, G. D. *Externally and eternally obese: The application of locus of control to the treatment of obesity*. Unpublished manuscript, Vanderbilt University, 1974.

Kaplan, G. D., & Cowles, A. Health locus of control and health value in prediction of smoking reduction. *Health Education Monographs*, 1978, *6*, 129–137.

Key, M. K. *Psychosocial and education factors surrounding compliance behavior of hypertensives*. Unpublished doctoral dissertation, George Peabody College for Teachers, 1975.

Kirscht, J. P. Perceptions of control and health beliefs. *Canadian Journal of Behavioral Science*, 1972, *4*, 225–237.

Krantz, D. S., Baum, A., & Wideman, M. V. Assessment of preferences for self-treatment and information in medical care. *Journal of Personality and Social Psychology*, 1980, *39*, 977–990.

Langer, E. J. The illusion of control. *Journal of Personality and Social Psychology*, 1975, *32*, 311–328.

Langer, E. J. The psychology of chance. *Journal for the Theory of Social Behavior*, 1977, *7*, 185–208.

Lauver, D. *Relevant factors of client responsibility: Health locus of control, value on health, and temporal orientation*. Unpublished master's thesis, University of Rochester, 1978.

Lefcourt, H. M. Internal versus external locus of control: A review. *Psychological Bulletin*, 1966, *65*, 206–220.

Lefcourt, H. M. *Locus of control: Current trends in theory and research*. Hillsdale, N.J.: Lawrence Erlbaum Associates, 1976.

Lefcourt, H. M. (Ed.). *Research with the locus of control construct* (Vol. 1). New York: Academic Press, 1981.

Levenson, H. Multidimensional locus of control in psychiatric patients. *Journal of Consulting and Clinical Psychology*, 1973, *41*, 397–404.

Levenson, H. Differentiating among internality, powerful others, and chance. In H. Lefcourt (Ed.), *Research with the locus of control construct* (Vol. 1). New York: Academic Press, 1981.

Levin, A., & Schulz, M. A. *Multidimensional health locus of control and compliance in low and high participation hemodialysis.* Unpublished master's thesis, University of Wisconsin, Madison, 1980.

Lewin, K. *Field theory in social science.* New York: Harper, 1951.

Lewis, F. M., Morisky, D. E., & Flynn, B. S. A test of construct validity of health locus of control: Effects of self-reported compliance for hypertensive patients. *Health Education Monographs,* 1978, *6,* 138–148.

Linn, L. S., & Lewis, C. E. Attitudes toward self-care among practicing physicians. *Medical Care,* 1979, *17*(2), 183–190.

Lowenstein, V. H. *The relationship between pregnant women's beliefs of health locus of control and reported health maintenance behavior.* Unpublished master's thesis, Pennsylvania State University, 1979.

Macri, L. M. *The relationship of personality type and health locus of control to delay in seeking medical care for chest pain.* Unpublished master's thesis, St. Louis University, 1980.

McCusker, J., & Morrow, G. The relationship of health locus of control to preventive health behaviors and health beliefs. *Patient Counseling and Health Education,* 1979, *1,* 146–150.

McGrath, D. M. *Relationship between mothers' locus of control and compliance with their children's anticonvulsant therapy.* Unpublished master's thesis, University of Washington, 1980.

Mechanic, D. Correlates of physician utilization: Why do major multivariate studies of physician utilization find trivial psychosocial and organizational effects? *Journal of Health and Social Behavior,* 1979, *20,* 387–396.

Mendelsohn, R. S. *Confessions of a medical heretic.* Chicago: Contemporary Books, 1979.

Nagelberg, D. B. *Evaluating the BGSU health risk reduction program: A comparison of differing methods of providing health information to college students.* Unpublished doctoral dissertation, Bowling Green State University, 1979.

National Clearing House for Smoking & Health. Smoking habits and attitudes of physicians, dentists, nurses, and pharmacists, 1975. *Morbidity and Mortality Weekly Report,* June 10, 1977, *26*(23), 185.

Nice, D. S. *The course of depressive effect in navy wives during family separation.* Paper presented at the annual meeting of the Western Psychological Association, Honolulu, 1980. (a)

Nice, D. S. *Navy family separation and physician utilization.* Paper presented at the annual meeting of the National Council on Family Relations, Portland, Or., 1980. (b)

Nicholson, J. *Childbirth events and changes in maternal health locus of control.* Paper presented at the annual meeting of the American Psychological Association, Montreal, 1980.

Olbrisch, M. E. Perceptions of responsibility for illness and health related locus of control in gonorrhea patients. Unpublished master's thesis, Florida State University, 1975.

Parcel, G. S., & Meyers, M. P. Development of an instrument to measure children' health locus of control. *Health Education Monographs,* 1978, *6,* 149–159.

Phares, E. J. *Locus of control: A personality determinant of behavior.* Morristown, N.J.: General Learning Press, 1973.

Phares, E. J. *Locus of control in personality.* Morristown, N.J.: General Learning Press, 1976.

Phares, E. J. Defensiveness and perceived control. In L. C. Perlmuter & R. A. Monty (Eds.), *Choice and perceived control.* Hillsdale, N.J.: Lawrence Erlbaum Associates, 1979.

Pill, R., & Stott, N. *The relationship between health locus of control and belief in the relevance of life style to health.* Unpublished manuscript, Welsh National School of Medicine, Cardiff, 1981.

Radloff, L. Sex differences in depression: The effects of occupation and marital status. *Sex Roles,* 1975, *1,* 249–265.

Roter, D. L. Patient participation in the patient-provider interaction: The effects of patient question asking on the quality of interaction, satisfaction and compliance. *Health Education Monographs,* 1977, *5,* 281–315.

Rotter, J. B. *Social learning and clinical psychology.* Englewood Cliffs, N.J.: Prentice-Hall, 1954.

Rotter, J. B. Generalized expectancies for internal versus external control of reinforcement. *Psychological Monographs,* 1966, *80*(Whole No. 609).

Rotter, J. B. A new scale for the measurement of interpersonal trust. *Journal of Personality,* 1967, *35*(4), 651–665.

Rotter, J. B. Some problems and misconceptions related to the construct of internal vs. external control of reinforcement. *Journal of Consulting and Clinical Psychology,* 1975, *43,* 56–67.

Rotter, J. B. Individual differences and perceived control. In L. C. Perlmuter & R. A. Monty (Eds.), *Choice and perceived control.* Hillsdale, N.J.: Lawrence Erlbaum Associates, 1979.

Rotter, J. B., Chance, J., & Phares, E. J. (Eds.), *Application of a social learning theory of personality.* New York: Holt, Rinehart & Winston, 1972.

Ryan, W. *Blaming the victim.* New York: Pantheon, 1971.

Ryman, D. H., Biersner, R. J., & LaRocco, J. M. Reliabilities and validities of the mood questionnaire. *Psychological Reports,* 1974, *35,* 479–484.

Safer, M. A., Tharps, Q. J., Jackson, T. C., & Leventhal, H. Determinants of three stages of delay in seeking care at a medical clinic. *Medical Care,* 1979, *17,* 11–29.

Saltzer, E. B. *Causal beliefs and losing weight: A study of behavioral intention theory and locus of control in prediction of health-related behavior.* Unpublished doctoral dissertation, University of California at Irvine, 1979.

Saltzer, E. B. Social determinants of successful weight loss: An analysis of behavioral intentions and actual behavior. *Basic and Applied Social Psychology,* 1980, *1,* 329–341.

Schiller, P. L., Steckler, A., Dawson, L., & Heyman, H. *Report of the evaluation of the McDowell County (West Virginia) health education program: Year II.* Chapel Hill, N.C.: University of North Carolina, Department of Health Education, School of Public Health, August, 1979.

Selltiz, C., Wrightsman, L. S., & Cook, S. W. *Research methods in social relations* (3rd ed.). New York: Holt, Rinehart & Winston, 1976.

Shipley, R. H. *Effect of followup letters on maintenance of smoking abstinence.* Paper presented at the annual meeting of the Midwestern Psychological Association, St. Louis, Mo., 1980.

Smith, R. A., Wallston, K. A., & Wallston, B. S. *Measuring desire for control of health care.* Unpublished manuscript, Vanderbilt University, 1981.

Sproles, K. J. *Health locus of control and knowledge of hemodialysis and health maintenance of patients with chronic renal failure.* Unpublished master's thesis, Virginia Commonwealth University, 1977.

Steele, J. L., & McBroom, W. H. Conceptual and empirical dimensions of health behaviors. *Journal of Health and Social Behavior,* 1972, *13,* 383–392.

Strickland, B. R. Internal–external expectancies and health-related behaviors. *Journal of Consulting and Clinical Psychology,* 1978, *46,* 1192–1211.

Stuart, R. B. *Health Locus of Control Scale: A dialogue in predictive compliance* (with K. A. Wallston). Presentation at the annual meeting of the American Psychological Association, New York, 1979.

Taylor, S. E. Hospital patient behavior: Reactance, helplessness, or control? *Journal of Social Issues,* 1979, *35,* 156–184.

Tolor, A. Some antecedents and personality correlates of health locus of control. *Psychological Reports,* 1978, *43,* 1159–1165.

Toner, J. B., & Manuck, S. B. Health locus of control and health-related information seeking at a hypertension screening. *Social Science and Medicine,* 1979, *13A,* 823.

Wallston, B. S., & Wallston, K. A. *Health care education programs: Training patient internality.* Paper presented at the annual meeting of the American Public Health Association, San Francisco, 1973.

Wallston, B. S., & Wallston, K. A. Locus of control and health: A review of the literature. *Health Education Monographs,* 1978, *6*(2), 107–117.

Wallston, B. S., & Wallston, K. A. Social psychological models of health behavior. In A. Baum, S. Taylor, & J. E. Singer, (Eds.), *Handbook of psychology and health, volume 4: Social aspects of health.* Hillsdale, N.J.: Lawrence Erlbaum Associates, in press.

Wallston, B. S., Wallston, K. A., Kaplan, G. D., & Maides, S. A. Development and validation of the health locus of control (HLC) scale. *Journal of Consulting and Clinical Psychology,* 1976, *44,* 580–585.

Wallston, K. A., Maides, S., & Wallston, B. S. Health-related information seeking as a function of health-related locus of control and health value. *Journal of Research in Personality,* 1976, *10,* 215–222.

Wallston, K. A., & McLeod, E. *Predictive factors in the adherence to an antihypertensive regimen among adult male outpatients.* Unpublished manuscript, Vanderbilt University, 1979.

Wallston, K. A., & Wallston, B. S. Health locus of control scales. In H. Lefcourt (Ed.), *Research with the locus of control construct* (Vol. 1). New York: Academic Press, 1981.

Wallston, K. A., Wallston, B. S., & DeVellis, R. Development of the Multidimensional Health Locus of Control (MHLC) Scales. *Health Education Monographs,* 1978, *6,* 161–170.

Weigel, R. H., & Newman, L. S. Increasing attitude-behavior correspondence by broadening the scope of the behavioral measure. *Journal of Personality and Social Psychology,* 1976, *33,* 793–802.

Wildman, H. E., Rosenbaum, M. S., Framer, E. M., Keane, T. M., & Johnson, W. G. *Smoking cessation: Predicting success with the health locus of control scale.* Paper presented at the annual meeting of the Association for the Advancement of Behavior Therapy, San Francisco, 1979.

Witt, R. *Medication compliance among psychiatric outpatients as a function of locus of control, value placed on health, and methods of patient education.* Unpublished doctoral dissertation, University of Texas at Austin, 1978.

Wortman, C. B., & Dunkel-Schetter, C. Interpersonal relationships and cancer: A theoretical analysis. *Journal of Social Issues,* 1979, *35,* 120–155.

Zung, A. Self-rating depression scale. *Archives of General Psychology,* 1965, *12,* 63.

II MEDICAL INFORMATION PROCESSING

4 The Psychology of Physical Symptoms and Sensations

J. A. Skelton
James W. Pennebaker
University of Virginia

It would be difficult to overestimate the impact on society of people's experiences of physical symptoms. Although catastrophic illnesses affect thousands of Americans each year, more mundane problems such as headaches, backaches, and nasal congestion are features of vitually everyone's life. American consumers spend billions of dollars annually seeking relief from physical symptoms ranging from the itch of athlete's foot to the annoyance of postnasal drip. According to the National Center for Health Statistics (1979a), 23% of Americans report using aspirin at least once a week, and another 25% use it at least occasionally. Americans restrict their activities because of symptomatic experiences an average of 9.7 days per year (NCHS, 1979b) and visit physicians an average of 2.7 times per year (NCHS, 1979c). Physical symptoms and their sequelae thus have a profound social and economic impact on our lives.

Clearly, the experience of physical symptoms is familiar and pervasive in our daily lives. For example, a national survey asking respondents to indicate whether they have been bothered by 12 common symptoms such as headache, palpitating heart, and dizziness found that 78% of Americans responded affirmatively to at least one symptom (NCHS, 1970); 70% of college students report that headaches, colds, or sore throats have occurred at least once during the preceding academic year (Comstock & Slome, 1973). Nearly 80% of students report experiencing at least one physical symptom on a 12-symptom checklist when completing such checklists in introductory psychology classes (Pennebaker & Skelton, 1978). In addition, they report experiencing an average of about 17 different physical symptoms per month on 55-item checklists (Skelton, 1980b; Skelton & Pennebaker, 1978).

What factors influence the perceptions of physical symptoms? Historically, two approaches have predominated: medical and motivational. Probably the most common way of thinking about symptomatic experiences is as manifestations of the body's reactions to injury or dysfunctional organic states. According to the biomedical model of disease (Engel, 1977), symptoms reflect abnormal physiological functioning. We do not disagree that symptomatic experiences can result from trauma, infections, and a variety of physical causes. However, a purely physiological or medical approach is insufficient to account for all symptomatic states across individuals and situations.

Another way practitioners and researchers have sought to account for symptomatic experiences is in terms of the social gains provided by being ill. According to the secondary gain perspective (see, e.g., Mechanic, 1978; Shontz, 1975), illness is a social role that people may adopt to obtain certain benefits. These benefits include increased attention from significant other persons; relief from social, financial, and work obligations; and the displaced expression of dissatisfaction with one's life circumstances. Any student who has ever become ill the night before a dreaded exam will recognize that illness can sometimes be beneficial. In this formulation, then, symptomatic experiences allow the person to claim legitimate occupancy of the illness role.

The secondary gain perspective certainly has much to offer in our thinking about the social character of physical symptoms and illness, and it has inspired much research and speculation. It adds a motivational dimension to symptomatic experiences, which supplements the purely physiological orientation. The major drawback of this approach, however, is that it fails to specify the psychological processes through which the person first achieves awareness of physical symptoms and then labels symptoms as indicators of illness. That is, there is very little specification of molecular cognitive processes that allow people to use the information provided by their bodily sensations and integrate this information with other knowledge to determine the meaning of their experience.

The study of how individuals obtain and use information about bodily sensations and symptoms is important if we wish to understand the basis of health-related behavior. People's perceptions and appraisals of bodily information are obvious preconditions for their decisions to curtail normal activities, to seek medical treatment, and to adhere to recommended treatment plans. Despite the formidable advances made by medical science in developing formal procedures and rules for diagnosing illness, such developments may bear very little relation to the ways medically untrained people evaluate and diagnose themselves. Thus, although the processes underlying self-diagnosis may be very different from those of formal, medical diagnosis, individuals nevertheless actively and systematically appraise themselves and assign diagnostic meaning to bodily experiences. So, when it happens that the individual's coping activities deviate from those recommended by a physician (as is frequently the case), such deviations may result not from the individual's ignorance, lack of motivation, or sheer perversity, but rather from the very different perspectives of patient and physician concerning the meaning of the patient's physical condition.

In addition to illuminating differences between the diagnostic processes of the layperson and the physician, the study of psychological processes mediating the perception and evaluation of bodily information has another important function. Medical diagnosis depends not only on signs of illness (e.g., laboratory test results) but also on patients' reports of symptoms and bodily complaints. Thus, formal diagnosis is itself dependent on patients' self-diagnosis, and so it is critical to understand how patients perceive bodily sensations and decide that these sensations are in fact symptomatic of some health problem worthy of reporting to the physician. As we have already noted, appraisals and reports of sensations and symptoms are only partly a function of physiological reactions to noxious stimulation or pathological events; much of the variation in bodily experience and symptoms is therefore psychologically mediated. It thus behooves us to try to understand these mediating processes.

The purpose of this chapter is to present a cognitively oriented psychological approach for thinking about the causes and effects of physical symptoms. Such an approach can aid in the understanding and ultimate control of a variety of phenomena in which symptoms are implicated. These include situational variations in people's reports of the intensity of symptoms, placebo effects, unusual symptomatic outbreaks such as mass psychogenic illness (MPI) and medical student's disease, and the effects of illness on the individual's general outlook. We hope to provide a useful supplement to physiological and motivational (e.g., secondary gain) accounts of symptomatic experiences. Finally, we wish to emphasize the important role of people's working hypotheses in their experiences of bodily sensations and symptoms and identify the social bases for such hypotheses.

SYMPTOMS AS PSYCHOLOGICAL EXPERIENCES

In this section, we argue that physical symptoms can be usefully conceived as psychological or perceptual experiences. We first outline some of the problems associated with thinking of symptoms in primarily physiological or medical terms. We then define the role of social contextual factors in our awareness and labeling of bodily sensations and discuss the general perceptual principles implicated by this approach.

Beyond the Physiological-Medical Orientation

As noted earlier, physical symptoms or sensations cannot be fully explained in purely physiological terms. The basis for this contention is that bodily sensations and physiological activities are not isomorphic. That is, there is no one-to-one corresondence between responses that occur at the physiological level (e.g., cutaneous stimulation, actions of the viscera, muscle movements) and our experiences of bodily sensations and symptoms.

First, individuals often experience bodily sensations and symptoms in the absence of detectable physiological change. For example, certain classes of neuroses are accompanied by bodily complaints having no specifiable physiological basis. In glove anesthesia, the individual loses all sensation and feeling in a particular body part in the absence of neurological impairment. Phantom-limb pain, in which people who have lost a limb through amputation continue to feel pain in the now-severed limb, is a frequent problem of amputees (see Leventhal & Everhart, 1979). Although manifesting themselves in different ways, both glove anesthesia and phantom-limb pain amount to bodily hallucinations. In outbreaks of mass psychogenic illness (MPI; sometimes called hysterical contagion), large groups of people experience symptoms and illnesses for which there exist no organic basis. Such outbreaks have led to the closing down of factories, businesses, and even schools (Colligan, Pennebaker, & Murphy, 1981). A purely physiological account of physical symptoms is difficult to reconcile with the phenomenon of symptoms unaccompanied by physiological change.

In addition to the problem of symptoms with no physiological concomitants, there is the problem of cross-cultural and subcultural variation in symptom reporting and pain experiences. For example, Zola (1966) found that Italian-Americans were more likely to seek medical attention for symptoms than Irish-Americans and that the most common symptomatic complaints of the two subcultures also differed. Several investigators (e.g., Sternbach & Tursky, 1965; Tursky & Sternbach, 1967; Zborowski, 1952, 1969) have found subcultural differences in responses to standardized, experimentally induced pain. Mead (1950) reported that among the Arapesh tribe pregnant women do not show signs of morning sickness. Raper (1958), another anthropologist, found that the incidence rate of peptic ulcers (determined by autopsy) in an African tribe he studied equalled that of Great Britain; yet tribe members never complained of symptoms associated with peptic ulcer. Taken together, these diverse findings seem to undermine a purely physiological interpretation of symptomatic experiences.

Finally, there is abundant evidence that people are not especially accurate perceivers of physiological events having known concomitants in bodily sensations. For example, Beecher (1959) pointed to the fact that combat soldiers' perceptions of pain were poorly correlated with the extent of injury due to wounds. Similarly, Stunkard and his associates have found that objective indicators of gastric motility (stomach contractions) are far from perfectly correlated with self-reports of feeling hungry, especially among the obese (Griggs & Stunkard, 1964; Stunkard & Koch, 1964). Our own research has substantiated these findings. In a recent study, subjects tracked their own heartbeats by pressing a button while, at the same time, actual heart rate was continuously measured. Within-subject correlations between perceived and actual heart rate averaged only + .20 (Pennebaker, 1981). Similarly, correlations between ratings of sweaty hands and skin conductance have ranged between + .10 and + .20 (Pennebaker, Gonder-Frederick, Stewart, Elfman, & Skelton, 1980; Skelton, 1979). Both between-subject and within-subject correlations among perceived and actual breathing rate, perceived and actual finger temperature, and perceived and actual nasal congestation have never exceeded .37 (Pennebaker & Skelton, 1978).

In summary, then, the evidence indicates that there often is a lack of correspondence between bodily sensations and symptoms, on the one hand, and the physiological processes that presumably form the basis for sensations and symptomatic experiences, on the other. One reason for this poor fit may simply be that we often lack the verbal labels needed to describe and localize certain bodily experiences (cf. Fisher, 1973). That is, our vocabulary for describing bodily sensations and symptoms may be more limited than our vocabularies for describing, say, the colors of light, the shape of external objects, and so forth. Another reason may be that we ordinarily do not attend to bodily experiences until they deviate sufficiently from a base-line level of background sensory stimulation. Hence, we receive little practice in accurately perceiving bodily states (Blascovitch, 1980). These diverse findings, then, indicate that symptomatic experiences reflect not merely the body's reaction to organic conditions but also a variety of psychological processes. It is to a more detailed consideration of these processes that we now turn.

Psychological Bases of Physical Symptoms and Sensations

The basic assumption underlying our approach in this chapter is that "perception" is a unitary phenomenon. That is, the processes responsible for the perception of visual or auditory information (which have been the primary foci of research by perceptual and cognitive psychologists) are the same processes that govern the perception of bodily information. We do not need to postulate separate perceptual systems for information having origins in the external environment versus information originating from our insides. Perception, in other words, does not depend on where information comes from; instead, it depends on what we do with that information once we have it (Neisser, 1976). To appreciate the parallels between the perception of external and internal information, consider the following examples:

1. You're walking down a deserted street late at night. In the distance, you see two pinpoints of light. You move to the side of the road to avoid what you believe is an oncoming car.
2. You go to your office one morning and notice you're having trouble concentrating on your work. You observe you're experiencing some un-

usual and/or unpleasant bodily sensations. You subsequently leave work early because you believe you've caught the flu.

Now, let's look at the processes responsible for perception and action in these examples.

Attending to the Available Information. Much perceptual research has dealt with the factors influencing the likelihood that available information will be noticed and encoded. Given a manifold of stimuli competing for our attention, how do we come to focus on a subset of the information available to us? Some very general characteristics of attended stimuli are novelty, complexity, and movement or change (Berlyne, 1960). If we use the Gestalt psychology distinction between *figure* and *ground* as components of the perceptual field, we see that stimuli that stand out from a background (i.e., are figural) tend to be unique, unusual, and characterized by change. In the approaching-car example, the perceiver could conceivably have attended to, say, the vague and hazy shapes of trees or the pattern of lines on the darkened street. What was attended to, however, was pinpoints of light against a relatively undifferentiated background of darkness. Likewise with the flu example: The perceiver's inability to concentrate constituted an interruption of the ongoing flow of activity and hence became a focus for attention (cf. Mandler, 1975). Moreover, the interruption directed attention to bodily sensations, which are ordinarily unattended (groundlike) in comparison to more attention-getting events such as overt behavior or thought (Brener, 1977; Shontz, 1975).

There now exists considerable evidence showing that the more we attend to stimuli originating outside ourselves (e.g., people or objects), the more extreme is our tendency to evaluate those stimuli (see review by Taylor & Fiske, 1978). An entirely analogous process seems to occur with internal, bodily stimuli. Pennebaker and Brittingham (1982) and Pennebaker and Lightner (1980) have shown that individuals report more intense physical symptoms and exhibit symptomatic behavior when information from the external environment is either minimal (i.e., nonnovel, redundant, boring) or overwhelming (i.e., blurs into an undifferentiated background because there is more than can be dealt with).

Thus, although our attention is usually directed outward, toward the external environment, there are certain conditions that draw attention to our bodies, including novel bodily sensations or lack of external information (cf. Matthews, Scheier, Brunson, & Carducci, 1980). Once attention has been attracted to bodily stimuli, these will be evaluated in an extreme fashion.

Adopting Hypotheses. Up to this point, we have portrayed perceivers as almost passive entities who respond to information that "jumps out" at them from an array of potential stimuli. Although orientation to various features of incoming information is a necessary prerequisite for integrated perception and action, perceivers do more than merely orient toward sources of information; they transform or process available information and actively give it meaning (Bruner, 1973; Neisser, 1976).

In the approaching-car scenario, for example, the raw information, or *data,* available to the perceiver's visual receptors was merely two pinpoints of light. Such data are, in themselves, insufficient to support the perceiver's behavior based on the conclusion that a car is approaching. Higher orders of data transformation and information processing are needed to explain the perceiver's perception and action. These higher order operations amount to what we call the perceiver's *hypotheses* about the meaning of the data. As we see later, such hypotheses guide the perceiver's subsequent information-gathering actions.

A particularly important issue deals with how hypotheses are adopted in the first place. Body-relevant hypotheses can be adopted from the perceiver's previous experiences (e.g., learning and development), contact with social information (e.g., hearing a person talk about illness, seeing another become ill, or even reading about illness; cf. Sanders, Chapter 5, this volume), and even logical deduction or inference. Along the same lines, there is strong evidence that certain individual-difference measures are related to hypothesis adoption.

Clearly, the perceiver's early experiences can serve as sources of hypotheses. Research by Mechanic (1979) indicates that the health of the child's mother when under stress is somewhat related to the types of symptoms the child acquires (see also Campbell, 1975). Presumably, children learn to chronically "search" their body for symptoms comparable to the parent, and/or the parent essentially trains the child to search for the symptoms. Other developmental research indicates that children who are considered to be lacking in sociability by either the parent or teacher are more likely to be absent from nursery school due to illness than are sociable children (Pennebaker, Hendler, Durrett, & Richards, 1981). This is possibly due to the fact that unsociable children are more likely to search actively for illness sensations in order to remove themselves from the school setting. Clearly, early developmental factors can influence the way children think about and use their symptom information.

Specific early experiences can also be important in the acquisition and use of hypotheses. An individual who has broken an arm may continue to be extremely attentive to any type of sensations in that arm long after it has healed. In other words, the person has learned to be chronically attentive to the arm due to previously adaptive hypotheses concerning the arm when it was broken. Memories, then, can provide a context in which current experience can be evaluated. The perceiver on a dark street knows that cars usually travel on streets and shine lights in the dark. Similarly, the perceiver whose concentration is disrupted and experiences unusual bodily sensations may link these events with prior bouts of flu. In other words, memory-based expectancies increase the subjective likelihood that the minimal raw data of points of light or odd sensations do, in fact, represent the information predicted by the perceiver's hypotheses.

Another potent source of hypotheses is social information such as comparisons with other people or suggestions made by others. Our hypothetical office worker might mention his or her odd feelings to a co-worker who might reply, "It sounds just like I felt last week when I had the flu." The co-worker's suggestion amounts to a socially derived hypothesis that the perceiver's disrupted concentration and bodily sensations represent "flu." As is discussed in greater detail later, suggestion-induced hypotheses can profoundly affect perceived bodily states and symptom-related behavior. For now, it is sufficient to note that perceivers actively generate hypotheses from a number of sources.

In addition to the learned or acquired ways of adopting hypotheses, there is strong evidence that certain individual-difference measures tap hypothesis use. For example, individuals who are privately self-conscious (e.g., Fenigstein, Scheier, & Buss, 1975) report more physical symptoms than individuals who are not self-conscious (Pennebaker & Skelton, 1978). Similarly, various studies have shown that sensitizers report more health problems and visit health centers more often than repressors (Byrne, Steinberg, & Schwartz, 1968). Those high in self-consciousness and sensitizers process more internal information and more readily notice signs of illness. Of course, several other individual-difference measures have been shown to correlate with symptom reporting (see Pennebaker & Brittingham, 1981, for details). The primary point is that some individuals are more likely to invoke a body-related hypothesis than others.

Hypotheses and the Search for Verification. Perceivers have available not only a certain amount of raw data but also certain hypotheses concerning the meaning of those data. However, there may exist more than one hypothesis capable of explaining the data, particularly if the data themselves are vague. Pinpoints of light on a dark street might represent automobile headlights, but they might also represent two people walking side by side carrying flashlights. Odd bodily feelings might represent the onset of flu, but they might also be signs of indigestion resulting from the perceiver's fast breakfast at a greasy-spoon diner on the way to work. In fact, our previous discussion of the lack of correspondence between bodily sensations and objective indicators of underlying physiological processes implies that the data available for the perception of bodily events are *often* vague, ill-defined, and ambiguous (Pennebaker, 1982; Pennebaker & Skelton, 1981; Skelton, 1980a), and hence can support a variety of interpretations. This is no trivial problem, for the behavior resulting from adopting the wrong hypothesis can produce tragic results. An excellent example is a finding by Hackett and Cassem (1969) that some heart attack victims mistake their bodily sensations for symptoms of indigestion and fatally delay seeking medical help.

This suggests that our attempts to verify perceptual hypotheses are *selective*. If the perceiver hypothesizes that pinpoints of light on a dark street represent an approaching car, he or she will be most sensitive to subsequent information supporting that hypothesis (e.g., the sound of an auto engine). Hypothesizing two pedestrians with flashlights, however, the perceiver might be more alert to information concerning the relative positions of the lights (e.g., do they move in unison?) or the sound of human voices. The same is true of the indigestion versus the flu hypotheses. Given the indigestion hypothesis the perceiver might seek additional information relevant to gastrointestinal disturbance (e.g., how does my stomach feel?), whereas under the flu hypothesis he or she might search for evidence of fever, nasal congestion, or other flu-related symptoms.

What we have, then, is a perceiver who orients to available information on the basis of its attention-getting properties, or salience, and then generates hypotheses from various sources that subsequently guide the search for additional data. The goal of the search is confirmation or verification of the hypothesis being considered. Given the inherent ambiguity of many of our bodily sensations, many plausible hypotheses could be generated. Of particular importance, however, is the fact that individuals exhibit a tendency for the hypothesis under consideration to be verified by subsequent information unless that information is extremely discrepant with hypothesis-induced expectations (see Snyder, 1979; Taylor & Crocker, 1981, on the persistence of hypotheses). In other words, if the incoming information possesses sufficient features predicted by the hypothesis, the hypothesis will be viewed as having been confirmed. Given the parallel we have drawn between perception of external and internal information, then, we expect that many of the same errors and biases that characterize the hypothesis-driven processing (Bobrow & Norman, 1975; Taylor & Crocker, 1981) of social information and other data obtained through the distally oriented receptive systems will also characterize our processing of bodily data. The following section presents evidence for this prediction.

HYPOTHESIS VERIFICATION AND SYMPTOMATIC EXPERIENCES

The information contained in bodily sensations is rarely given directly. Instead, it must be extracted from a total field of stimulation and synthesized into a causal explanation or symptom label. The processing of bodily information may be facilitated by the adoption of tentative hypotheses against which perceived somatic activity may be compared for goodness-of-fit (cf. Leventhal, Nerenz, & Straus, 1980). For example, causal analysis of our sensations of nausea, headache, and dehydration is aided by our knowledge that such sensations are frequently the morning-after concomitants of overindulging in alcohol. Given a match between our present sensations and those predicted by the hangover hypothesis, if we also recall that we lost count of the number of beers we consumed at last night's party, we are likely to feel our hypothesis has been confirmed. Our tendency to adopt a tentative hypothesis, which we then seek to verify, is no doubt aided by the fact that most of our bodily sensations are not novel. Most of us know how it feels to have the flu, a hangover, or to experience pain, and our memories of the context in which sensations associated with such experiences have occurred provide us with a basis for our tentative hypotheses.

Often, our adoption of a hypothesis-verification strategy will lead to accurate labeling of symptoms and appropriate action. However, the selective information search generated by this strategy may interfere with accurate perception and labeling of bodily states. A central problem is that the data provided by bodily sensations may support more than one interpretation. A feeling of queasiness in the stomach, for example could reflect hunger, anxiety, indigestion, an infection of the stomach lining, or even a malignant tumor. The interpretation we adopt will depend in part on its plausibility in light of the current situation. Furthermore, the selective search for additional data that confirms the tentative hypothesis will, by definition, tend to bias us in favor of the hypothesis being considered because it will tend to make disconfirming evidence less salient to us. In short, hypotheses generated through recalled experiences or through comparison with others can sometimes create real problems in our arriving at accurate characterizations of our bodily states.

The remainder of this section examines the effects of experience-based and socially induced hypotheses on our perceptions of bodily sensations and the labeling of symptoms.

Suggestion and Social Factors in Symptomatic Experience

Labeling Pain and Pleasure. Anderson and Pennebaker (1980) performed a study showing that pain and pleasure may function as alternative interpretations of identical sensory data. In their experiment, 49 students placed their middle fingers for 1 second on a small emery board, which was attached to a vibrator. Prior to the experiment, subjects had signed a consent form that conveyed a manipulation of the sensations subjects might expect to experience while touching the emery board. Subjects were divided into three groups depending on whether the consent form contained the statement: "I understand I will come into contact with a stimulus which has been found to produce a degree of pain" (Pain interpretation), an identical statement in which the word "pain" was replaced by the word "pleasure" (Pleasure interpretation), or no statement concerning the painfulness/pleasurableness of the stimulus (No Interpretation control).

After touching the vibrating emery board, subjects rated the stimulus on a 13-point pain–pleasure scale, where lower ratings indicated the stimulus was experienced as painful. The differences in the pain–pleasure ratings of the three groups were modest but highly significant. The mean rating of the Pain group was -1.00, that of the Pleasure group was $+1.01$, and that of the No Interpretation group was + .13 (i.e., very close to the neutral, zero point). Postexperimental interviews with the subjects revealed that none thought the sensations created by contact with the stimulus could have been differently perceived from the way subjects perceived them. That is, Pain subjects did not believe the stimulus could have felt pleasurable, and Pleasure subjects did not believe it could have hurt. Clearly, then, subjects' expectations about the stimulus affected the way in which the stimulus was perceived, and their perceptions confirmed their expectations.

Obviously, there are limits to the degree to which bodily data may be interpreted as painful versus pleasurable. The limits might not be as strict as we suppose, however. Consider the sexual deviation known as masochism. Here, the individual has come to associate painful stimulation, often induced by a variety of torture-chamber devices, with feelings of intense sexual pleasure. Though we know of no research to document this assertion, we expect that the association of pain with sexual arousal in masochism is highly dependent on context. That is, we doubt that people having a masochistic orientation would find cutting themselves with a kitchen knife while preparing dinner to be sexually arousing; the interpretation of pain as sexually enjoyable is very likely restricted to explicitly sexual contexts. Thus, the context in which sensory data occur will affect the person's hypotheses and interpretations of those data.

Selective Monitoring of Illness-Related Symptoms. We have proposed that hypotheses concerning the meaning of bodily states generate selective search for information capable of verifying specific hypotheses. Burnam and Pennebaker (1977) performed a study that nicely illustrates the effects of suggestion-induced selective monitoring on perceptions of symptoms related to a specific illness. Subjects completed a checklist of 12 common physical symptoms either after running in place for 2 minutes or after merely walking in place for 2 minutes. The symptom checklist contained a mix of items that might plausibly be associated with flu (e.g., headache, nasal congestion, upset stomach) and with physical exercise (e.g., racing heart, shortness of breath). In addition, the experimenter who administered the checklists casually commented to half the subjects, "As you know, this is the time of year when we are surrounded by cold and flu-producing viruses, and many people aren't feeling well." Subjects then completed the checklist, rating the extent to which they were experiencing each of the 12 symptoms at that moment. Among subjects who had run in place, exercise-related symptoms were rated much more strongly than flu-related symptoms. Among those who had walked in place, however, ratings of exercise-related symptoms did not differ from ratings of flu-related symptoms. In addition, when differences in subjects' systolic blood pressure were partialled out, the flu suggestion tended to increase ratings of flu-related symptoms relative to exercise symptoms. These data indicate that the flu suggestion resulted in the selective monitoring and reporting of flu-related symptoms. This suggests that a given illness or other body-relevant hypothesis will cause the subject to report a constellation of relevant symptoms rather than only one specific sensation.

The work of Leventhal and his associates (Chapter 7, this volume) is also pertinent to the selective monitoring of illness-related symptoms. Meyer, Leventhal, and Gutmann (1980) extensively interviewed patients suffering from hvpertension (high blood pressure) and found that these patients have difficulties believing medical opinion, which defines hypertension as asymptomatic. ''Illness'' requires the occurrence of illness symptoms, as these patients see it, and they monitor specific symptoms that they feel should be associated with hypertension. Some patients, for example, construe hypertension as a form of heart disease and thus monitor cardiac sensations for signs of blood pressure elevations. Others, who regard hypertension as a vascular disease, are particularly sensitive to vascular symptoms such as headaches or vasoconstriction-induced coldness in their extremities. Still others view the disease as stress induced and so monitor themselves and their environments not for physical symptoms but for signs of increased psychological stress. Thus, patients' hypotheses concerning the ontogeny of hypertension lead to highly specific monitoring of bodily data. Furthermore, most patients believe they can accurately detect elevated blood pressure by monitoring the symptoms they associate with the disease.

Selective Monitoring of Benign Sensations: Coughing and Scratching. The studies discussed thus far have dealt with self-reported symptoms associated with illness. A natural problem with self-reports is that such measures are dependent on various experimental demands and may not truly reflect the degree to which subjects are aware of internal states. Two recent naturalistic studies attempted to assess the degree to which selective monitoring occurred with relatively benign sensations: perceptions of tickling throats and itching. Rather than relying on self-reports, we measured the spontaneous behaviors of coughing and scratching, which were assumed to be automatic and reflexive behaviors associated with perceptions of internal state. Whereas the coughing study simply sought to demonstrate that hearing another person cough caused subjects to monitor their own throats and thereby increased the probabilities that they, too, would emit a cough, the scratch study investigated the roles of different types of potential causal ''itching'' hypotheses that would affect scratching behavior.

In the coughing study, the number of spontaneously occurring coughs was counted in large lecture classes during exams. We assumed that hearing a person cough would cause others to monitor their own throats for tickling or itching sensations. The mere awareness of cough-related sensations, then, should result in the increased likelihood of coughing. This reasoning was supported in two ways. First, we found that coughing occurs in bunches. That is, there would be several seconds of silence and then a large number of coughs from different people would be emitted within a short period of time (3–5 seconds). Second, we found that the closer a person was to a cougher, the greater the probability that that person would also cough (Pennebaker, 1980). These findings, then, suggest that the hypotheses set up by others' behavior results in monitoring one's own bodily sensations.

Our experiment dealing with scratching behavior attempted to learn if manipulated causal hypotheses in addition to observable scratching by a confederate would affect scratching behavior. In the study (which took place in the university library), two confederates sat next to a person who was reading. After 1 minute, one of the confederates did and said one of four things: (1) she began scratching and announced to the other confederate that she was just bitten by a mosquito; (2) she scratched and said that she received sun poisoning at a lake the previous day; (3) she scratched and said she wanted to leave to get something to eat; (4) she did not scratch and said she wanted to get something to eat. The two confederates then left while an observer watched the subject for 1 minute to see if he or she scratched. In other words, the confederate scratched and gave a possible contagious cause (mosquito), noncontagious cause (sun poisoning), or no cause at all. Of the 16 subjects in each condition, 50% scratched in the mosquito and sun poison cells, 32% scratched in the no cause cell, and no subjects scratched in the no scratch condition. These results are of interest because they demonstrate that merely observing another person scratch—irrespective of the presumed cause—results in awareness of itching (and subsequent scratching) in others. In other words, our selective monitoring of benign sensations is highly dependent on the body-relevant behavior of others.

Selective Monitoring of Specific Bodily Changes. One important implication of our earlier discussion of the role of attention and novelty in the perception and labeling of bodily data is that people are most attentive to *change* in their bodily states rather than to absolute levels of sensory stimulation. Gestalt notions of figure and ground carry a similar implication. Indeed, some psychologists (e.g., Newtson, 1976) maintain that what we typically perceive are successive changes in the states of the objects of perception. How may we apply these insights to the problems of perceiving and labeling physical symptoms?

Based on the idea that our perception of somatic activity reflects selective search for hypothesis-verifying data, we have proposed that the very act of monitoring sensations for signs of change increases the probability that the expected change will be perceived (Pennebaker & Skelton, 1981). For example, expecting a drug to produce changes in symptom *X* will produce selective monitoring of data consistent with that expectation and an increased likelihood of perceiving the expected change in *X*. Underlying the proposal is the assumption that bodily data are encoded in a manner consistent with the hypothesis the individual seeks to verify. Thus, the individual will tend to judge ambiguous bodily sensations as confirming instances of his or her tentative hypothesis rather than as disconfirming instances. A series of studies was conducted to test this proposal and its underlying assumption.

In the first study (Pennebaker & Skelton, 1981, Experiment 1), subjects were told that exposure to (bogus) ultrasonic noise might affect skin temperature. For some subjects, the experimenter noted that ultrasonic noise might cause skin temperature to increase (Increase group), whereas others were told that decreased skin temperature might result from their exposure (Decrease group). Both groups received elaborate rationales concerning the effects of ultrasonic vibrations on vasodilation/constriction and how such physiological effects were translated into skin temperature sensations. A third group was simply told that their skin temperatures would be monitored but received no suggestion concerning ultrasonic noise effects (Control group). All subjects were told that the experiment concerned effects of ultrasonic noise on subsequent task performance and so expected to perform an unspecified task following exposure.

Following delivery of the expectancy manipulations, subjects were escorted to a second experimenter who was blind to their condition. He attached a thermistor (heat sensor) to subjects' hands. After 2 minutes of base-line recording of skin temperatures, he told subjects the noise would be delivered through headphones connected to a tape recorder. Subjects actually heard a low volume pure tone of 62 db (A), which began at 2000Hz and gradually increased in pitch for 15 seconds, until it was no longer audible. The remaining 1 minute 45 seconds of the tape was blank. At tape's end, subjects were asked to complete a short questionnaire, "before we begin the task." The subject was then escorted to a third experimenter who explained that the experiment was completed.

One postnoise questionnaire item showed that Increase and Decrease subjects had, in fact, formed tentative hypotheses about the effects of ultrasonic noise on skin temperature based on the first experimenter's suggestion. Increase subjects expected their finger temperatures to become warmer than did Decrease subjects (means = 85 and 18, respectively, on a 100-point scale where 1 = "I expected my finger temperature to become cooler"; 50 = "I expected no change"; 100 = "I expected my finger temperature to become warmer"). Control subjects' expectations were close to the midpoint of the scale (mean = 60). Ratings of expectations were significantly different among the three groups.

The role of subjects' tentative hypotheses in guiding their search for verifying information was assessed in two ways. First, two questionnaire items asked subjects to indicate how much they had attended to sensations of increasing and decreasing skin temperature (1 = "not at all"; 100 = "a great deal" for both items). Increase subjects reported attending significantly more to sensations of increasing skin temperature and less to sensations of decreasing skin temperature than did Decrease subjects (means for the increasing-temperature item were 67 vs. 34; means for the decreasing-temperature item were 21 vs. 43). Moreover, Control subjects reported attending about equally—and very little—to sensations of either increasing or decreasing temperature (means = 30 and 25 for increasing- and decreasing-temperature items, respectively). Without a tentative hypothesis concerning effects of ultrasonic noise on skin temperature, then, Control subjects failed to monitor skin temperature-related sensations to any great extent, whereas Increase and Decrease subjects tended to monitor only those sensations consistent with their suggestion-induced hypotheses.

A far more interesting way to examine the selective monitoring/search notion is to compare our recordings of subjects' actual skin temperatures with their ratings of perceived skin temperature. Actual skin temperatures did not differ as a function of condition and failed to correlate with subjects' ratings of how warm or cool their fingers felt. We then counted the number of times each subject's skin temperature fluctuated across the experimental session (i.e., the number of times the subject's temperature increased then decreased, and vice versa). A fluctuation, according to this definition, indicates a subject has potential sensory data concerning both the fact of temperature change and the direction of that change. If selective monitoring of changes in bodily sensations amounts to hypothesis-guided use of available data, we would expect subjects to use the change information available in a fluctuation that was consistent with their hypothesis and ignore hypothesis-inconsistent information.

This is precisely what occurred. Collapsing over groups, the correlation between number of temperature fluctuations and ratings of perceived skin temperature was negligible and nonsignificant. Correlations calculated within each group, however, showed that subjects were interpreting temperature fluctuations in very different ways depending on their tentative hypotheses. The Increase subjects' correlation between number of fluctuations and self-reported skin temperature was + .48 (i.e., the more fluctuations subjects experienced, the warmer they rated skin temperature); the Decrease subjects' correlation was virtually the mirror image of Increase subjects' ($r = -.49$, i.e., the more fluctuations subjects experienced, the cooler they rated skin temperature). These correlations differed significantly ($p = .02$, two-tailed). Fluctuations in temperature were unrelated to finger temperature ratings for Control subjects ($r = .11$). Thus, subjects who held a suggestion-induced hypothesis about ultransonic noise effects on skin temperature used available information selectively to support their respective hypotheses.

Finally, subjects rated their perceived skin temperatures in a manner consistent with their tentative hypotheses. Table 4.1 shows that Increase subjects rated their finger temperatures as becoming warmer than did Decrease subjects, whereas ratings made by the Control group fell between those of the other subjects. Thus, subjects' perceptions of skin temperature verified their tentative hypotheses.

Two partial replications of this experiment (also reported in Pennebaker & Skelton, 1981) extended the effect of selective monitoring of sensations to two other perceived bodily states: nasal congestion and ratings of heart rate. In both

TABLE 4.1
Summary of Measures in Skin Temperature Study[a]

	Measures			
Condition	(1) Self-Reported Temperature[b]	(2) Attention to Warmth[c]	(3) Attention to Coolness[c]	(4) r, (1) with Fluctuations
Increase	69.6	66.5	21.3	+.48
Decrease	48.1	33.5	42.5	−.49
Control (No Suggestion)	57.8	29.9	24.8	+.11

[a]From Pennebaker and Skelton, 1981, Experiment 1.

[b]Self-reported temperature scale ranged from 1 = "finger became cooler," to 50 = "no change," to 100 = "finger became warmer."

[c]The attention scales ranged from 1 = "not at all" to 100 = "a great deal."

studies, the experimenter imposed selective monitoring strategies on subjects rather than merely providing a suggestion. In one study, subjects were told to attend to sensations of nasal stuffiness and congestion, sensations of free and unobstructed breathing through the nose, sensations occurring while breathing through the nose with no further specification, or a nonbodily distractor. Analyses of mean change in ratings of nasal congestion from pretest ratings showed that subjects who attended to congestion sensations evinced increased perceived congestion, subjects who attended to free breathing sensations evinced decreased perceived congestion, and the remaining groups showed very little change in congestion ratings. Interestingly, three subjects actually blew their nose during the postexperimental interview: All had been in the attend-to-congestion group. The odds are less than 1 in 50 that such behavior would be exhibited by chance alone in only this one group.

In the other partial replication, subjects were told to monitor sensations of an increasing heart rate, a decreasing heart rate, or simply to attend to heart rate with no directional specification. For example, those in the increase condition were told to "attend to any sensations indicating an acceleration or increase in your heart rate." Differences between pre- and postexperimental ratings of perceived "racing heart" showed that subjects who monitored increase sensations perceived their heart rates as increasing, those who monitored decrease sensations perceived their heart rates as decreasing, and the remaining group perceived no change. In addition, subjects' actual heart rates did not change during the experiment as a function of condition.

These studies provide strong support for the selective search notion and its implications for perceptions of symptomatic experience. In the skin-temperature study, subjects adopted suggestion-induced strategies of monitoring for specific bodily sensation . In all studies, the effect of such selective monitoring was to verify whatever hypotheses were implied by subjects' selective search strategies. An important implication of these findings is that when bodily data are vague and ambiguous, individuals use such data quite selectively to attain integrated perception of their bodily states. This insight, in turn, offers an explanation for such phenomena as placebo effects, mass psychogenic illness (MPI), and medical student's disease.

IMPLICATIONS OF SELECTIVE MONITORING: PLACEBOS, MPI, AND MEDICAL STUDENT'S DISEASE

When a physician gives a patient medication that is described as having an effect on some physical condition or its sensory representation, the patient has in effect acquired a hypothesis concerning the expected outcome of using the medication. The strength of this expectation can be understood by considering the *placebo effect.* A placebo is an inert, nonactive agent described to the patient as effective. Across a remarkable variety of somatic and psychological conditions, placebos have been found to reduce symptom reporting (Rickels, 1968). In fact, the placebo effect is so pervasive that experimental tests of new drugs typically include at least one placebo group to permit assessment of the "true" versus the "suggestion" effect of the drug.

Our perspective argues that placebo effects result from selective monitoring of bodily data that verifies the suggestion-induced hypothesis. People ordinarily place great faith in the pronouncements of medical practitioners, so their willingness to accept placebo-related suggestions is quite strong. So long as the patients' bodily data do not radically disconfirm their expectations, they will be likely to perceive the placebo as effective. Given the selective search for confirming data implied by the practitioner's statements concerning the placebo, it is no surprise that placebo effects are so common.

Mass psychogenic illness (MPI) is the phenomenon of widespread symptom reporting and illness-related behavior among large groups of people, even though the reported symptoms have no basis in detectable pathology. MPI generally occurs in relatively isolated social environments (e.g., schools, factories) where people are frequently under high stress. In a classic study, Kerckhoff and Back (1968) reported one outbreak of MPI, which occurred in a Southern textile mill. The mill was eventually closed when a large number of workers fell prey to a mysterious disease said to be caused by a "June bug" infesting the materials with which the employees worked. It is very important to note that employees were suffering from high levels of both psychological and physical stress because it was the height of the production season.

Psychoanalysts label MPI "mass hysteria" or "hysterical contagion" and described it as a *conversion reaction*. That is, people's unexpressed stresses are converted into physical symptoms. This perspective, however, is really only a description, not an explanation, and it fails to detail the role of bodily data and their interpretation. The selective monitoring perspective, on the other hand, views MPI as an outcome of hypothesis-guided search. The stress resulting from the exhausting working conditions in the factory manifested itself in part through a variety of ambiguous and unpleasant bodily sensations. With the collapse of the first few workers, the remaining employees formed an illness hypothesis linked to the presumed insect infestation. Their stress-related bodily complaints now had a legitimate interpretation—the June bug virus. This hypothesis was reinforced through the mechanisms of rumor transmission and the vivid evidence of workers collapsing, and thus resulted in the rapid spread of the symptoms.

A very similar process explains medical student's disease, which occurs individually rather than on a mass basis. Like Kerckhoff and Back's (1968) factory workers, medical students often experience high levels of physical and psychological stress. Not infrequently, such students will attain the conviction of having contracted a rare and exotic disease about which they have recently read in their course of studies (Mechanic, 1972). By its very nature, medical education provides the student with a variety of detailed hypotheses concerning the meaning of bodily data. When the student experiences bodily sensations that are actually stress induced, he or she may then selectively monitor these sensations for data to confirm a particular illness hypothesis. As we have argued, such hypotheses are very likely to be verified.

It must be noted that these explanations for MPI and medical student's disease are similar to those advanced by Schachter and Singer (1962) as well as those interested in misattribution (e.g., Nisbett & Valins, 1971). These approaches assume that the individual feels physically aroused and then searches for an appropriate emotion or illness label for arousal sensations. Our approach differs in the sense that the label or hypothesis actually is presented first and then produces the selective search for confirming sensory data. In truth, both processes probably occur (cf. Leventhal et al., 1980). In some cases the person may first notice the arousal, become worried, and then seek out a handy explanation. In other cases the person may first hear, see, or read about something that would cause selective search. In both cases, however, we must assume that the individual is actively involved in the search process in order to learn more about the environment and the arousal symptoms.

So far, we have concentrated largely upon hypotheses induced by specific suggestions and social information. However, as pointed out in the introduction to this section, our own experiences can serve as yardsticks for analyzing bodily data as well. Let us now briefly consider some research that examines this issue.

Self-Induced Hypotheses and Symptomatic Experiences

In many cultures, women experience a variety of physical (e.g., abdominal cramps) and psychological symptoms (e.g., depression) associated with different phases of their menstrual cycles. Recently, some controversy has arisen concerning the extent to which such symptoms have an underlying, physiological basis as opposed to being effects of culture-specific, learned expectations. Many women report anecdotally, for example, that their mothers described the onset of menses in highly negative terms (e.g., "the curse") and that their own experiences have tended to verify this description.

Ruble (1977) conducted an important study showing that symptom reporting associated with the menstrual cycle is affected by the stage of the cycle at which a woman perceives herself to be, relatively independently of the woman's actual location in that cycle. Forty-four women underwent a simulated electroencephalographic (EEG) examination purported to be able to pinpoint a woman's location in the menstrual cycle with a high degree of accuracy. A third of the subjects were informed that they were within 1 to 2 days of beginning menstruation (Premenstrual group), another third were told not to expect onset of menstruation for 7 to 10 days (Intermenstrual group), and a final third received no information. Subjects then completed a questionnaire that tapped physical, psychological, and behavioral symptoms associated with menstruation. Although none of the groups actually differed in the day of menstruation onset, there were several interesting differences in their symptom reports. Women in the Premenstrual group rated themselves as experiencing more water retention and pain than did women who believed themselves to be intermenstrual. The former also indicated a greater degree of change in their eating habits and level of sexual arousal than the Intermenstrual group.

Ruble (1977) interpreted her results as meaning that strictly physiological interpretations of menstrual symptoms were insufficient to account for differential symptom reporting. Although not denying that there is a physiological component to menstrual complaints, she argued that an individual's beliefs concerning the association between cycle location and symptoms must also be taken into account. In the terms employed in the present paper, women's prior experiences of menstrual difficulties, along with the manipulation, provided them with a hypothesis for evaluating any bodily data they experienced while completing the symptom questionnaire. Ruble's results are thus highly consistent with those we have reported here for judgments of pain, illness-related symptoms, and specific bodily sensations.

The work of Meyer et al. (1980), which we reviewed earlier in a different context, also points out the importance of self-generated hypotheses in the evaluation of symptomatic experiences. Recall that hypertensives monitor specific bodily sensations that are associated with their beliefs concerning the causes of hypertension. Such beliefs can be viewed as providing hypotheses having both suggestion- and experience-based components, which guide the search for specific, confirming information.

Summary

In this section, we have demonstrated the important role played by selective hypothesis-verification strategies in our evaluations of bodily data and subsequent symptomatic experiences. Such selective search strategies affect which data are monitored and also the way in which bodily sensations are experienced. Moreover, some of the sources of these hypothesis-guided selection strategies have been outlined. In the next section, we change our focus from the perceptual and environmental influences on bodily experiences to the effects of symptomatic experiences on subsequent perception of externally originating or nonbodily information.

PERCEPTUAL EFFECTS OF SYMPTOMATIC EXPERIENCES

Up to this point, we have been principally concerned with the question of how people perceive their own bodily states and label them as symptomatic. We have focused on the cognitive and social factors that play a causal role in the perception of physical symptoms. However, it is equally important to recognize that symptomatic experiences can themselves function as causes for behaviors such as seeking medical attention for illness-related symptoms (cf. Rodin, 1978). The research to be reported here concerns the effects of symptomatic experiences on our perception of information from the external environment. Our work in this area has only recently begun, but it already appears that symptomatic experiences can affect judgments and perceptions of several classes of externally originating information.

When we feel ill, not only is our capacity to perform routine activities impaired, but we may also view information from the external environment very differently than when we feel healthy. This altered view of the outside world can be reflected in a variety of ways (e.g., in mood changes that affect our relations with other people). In addition, we may become especially sensitive to the implications of health-related external information. For example, when we feel ill we may show greater than usual interest in medication or diets, expose ourselves more than usual to information relating to health, and so forth. Skelton (1980b) has argued that our increased attentiveness to the health dimension of external information during times of salient symptomatic experiences may reflect the operation of a cognitive *availability* heuristic (Tversky & Kahneman, 1974). That is, being in a symptomatic state makes it easier for us to "see" the health implications of external information because our own state makes cognitions concerning health more available to affect our judgments and perceptions. The theoretical bases and limits of this argument are not yet fully developed. Nevertheless, we have performed several studies illustrating that such availability effects do, in fact, occur.

Judgments of "Second-Hand" Bodily Data

We performed an experiment (Pennebaker & Skelton, 1981, Experiment 2) that shows how individuals' own bodily reactions can affect their judgments of the bodily reactions of hypothetical, other persons. College students received copies of a heart rate chart of a hypothetical person who was said to have received a drug affecting heart rate at a designated point on the chart. The subjects' task was to determine whether the chart indicated the hypothetical person's heart rate had increased, decreased, or showed no change in response to the drug and to indicate the information they used in arriving at their judgment (see Fig. 4.1).

A few minutes before evaluating the heart rate chart, all subjects had completed a short symptom checklist and had indicated the degree to which they were themselves experiencing a fast pulse. Responses to the fast pulse item were used to divide subjects into a Fast Pulse group and a No Fast Pulse group for subsequent analysis. The hypothetical heart rate chart contained one of three clues concerning the drug's supposed effect, and these clues were intended to manipulate subjects' expectations concerning the drug. The procedure was relatively simple. Subjects received a copy of the chart with the following information:

> Assume the drug is administered directly into the bloodstream during the time that is boxed [on the chart]. The periods before and after the box are times when the drug is not in the bloodstream. Further assume that the drug works immediately and has no aftereffects.
>
> After you have rated the effectiveness of the drug below the diagram, circle the parts of the boxed area which were related to your assumptions about the effectiveness of the drug.

The chart included the manipulation of subjects' expectations and stated: "The drug that was used was supposed to cause a subtle *effect (increase, decrease)* on/in the person's heart rate." The three sets of clues, then, were intended to sensitize subjects to the possibility that the drug might cause directional changes in heart rate (Increase and Decrease instructions) or a nonspecific change in heart rate. Figure 4.1 shows that although the boxed area of the chart was constructed to show considerable variability in the hypothetical person's heart rate, it shows no overall change in average heart rate.

Both subjects' own bodily states and the expectancy-inducing clues affected their ratings of the effects of the drug on heart rate. As can be seen in Table 4.2,

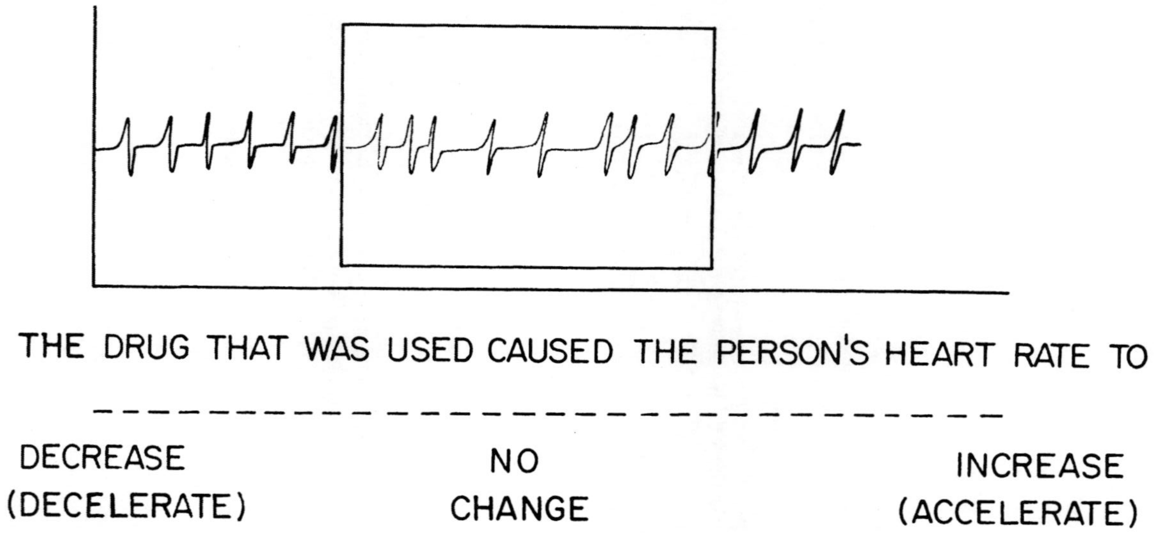

FIG. 4.1 Hypothetical heart rate chart from the "second-hand" bodily data study. From Pennebaker and Skelton, 1981, Experiment 2.

TABLE 4.2
Mean Ratings of Heartbeat Chart[a]

	Pulse Group		
Condition	*No Fast Pulse*	*Fast Pulse*	*Totals*
Increase	5.9	8.0	7.0
Control	7.1	8.2	7.4
Decrease	5.5	5.9	5.7
Totals	6.3	7.3	

Note: Marginal means are weighted by the number of subjects in each cell. Higher means indicate heartbeat is perceived as increasing.
[a]From Pennebaker and Skelton, 1981, Experiment 2.

Fast Pulse subjects saw the charted heartbeat as increasing significantly more than did No Fast Pulse subjects. Consistent with our previous research, subjects receiving the increase suggestion rated the heartbeat as increasing significantly more than subjects receiving the decrease suggestion. Subjects who received the nonspecific suggestion also tended to see the charted heartbeat as increasing, which might reflect a bias to assume physiological responses such as heart rate will tend to change in an increasing direction.

Subjects' own perceived heart rate and the suggestions also affected the information they used to make their judgments. Independent raters, blind to subjects' conditions, counted the number of times subjects circled parts of the chart indicating increased and decreased heart rates. If a subject circled one or more of the sets of closely grouped spikes in the boxed area of the chart shown in Fig. 4.1, he or she received an acceleration score equal to the number of times increase-relevant data were circled. Similar scores were derived for decrease-relevant data (deceleration score). If a subject circled closely grouped *and* separated spikes on the chart, he or she received a score of 1 on acceleration and deceleration measures. Interrater reliability for both measures was over .90.

Fast Pulse subjects used heart rate increase data significantly more than did No Fast Pulse subjects. Conversely, scores on the deceleration measure tended to be higher for subjects in the No Fast Pulse group. Also consistent with our selective monitoring hypothesis, subjects receiving the increase suggestion made significantly more use of increase data and marginally less use of decrease data than did subjects receiving the decrease suggestion. Acceleration and deceleration scores for subjects receiving the nonspecific suggestion were closer to those of the increase suggestion group than the decrease suggestion group, which seems to support our earlier speculation concerning a bias to assume heart rate changes tend to be manifested as increases. Perhaps the strongest evidence for selective monitoring comes from the fact that 92% of the subjects circled only the data on the chart that were consistent with the direction in which they had rated the charted heartbeat. That is, subjects who rated the heartbeat as increasing in rate circled only closely grouped spikes, whereas those rating the heartbeat as decreasing circled only separated spikes.

The findings of this study, then, support our earlier account of selective monitoring and extend it to second-hand bodily data. Perhaps most interesting is the finding that one's own bodily state appears to be "projected" onto judgments of others' bodily reactions. The mediator of this effect may be the availability heuristic. That is, cognitions concerning increased heart rate may have been more salient to Fast Pulse subjects, whereas cognitions concerning decreased heart rate may have been more salient to No Fast Pulse subjects. Thus, the possibility that the hypothetical drug would produce an increase versus decrease in heart rate may have been differentially available to the two groups of subjects. If this is so, it also implies that availability effects are mediated through selective monitoring of data that are consistent with the available hypothesis.

Judgments of Stimulus Health Relevance

Another set of studies (Skelton, 1980b) produced results consistent with the availability interpretation of the previously reported experiment. In addition, these studies showed that one's own bodily state can affect perceptions of a seemingly unlikely class of variables, namely, simple words. Individual differences in symptom reporting were operationalized in two different ways. In one study, subjects completed a 55-item inventory of common physical symptoms and bodily sensations by indicating how often each was experienced each month. This procedure produced High and Low Symptom groups based on whether subjects reported experiencing more or less than the median number (17.5) of symptoms per month. In the second study, subjects were classified into Ill or Not Ill groups depending on whether they reported an episode of actual illness within the preceding 2 days; many of the subjects in the Ill group were seen at the university's Student Health Center during regular, sick-call hours.

In both studies, subjects received a list of 65 common words and were asked to rate each word for its health relevance, that is, "the extent to which the word brings thoughts of health or illness to your mind" (1 = "Never related to health"; 5 = "Always related to health"). The lists were subsequently divided into health-related, ambiguous, and nonhealth-related subscales according to the median rating each word received. Health-related words included such items as *pain, ache,* and *pill;* the ambiguous subscale included *sweat, pull,* and *twist;* nonhealth-related items included *friend, dominate,* and *green.*

The results of the two studies are summarized in Table 4.3. High Symptom and Ill subjects rated the words as significantly more health related than did Low Symptom and Not Ill subjects. In addition, differences in health-relevance ratings between the groups of subjects were relatively uniform across all three

TABLE 4.3
Mean Ratings of Health Relevance of Three Word Classes[a]

	Item Type		
Group[b]	*Nonhealth*	*Ambiguous*	*Health-Related*
High Symptom/Ill	1.8	2.7	3.8
Low Symptom/Not Ill	1.6	2.4	3.6

Note: Higher means indicate items are rated as more health relevant.
[a]From Skelton, 1980b.
[b]Cell means are averaged over both studies.

subscales: Subjects for whom symptomatic experiences were salient (i.e., High Symptom and Ill subjects) tended to view all types of words as more health relevant than did subjects for who symptoms were nonsalient (i.e., Low Symptom and Not Ill subjects).

Similar to the study of second-hand bodily data, then, subjects in these two studies seemed to project their symptomatic experience onto judgments of externally originating information. Salient physical symptoms seem to produce comparative overestimates of stimulus health relevance, perhaps by making the health–illness dimension more available to the individual. What is most surprising, of course, is the extent to which such effects generalize across classes of stimuli. Both judgments of other people's bodily reactions and of common lexical items appear to be affected by one's own symptomatic status. We thus have come full circle. Just as environmental information influences the hypotheses about our bodies and the ultimate perception of physical symptoms, our awareness of symptoms can alter the way in which we perceive the external environment. Certain settings will cause us to monitor our bodies selectively; certain body states will cause us to monitor our behavior settings differently.

APPLICATIONS OF THE COGNITIVE APPROACH

One of the most obvious questions concerns the practical applications of the approach that has been advanced in this chapter. How might this perspective help the physician, patient, or even employer? This turns out to be an extremely complicated question for several reasons. First, we know that people often misinterpret sensory information. For example, they may believe that their heart attack is indigestion (Hackett & Cassem, 1969) or that their indigestion is a heart attack. In the first case, death may ensue; in the second, a waste of time for medical personnel as well as the patient will be the result. A related problem concerns cases wherein individuals are either overattentive to internal sensory information, and consequently overuse medical facilities, or are inattentive to internal information. From the physician's or therapist's perspective, each of these cases must be dealt with differently. Further, each case requires training the patient to reinterpret internal sensory information.

For example, a large number of people either interpret potentially dangerous symptoms as benign or actively try to suppress or distract themselves from these symptoms. Men and women illustrate differences in this regard. Across all age groups men visit physicians less and take fewer over-the-counter medications than women. Nevertheless, men have a life expectancy that is 5 years shorter than women. These data suggest that men are not attentive enough to internal sensory information.

How does the medical establishment induce a person to be more attentive and/ or interpret certain symptoms as dangerous? Clearly, a process such as this must start at an early age. Individuals should be told explicitly when sensations signal danger. This would especially be true of individuals at risk for specific diseases. For example, it would be to a company's advantage to assemble its hard-driving executives with high blood pressure and explain what sensations are indicative of a heart attack.

A different kind of problem exists for the person who is prone to interpret benign sensations in illness-related ways. The hypochondriac or "crock" is a persistent problem in the medical profession. Physicians are likely to refer such patients to someone else or simply tell them that nothing is wrong. But first it must be realized that these patients honestly believe that they are sick. They have adopted a hypothesis about certain physical sensations. Further, the hypothesis is probably confirmed in that there are certain sensations that are present that substantiate the patient's interpretation. Rather than dismissing the patient as a crock or crazy, the physician must provide alternative interpretations for the sensations. For example, if the patient complains of having malady *X* with symptoms *A*, *B*, and *C*, it would be incumbent on the physician to point out that symptoms *A* and *B* are irrelevant and that it is also necessary to have symptom D. Further, it is imperative to explain to the patient how sensations can be interpreted in a variety of ways.

These problems are far more difficult than has been implied. Old sets are extremely difficult to break. As work on perseverence has indicated (e.g., Ross, Lepper, & Hubbard, 1975), simply informing people about their false hypotheses is insufficient in bringing about lasting changes. Rather, it is necessary to alter the hypothesis as well as have the individual actively encode information within the framework of the "restructured" hypothesis (Massad, Hubbard, & Newtson, 1979). In each of the foregoing instances, then, the medical personnel should offer an alternative interpretation of the sensations and see to it that the person can and does encode new information in line with the new hypothesis.

CONCLUSION

Throughout this chapter, we have placed heavy emphasis on the role of our expectations and tentative hypotheses in symptomatic experiences. We have modeled perception as arising from the interplay of data and a hypothesis-guided search for additional, confirming data. Selective search or monitoring strategies may be likened to attempts to verify hypotheses, and the very selectivity of the search process increases the likelihood of verification. It has already been noted that our perspective can account for placebo effects, MPI, and medical student's disease. We have tended to downplay motivational factors in the perception and labeling of physical symptoms in favor of a more cognitively oriented approach.

Nevertheless, we feel that a fully adequate account of symptomatic experiences must address the role of motivational factors and their effects. As a starting point, it is important to recognize that bodily data and symptoms necessarily have motivational significance for the individual. Such experiences are maximally proximal to the person, and they clearly have implications that can be profoundly emotion evoking. It is this evocative character of symptomatic experiences that provides the energy in the guided search for verifying information. Furthermore, although we have focused largely on what might be viewed as errors or biases resulting from selective search for verification, such a strategy often gives us an accurate picture of the meaning of bodily sensations. Obviously, we would be poorly adapted for survival if our methods for evaluating bodily experience consistently produced incorrect results. Given the motivation to survive as individuals, most people would find it unnecessarily conservative and time-consuming to enumerate and test all the potential hypotheses that might be available to them.

Another motivationally relevant issue we have left unaddressed concerns the role of such states as fear or anxiety in symptomatic experience. Our work to date has focused almost exclusively on a relatively rational process of perception, which occasionally results in the comparative overreporting of symptoms. Thus, we have presented evidence showing that suggestion-induced hypotheses, social factors, and recalled experiences may cause us to mislabel mild or ambiguous bodily data as signs of illness. However, mislabeling can occur in the opposite direction as well, with tragic consequences. Although incorrect labeling of relatively benign bodily sensations has enormous social and economic costs by channelling people into the health-care system unnecessarily, the mislabeling of bodily experience having a pathological basis as benign can be disastrous for the individual. Certainly, the fear and anxiety associated with some of the tentative hypotheses people entertain (e.g., cancer) may lead people to deny their experience is symptomatic. It is possible, for example, that certain hypotheses are so threatening to the person that he or she will fail even to initiate attempts to verify them. A complete account of the psychology of physical symptoms will need to make room for such issues as the emotional and motivational relevance for the individual of the tentative hypotheses at his or her disposal.

REFERENCES

Anderson, D. B., & Pennebaker, J. W. Pain and pleasure: Alternative interpretations of identical stimulation. *European Journal of Social Psychology*, 1980, *10*, 207–212.

Beecher, H. K. *Measurement of subjective responses: Quantitative effects of drugs*. New York: Oxford University Press, 1959.

Berlyne, D. *Conflict, arousal, and curiosity*. New York: McGraw-Hill, 1960.

Blascovich, J. *Visceral perception and social behavior*. Paper presented at the annual meeting of the American Psychological Association, Montreal, 1980.

Bobrow, D. G., & Norman, D. A. Some principles of memory schemata. In D. G. Bobrow & A. Collins (Eds.), *Representation and understanding*. New York: Academic Press, 1975.

Brener, J. Visceral perception. In J. Beatty & J. Legewie (Eds.), *Biofeedback and behavior*. New York: Plenum, 1977.

Bruner, J. S. *Beyond the information given*. New York: Norton, 1973.

Burnam, M., & Pennebaker, J. *Cognitive labeling of physical symptoms*. Paper presented at the annual meeting of the Eastern Psychological Association, Boston, 1977.

Byrne, D., Steinberg, M., & Schwartz, M. Relationship between repression-sensitization and physical illness. *Journal of Abnormal Psychology*, 1968, *73*, 154–155.

Campbell, J. Illness is a point of view: The development of children's concepts of illness. *Child Development*, 1975, *46*, 92–100.

Colligan, M. J., Pennebaker, J. W., & Murphy, L. (Eds.). *Mass psychogenic illness: A social psychological analysis*. Hillsdale, N.J.: Lawrence Erlbaum Associates, 1981.

Comstock, L., & Slome, C. A health survey of students, 1: Prevalence of problems. *Journal of American College of Health Associations*, 1973, *22*, 150–155.

Engel, G. The need for a new medical model. *Science*, 1977, *196*, 129–136.

Fenigstein, A., Scheier, M., & Buss, A. Public and private self-consciousness: Assessment and theory. *Journal of Consulting and Clinical Psychology*, 1975, *43*, 522–527.

Fisher, S. *Body consciousness*. Englewood Cliffs, N.J.: Prentice-Hall, 1973.

Griggs, R. C., & Stunkard, A. The interpretation of gastric motility, II. *Archives of General Psychiatry*, 1964, *11*, 82–89.

Hackett, T. P., & Cassem, N. H. Factors contributing to delay in responding to the signs and symptoms of acute myocardial infarction. *American Journal of Cardiology*, 1969, *24*, 651–658.

Kerckoff, A., & Back, K. *The June bug: A study of hysterical contagion*. New York: Appleton, 1968.

Leventhal, H., & Everhart, D. Emotion, pain, and physical illness. In C. Izard, (Ed.), *Emotions and psychopathology*. New York: Plenum, 1979.

Leventhal, H., Nerenz, D., & Straus, A. Self-regulation and the mechanisms for symptom appraisal. In D. Mechanic (Ed.), *Psychosocial epidemiology*. New York: Neal Watson, 1980.

Mandler, G. *Mind and emotion*. New York: Wiley, 1975.

Massad, C. M., Hubbard, M., & Newtson, D. Selective perception of events. *Journal of Experimental Social Psychology*, 1979, *15*, 513–532.

Matthews, K., Scheier, M. F., Brunson, B. I., & Carducci, B. Attention, unpredictability, and reports of physical symptoms. *Journal of Personality and Social Psychology*, 1980, *38*, 525–537.

Mead, M. *Sex and temperament in three primitive societies.* New York: Mentor, 1950.
Mechanic, D. Social psychologic factors affecting the presentation of bodily complaints. *New England Journal of Medicine,* 1972, *286,* 1132–1139.
Mechanic, D. *Medical sociology* (2nd ed.). New York: Free Press, 1978.
Mechanic, D. Development of psychological distress among young adults. *Archives of General Psychiatry,* 1979, *36,* 1233–1239.
Meyer, D., Leventhal, H., & Gutmann, M. *Symptoms in hypertension.* Unpublished manuscript, Department of Psychology, University of Wisconsin, Madison, 1980.
National Center for Health Statistics. *Selected symptoms of psychological distress.* Public Health Services Series 11, Number 37: Washington, D.C.: Government Printing Office, 1970.
National Center for Health Statistics. *Acute conditions: Incidence and associated disability, United States, July 1977–June 1978.* Public Health Services Series 10, Number 132. Washington, D.C.: Government Printing Office, 1979. (a)
National Center for Health Statistics. *Physician visits: Volume and interval since last visit, United States—1975.* Public Health Service Series 10, Number 128. Washington, D.C.: Government Printing Office, 1979. (b)
National Center for Health Statistics. *Use habits among adults of cigarettes, coffee, aspirin, and sleeping pills.* Public Health Series 10, Number 131. Washington, D.C.: Government Printing Office, 1979. (c)
Neisser, U. *Cognition and reality.* San Francisco: Freeman, 1976.
Newtson, D. Foundations of attribution: The perception of ongoing behavior. In J. Harvey, W. Ickes, & R. Kidd (Eds.), *New directions in attribution research* (Vol. 1). Hillsdale, N.J.: Lawrence Erlbaum Associates, 1976.
Nisbett, R., & Valins, S. Perceiving the causes of one's own behavior. In E. Jones, D. Kanouse, H. Kelley, R. Nisbett, S. Valins, & B. Weiner (Eds.), *Attribution: Perceiving the causes of behavior.* Morristown, N.J.: General Learning Press, 1971.
Pennebaker, J. W. *The psychology of physical symptoms.* New York: Springer-Verlag, 1982.
Pennebaker, J. W. Perceptual and environmental determinants of coughing. *Basic and Applied Social Psychology,* 1980, *1,* 83–91.
Pennebaker, J. W. Stimulus characteristics influencing estimation of heart rate. *Psychophysiology,* 1981, *18,* 540–548.
Pennebaker, J. W., & Brittingham, G. L. Environmental and sensory cues affecting the perception of physical symptoms. In A. Baum & J. Singer (Eds.), *Advances in environmental psychology* (Vol. 4). Hillsdale, N.J.: Lawrence Erlbaum Associates, 1982.
Pennebaker, J. W., Gonder-Frederick, L. A., Stewart, H., Elfman, L., & Skelton, J. A. *Physical symptoms associated with blood pressure.* Paper presented at the annual meeting of the American Psychological Association, Montreal, 1980.
Pennebaker, J. W., Hendler, C. S., Durrett, M. E., & Richards, P. Social factors influencing absenteeism due to illness in nursery school children. *Child Development,* 1981, *52,* 692–70.
Pennebaker, J. W., & Lightner, J. M. Competition of internal and external information in an exercise setting. *Journal of Personality and Social Psychology,* 1980, *39,* 165–174.
Pennebaker, J., & Skelton, J. Psychological parameters of physical symptoms. *Personality and Social Psychology Bulletin,* 1978, *4,* 524–530.
Pennebaker, J. W., & Skelton, J. A. Selective monitoring of bodily sensations. *Journal of Personality and Social Psychology,* 1981, *41,* 213–223.
Raper, A. The incidence of peptic ulceration in some African tribal groups. *Transactions of the Royal Society of Tropical Medicine and Hygiene,* 1958, *152,* 535–546.
Rickels, K. *Non-specific factors in drug therapy.* Springfield, Ill.: Thomas, 1968.
Rodin, J. Somatopsychics and attribution. *Personality and Social Psychology Bulletin,* 1978, *4,* 531–540.

Ross, L., Lepper, M., & Hubbard, M. Perseverence in self-perception and social perception: Biased attributional processes in the debriefing paradigm. *Journal of Personality and Social Psychology*, 1975, *35*, 880–892.

Ruble, D. Premenstrual symptoms: A reinterpretation. *Science*, 1977, *197*, 291–292.

Schacter, S., & Singer, J. Cognitive, social, and physiological determinants of emotional state. *Psychological Review*, 1962, *69*, 379–399.

Shontz, F. *The psychological aspects of physical illness and disability*. New York: Macmillan, 1975.

Skelton, J. A. *Suppression of facial responses and directional consistency among subjective, physiological, and expressive indices of emotion*. Unpublished masters thesis, University of Virginia, Charlottesville, 1979.

Skelton, J. A. *Data, theory, and the perception of bodily states*. Unpublished manuscript, Department of Psychology, University of Virginia, Charlottesville, 1980. (a)

Skelton, J. A. *Symptomatic experience and judgments of the health-relevance of verbal stimuli*. Paper presented at the annual meeting of the American Psychological Association, Montreal, 1980. (b)

Skelton, J., & Pennebaker, J. Dispositional determinants of symptom reporting: Correlational evidence. Paper presented at the annual meeting of the American Psychological Association, Toronto, 1978.

Snyder, M. Self-monitoring processes. In L. Berkowitz (Ed.), *Advances in experimental social psychology* (Vol. 12). New York: Academic Press, 1979.

Sternbach, R., & Tursky, B. Ethnic differences among housewives in psychophysical and skin potential responses to electric shock. *Psychophysiology*, 1965, *1*, 241–246.

Stunkard, A., & Koch, C. The interpretation of gastric motility, I. *Archives of General Psychiatry*, 1964, *11*, 74–82.

Taylor, S. E., & Crocker, J. Schematic bases of social information processing. In E. T. Higgins, C. P. Herman, & M. P. Zanna (Eds.), *Social cognition: The Ontario Symposium*, Volume 1. Hillsdale, N.J.: Lawrence Erlbaum Associates, 1981.

Taylor, S. E., & Fiske, S. T. Salience, attention, and attribution: Top of the head phenomena. In L. Berkowitz (Ed.), *Advances in experimental social psychology* (Vol. 11). New York: Academic Press, 1978.

Tursky, B., & Sternbach, R. Further physiological correlates of ethnic differences in responses to shock. *Psychophysiology*, 1967, *4*, 67–74.

Tversky, A., & Kahneman, D. Judgment under uncertainty: Heuristics and biases. *Science*, 1974, *185*, 1124–1131.

Zborowski, M. Cultural components in responses to pain. *Journal of Social Issues*, 1952, *4*, 16–30.

Zborowski, M. *People in pain*. San Francisco: Jossey-Bass, 1969.

Zola, I. Culture and symptoms: An analysis of patients presenting complaints. *American Sociological Review*, 1966, *31*, 615–630.

5 Social Comparison and Perceptions of Health and Illness

Glenn S. Sanders
State University of New York at Albany

One of the most striking features of the journey from health to illness and back again to health is the nearly constant presence of uncertainty. What caused the problem? Is it serious? Is treatment necessary? Is a given diagnosis accurate? How long will recovery take? How effective is this treatment? These are but a handful of the questions that have likely demanded the attention of anyone in physical distress. Presumably, the best answers to such questions are provided by health professionals. Nonetheless, it is far from uncommon to observe these queries being directed to and answered by family, friends, and even strangers, few of whom have any well-founded idea of what they are talking about. Furthermore, it does not tax the imagination to assume that the practice of having laypeople reduce each other's illness-related uncertainty can have serious consequences. People may exacerbate a problem by persisting in behaviors condoned or encouraged by others; they may postpone treatment until it is too late, having been told by others that treatment is either hopeless or unnecessary; they may discontinue an effective therapy, impressed by the negative reactions of their friends; and so forth.

The following material is an initial exploration into the dynamics of acquiring medically relevant information from unqualified sources. Chief among the issues to be considred are: (1) How common is the use of nonexpert opinions for clarifying illness-related uncertainty? (2) Why do people seek nonexpert opinions, and why are others willing to provide them? (3) What are some determinants of the likelihood of seeking nonexpert information? (4) What are the *possible* influences of nonexpert information at various stages of illness and recovery? (5) What determines the *actual* content of nonexpert information? and (6) How does the influence of nonexpert information interact with attempts to modify health care behavior?

Due to the scarcity of previous research specifically aimed at these issues, much of the discussion is somewhat speculative, although relevant data and theory are supplied when possible. Consequently, the reader is advised to approach the material with the aim of uncovering problems that may otherwise have remained hidden, rather than of finding firm answers to long-standing questions. This is not to say, however, that this chapter is simply fuel for future research. The ideas presented often have direct implications for layreaders and students as they are involved in the process of nonprofessional information exchange and for health professionals as they are affected by it. These implications are spelled out at the end of each section.

As an organizing framework, the issues to be explored are viewed as instances of the general process of *social comparison* (cf. Festinger, 1954; Suls & Miller, 1977). This term refers to the tendency of people to evaluate various aspects of themselves through a comparison of their own characteristics (opinions, feelings, behaviors) with those of other people. In the following discussion, it is assumed that people often have mixed feelings concerning their health status and what to do about it. The resulting ambiguity and ambivalence can be resolved by hearing others' opinions and deciding that those feelings shared by others are more valid than the remaining nonshared impulses. For example, a person may want to see a doctor but be afraid of the cost. The cost factor will play more (or less) of an inhibiting role to the degree it is emphasized (or overlooked) by others. Thus, the appropriateness of being concerned about cost has been clarified through social comparison. In general terms, then, the act of seeking medical information from nonexpert others can be seen as yet another example of the pervasive practice of using comparison information for self-evaluation and self-direction.

FREQUENCY AND IMPACT

The concept of a "lay referral structure" (Friedson, 1961) or "lay conferral system" (Elder, 1968) has attracted the attention of medical sociologists for the last 2 decades. This concept describes an informal community-based network of individuals, most of whom are not medical professionals, whose function is to provide medically relevant information in the form of diagnoses, treatments, and professional referrals. Available data indicate that this is a very active and influential network.

Suchman (1965) reported that unusual physical symptoms were followed by lay consultation in 74% of his sample and that 16% of the sample talked with two or more nonexpert others. Lay conferrals were felt to have provided a fairly clear course of action by 78% of the respondents, and over 70% described others' opinions as highly influential in determining subsequent action. Similarly, Miller (1973) found that early signs of head and neck cancer prompted discussion with medically uninformed consultants 62% of the time and that in 55% of these instances others' opinions became the guide to action. Davis and Eichorn (1963) asked cardiac patients whether they had asked for others' opinions of their doctor-prescribed recovery and prevention regimen. Over 90% of the sample answered in the affirmative, and 52% said they were more influenced by the opinions of family and friends than by their physician's advice. Twaddle (1969) observed that symptoms resulting in great pain or sudden disability prompted doctor visits without lay consultation, but that other symptoms, constituting the majority of cases, triggered a series of nonexpert discussions, with the typical subject consulting others until finding one that recommended professional attention. If no such advice was received, the symptoms were usually ignored until they became much worse. Heinzelmann and Bagley (1970) studied the decision of potential cardiac victims to participate in a preventive physical activity program. They noted an 80% participation rate for subjects whose spouse had a positive opinion of the program, whereas only 40% participated if their spouse's attitude was neutral or negative. Osterweis, Bush, and Zuckerman (1979) found that the best predictor of patients' adherence to prescribed medicine-taking was the extent to which other family members used medicine. If others did not believe in the validity of taking medicine, adherence was extremely limited.

In order to get an even clearer idea of the magnitude of the lay referral system, I had 220 undergraduates complete a health questionnaire. It first asked how often in the last year they had experienced unusual physical symptoms with mixed feelings and no ready explanation. The main response was 2.4, or about once every 5 months, with only 6% indicating no such occurrences. On the average, each time uncertainty-provoking symptoms were experienced, 2.7 nonexperts were consulted, and their advice or opinions had a strong directive influence on reactions to symptoms in 68% of such discussions. Furthermore, subjects had an average of 1.8 instances in the last year of being given medical advice by laypersons without having asked for it. The typical subject reported having offered medical opinions and advice to 3.2 others a total of 5.5 times in the last year (the distribution on this item was sharply bimodal, with roughly a third of the sample rarely or never giving advice and the remainder doing so every 1 or 2 months). Only 13% of the sample reported they would not offer any opinion due to their lack of expert information if consulted by others with medically related questions.

In general, subjects reported seeing a doctor to inquire about symptoms .9 times, or about once every 14 months. Whereas professional advice concerning home treatment, recovery, and/or future prevention was obtained in 74% of these cases, nonexpert opinions were sought 88% of this time, and unsought advice and opinions were offered by others in 5 out of every 10 instances. Additionally, subjects felt that lay information was *at least* as influential as professional information in determining their feelings and actions in 65% of their postdoctor-visit experiences.

Finally, on an overall basis, 81% of the subjects said that they consulted with others in order to clarify their own feelings and decide on a course of action, as opposed to just wanting to vent their own feelings, obtain reassurance, or gather support for decisions they had already made. This last finding again suggests that the lay conferral system plays an active and influential role in shaping perceptions of health and illness. There seems to be little doubt, then, that consultation with nonexpert others is both a common and important aspect of the experience of illness.

Implications

Laypersons. Seeking and offering medical advice is apparently commonplace among the medically uninformed. As such, these activities are most likely acceptable and perhaps even expected. People should therefore not hesitate to seek the opinions of lay consultants because these opinions will usually be readily offered and failure to accept them will typically result in prolonged ambivalence and inaction. Similarly, laypersons need not be too hesitant about offering medical advice to others (particularly if one has special experiences that may be relevant) because such advice is probably desired and will probably be obtained from others if not from oneself. People should also be aware that failure to engage in lay consultation may be interpreted as indifference, lack of respect, and so forth (rather than prudent silence in the face of ignorance) due to the readiness of most people to participate in the lay conferral system.

Health Care Professionals. These data should make it clear that medical personnel and their patients do not interact in a vacuum. The factors that bring patients to professionals and mediate recovery and prevention are by no means confined to a strictly medical domain (cf. e.g., the findings of Zola, 1973, that various types of physical symptoms are in and of themselves unrelated to the decision to see a doctor). Rather, the health care professionals must take into account the fact that their patients' feelings and behavior are strongly influenced by information received from nonexperts and that such information can obviously be at odds with the professional's intentions. Particularly in troublesome cases, some effort should be devoted to determining what information, if any, the patient is receiving from uninformed others and to understanding that the patient is being influenced by this information rather than by medical factors alone.

THE IMPETUS FOR LAY CONFERRAL

Although lay consultation is clearly an extensive and influential practice, it is not readily apparent as to why this is the case. Few people would deny that good health is one's most important asset and that improper health care can create life's greatest disasters. It is also clear that medicine is an enormously complex discipline, requiring more years of intense study and practice than most other professions. How, then, can people be interested in and influenced by the medical opinions of others who have no such training and who are capable of delivering a large variety of potentially harmful or even fatal misinformation? At least intuitively, one would be rather hesitant to seek or heed the advice of an uninformed layperson if it pertained to investing life savings or fixing electrical malfunctions. Yet people seem ready to literally play with their lives and well-being in a game of unfounded medical opinions.

By the same token, it is also odd that people are willing to *offer* medical advice. Again intuitively, it seems that if one knew nothing about cars and was consulted about a problematic carburetor, the most likely response would be to claim ignorance, not to suggest a gas-treatment product or urge a costly and time-consuming visit to a mechanic. Nonetheless, even deeper ignorance of the causes and implications of symptoms, of the validity of treatment techniques, and so forth fails to inhibit people from offering health care suggestions with sufficient confidence to render them influential.

The following sections attempt to explain the high frequency of lay consultation, although the absence of much relevant data results in a good deal of pure speculation. Attention is first focused on the recipients of nonexpert information and then on its providers.

One of the central points made by Festinger's (1954) theory of social comparison is that when an objective basis for defining reality is not easily available, people will rely on a social definition of reality produced by mutually shared opinion. For example, it would be difficult to decide via purely objective evidence that one is creative, so one either "is" or "is not" creative as a function of a social consensus. In this manner, it may be that the great complexity of the medical domain, which should remove it from the influence of uninformed opinion, instead gives it the appearance of being difficult to define objectively, and thus leaves it susceptible to social definition. If it is felt that there is no definitive objective basis for knowing the meaning of a symptom or the efficacy of a treatment in any single case, then these matters will tend to be "known" by the opinions of others. That is, if *no* person can prove medical reality objectively, then *every* person is entitled to his or her say. In contrast, less involved matters, such as investment plans, electrical systems, or auto mechanics, are probably viewed as subject to objective definition—there is a right and a wrong, and it can be proved which is the case—and therefore, nonexpert opinions would be neither sought nor heeded. This reasoning leads to the expectation that other highly complex areas, such as interpersonal relations and mental disorders, would likewise be seen as defying objective definition and consequently susceptible to lay consultation. The bottom line here is that nonexpert opinions may be sought and heeded in medical matters because health care professionals themselves are viewed as nonexperts in the sense of lacking objective bases for their opinions.

A second reason for initiating and responding to lay consultation could involve the frequently high costs of relying on expert information. These costs can include: (1) time and effort (e.g., it will usually be easier and faster to consult family, friends, or colleagues than to see a doctor); (2) ease of disclosure (e.g., it will usually be more comfortable to discuss personal problems with familiar others than with a relatively unknown and possibly unsympathetic health professional); (3) pain and discomfort (e.g., lay consultants will probably be far less likely than professionals to recommend painful or difficult medical tests and curative or preventive procedures); (4) bad news (e.g., nonexpert others are probably motivated to avoid giving unpleasant information, cf. Tesser & Rosen, 1975, whereas professionals are bound to do so if the case merits it); (5) recrimination (e.g., familiar others are probably less likely than professionals to chide the subject for bad health habits or failure to follow advice); (6) commitment (e.g., people may feel at liberty to disregard the opinions of lay consultants if they are not pleased with what they hear, whereas seeking professional information tends to commit one to abiding by their opinions); (7) individuality (e.g., people are likely to feel they are a unique and important object of concern when presenting their problems to familiar others, whereas the constant stream of cases handled by professionals may produce in people a sense of being a mere slot in the schedule book and of no great moment, lost in the crowd of patients rather than the center of attention); and, last but not least (8) money (e.g., seeking professional information often introduces the vivid possibility of major or even ruinous expenses). In short, cost considerations suggest that people may use lay consultants to reduce medically related uncertainty not because they necessarily value such opinions but because they fear the consequences of consulting professionals.

A third factor promoting lay consultation may be a desire to avoid or minimize responsibility for important decisions. There are many ways in which people can appear foolish (or worse) to themselves and others when subjected to possible or real illness. If they take too much action, they may appear hysterical or hypochondriacal. Too little action would constitute negligence, making them "responsible" for their problems and removing them from entitlement to sympathy and support. A decline in health following abandonment of a prescribed regimen could lead to charges of stupidity or self-destructive tendencies, whereas a sudden decline in health following adoption of a treatment program could reflect a lack of common sense in choosing the program and/or being the dupe of a physician's desire to push a pet theory. The basic problem confronting people is that there are a variety of unforeseeable consequences that could make their health-related decisions seem unwise in retrospect. A considerable amount of protection from the implications of negative consequences would be gained by seeking and responding positively to others' opinions. Family, friends, and colleagues would be far less likely to point an admonishing finger if they were directly involved in the questionable decisions. Additionally, people could ease their self-recrimination if they knew that other nonexperts shared their opinions and would bave acted similarly.

One final impetus for initiating lay consultation may be the sense of helplessness and passivity imposed by physical impairment and high levels of uncertainty. As discussed by Parsons (1958), a major component of the "illness role" is the relinquishment of personal responsibility. People with physical problems are not generally expected to cure themselves or to choose courses of action independently, but rather are properly passive and malleable objects entrusting themselves to the guardianship of well, strong others. The origins of this concept of "proper" behavior is beyond our focus here, but the illness role does seem to be widely accepted both within and across most cultures. An obvious consequence of this general linkage of dependence with illness is that people who feel or suspect themselves to be ill will be obliged to consult with others before making decisions. For the other reasons reviewed earlier, this consultation will not be limited to or even centered on health care professionals.

Having at least made intelligible the high frequency of initiating lay consultation, let us now turn to the other side of the coin—the fact that nonexperts are virtually always willing to offer medical opinions when consulted and will even do so frequently when not explicitly asked about their feelings. For example, Miller (1973) reports that a woman with a persistent sore throat (which turned out to be sympotomatic of neck cancer) was told in strong terms by her family that she was malingering and should ignore the problem because it would certainly fade away. One explanation for this seemingly irresponsible behavior stems from the illness-role concept just discussed. In the same way that people with physical problems feel obliged to consult with others, the consultants themselves may feel it is their duty to provide some basis for action. Failure to offer an opinion would be tantamount to shrugging one's shoulders when told by a child that she cannot find her parents.

The obligation to respond produced by the illness role may be intensified by the highly self-revealing nature of seeking medical opinion. To discuss one's real or potential infirmities is a major act of self-disclosure—of opening oneself up for others' inspection. This form of giving of oneself probably induces a pressure for reciprocity—an implicit demand that the consultant give something in return. It is as if the initiator were saying, "I have revealed something important, made myself vulnerable, and taken a real chance that you won't dangerously mislead me—the least you can do is to get involved in my problem and take a chance in offering some basis for action."

Another force operating on the consultant could be the implicit flattery of being asked for opinions on important matters and the resultant reluctance to forego the status of being "doctor-for-a-day." Health care professionals are almost universally regarded as having the highest occupational prestige, and to be consulted on even a casual basis is to ascend to that level instantly. The role of medical expert is offered to the consultant, and it is a difficult role to refuse. A desire for this role may also underlie the frequent offering of unsolicited information.

The complexity and ambiguity of medical processes and outcomes may also make it easier for consultants—prompted and tempted by the factors just reviewed—actually to go out on a limb and offer potentially dangerous information. The idea here is that it is usually very difficult to know whether one's medical opinions are helpful or harmful, involving as they do a one-subject sample with no control groups. When someone's health gets worse following action precipitated by a consultant's opinions, who is to say that alternate courses of action would have been any better? If a relapse follows discontinuation of a therapy triggered by a consultant's opinion, how can one know if the relapse wasn't inevitable anyway or if it wouldn't have been even worse had therapy been allowed to proceed? If a friend's suggested home remedy is ineffective, how was he or she to know that you were one of those rare individuals unreceptive to its powers? In many cases, if not most, the consultant can effectively deny responsibility for negative consequences because what constitutes proper and accurate information versus dangerous misinformation is frequently seen as a matter of debate even among professionals (of course, some opinions lend themselves more readily than others to denial of responsibility and therefore should more likely be offered, as is discussed in a later section of this chapter).

Finally, there is some evidence that many people, and perhaps most, have intuitive theories of illness that are fairly systematic and internally consistent. Harwood (1971), for example, described a hot–cold theory espoused by many Puerto Ricans in New York City. Essentially, various symptoms and treatments were seen as either hot (e.g., rashes and penicillin) or cold (e.g., colds and fruit juices), and treatment consisted of prescribing cold-type cures for hot-type problems or vice versa. There are doubtless many other cultural and idiosyncratic medical belief systems, and their existence probably serves to facilitate the offering of opinions greatly. That is, it is not as if the lay consultant has to grab advice out of thin air due to a lack of expertise; rather, the opinions are often dictated by a well-established, readily available, and possibly compelling medical theory. It may also be supposed that people who possess a coherent intuitive theory would be less likely to experience confusion when experiencing a physical difficulty and thus less likely to seek clarification through the lay conferral system.

Implications

Laypersons. Both recipients and providers of lay consultation should realize that there are strong pressures acting on people to offer information with confidence and to be significantly influenced by that information. It is not safe to assume that ignorance of the facts will prevent a consultant from readily offering opinions, nor is it safe to assume that one's opinions will be taken with a large grain of salt due to obvious lack of expertise. Great care should be taken in the choice of consultants and in the consultant's choice of words.

Health Care Professionals. It is important to realize that patients have a strong need for information. Any tendency to keep them in the dark, for practical or ethical reasons or because of personal discomfort, will probably intensify a preexisting tendency for lay consultation. Concerns with patients' emotional reactions to bad news or feelings that it is pointless or too much effort to inform them of details need to be balanced by the fact that professional silence could well be replaced by the uninformed but influential opinions of family and friends. Care should also be taken to present information in a coherent, systematic fashion, rather than as isolated fragments, in order to compete favorably with the potentially well-developed intuitive theories offered by lay consultants. Furthermore, professionals should try, when feasible, to minimize the costs (reviewed earlier) of seeking and heeding their opinion. Perhaps the easiest ways to cut these costs is to assume an informal and approachable manner, to convince patients that they are unique and important, to avoid stern lectures and recrimination, and to adopt a flexible, bargaining style in giving information, rather than trying to instill a sense of absolute commitment to prescriptions. In brief, the most successful professional consultation may be that which comes closest to simulating the atmosphere of lay consultations.

SOURCES OF VARIATION IN FREQUENCY AND IMPACT

Despite the pressures operating on people to engage in lay consultation, it is still the case that there is significant variation in both its frequency and impact. For example, Suchman (1965) observed that 26% of his sample did not discuss symptoms with nonexpert others and that 22% of those who initiated lay consultation felt the discussion had not provided a clear course of action; Miller (1973) reported that 45% of his sample rejected as invalid the opinions of their lay consultants; and I found that almost 25% of the respondents to my health questionnaire indicated that they never offered medical opinions. The following discussion highlights some of the major sources of individual differences in lay consultation.

Inasmuch as medical discussions with nonexpert others can be seen as a form of social comparison, we can begin with one of the central postulates of comparison theory—the similarity hypothesis. Festinger (1954) proposed that comparison information would be most desired and most influential when it was available from others who were similar to the subject. His reasoning was that dissimilar others may have motives or viewpoints that the subject does not share, and consequently, differences of opinion may signify differences in motives or in orientation to the issue rather than the possibility that one's feelings are invalid. The similarity hypothesis in essence supposes the subject to say, ''How can you know what is right for me if you are not like me?'' For example, Democrats would not try to clarify their feelings about a political candidate by comparing opinions with Republicans because their definition of what constitutes a good candidate may be so dissimilar that either agreement or disagreement would be highly ambiguous. As discussed by Goethals and Darley (1977), the emphasis on similar others is particularly strong when one is concerned with deciding on a course of action or with evaluating personal attributes such as capacities and emotions—the most likely topics in lay consultation.

When applied to the clarification of medical issues, the similarity hypothesis suggests that the absence of lay consultants who share the subjects' basic concerns and general outlook will inhibit the desire for and impact of nonexpert information. In two illustrations of this principle, I had subjects play the role of a student with physical problems and then react to comparison information from different types of sources (Sanders, 1980). The first situation assessed the impact of lay opinions on the decision to see a doctor about the appearance of unusual but nondebilitating symptoms. Lay consultation was much more influential if the source was fellow students rather than inner-city housewives. Presumably, this result was due to the fact that other students would be fairly attuned to the meaning of the symptoms for the subject—a student—and to the problems associated with a student's decision to see a doctor. In contrast, the housewives may have had peculiar theories of disease, may have been insensitive to the problems created for a student by the symptoms, or may have used irrelevant criteria for determining when a visit to the doctor was needed.

The second situation involved playing the role of a patient who had just been urged by a physician to enroll in a difficult and painful treatment program. In this case, the opinions of inner-city housewives who had physical problems similar to the subject were much more influential than the opinions of fellow students and friends who were in good health. Here it was the housewives who were most similar to the subject by virtue of their common ailments. Whereas the opinions of healthy fellow students may be based on general principles or unskilled imagination of the subject's circumstances, the afflicted housewives are likely to have more meaningful opinions based on careful consideration of and full exposure to the same uncertainties experienced by the subject.

Another illustration of the importance of similarity between subject and consultant in determining perceptions of health and illness is provided by Fillenbaum (1979). He found that elderly males' perceptions of how well they were could be predicted from the relationship of their actual health (according to professional diagnosis) with that of other elderly males; but these perceptions were unrelated to their standing within more general populations. That is, subjects felt thay were in good health if they were doing better than similar others, but they were uninfluenced by the superior or inferior health of dissimilar others. It seems that they were concerned not with "good health" but with "good health considering that one is an elderly male." In the same manner, my role-playing subjects were concerned not with "appropriate behavior" but with "appropriate behavior considering that one is a student or that one has received this diagnosis." The overall point of this discussion of the similarity hypothesis is that lay consultation will have a frequency and impact proportional to the consultants' ability to place themselves in the subject's position and offer self-relevant information.

A second potential mediator of lay consultation resides in the nature of the medical difficulties themselves. For one thing, some symptoms or treatments or difficulties with professionals, and so on, are more likely to be talked about than others. It is more probable, for instance, that the appearance of blotches on the arm will be brought to the attention of others than will a genital rash; resistance to a doctor's advice will become the subject of lay consultation more often if it is based on the doctor's self-contradictions than if it stems from the physician's facial resemblance to an incompetent uncle; one's degree of success at recovery will less likely be a matter of lay discussion for serious cases, when one still looks and feels awful despite improvement, than for mild ills, when it is a less painful topic even without improvement (cf. the discussion of communication with cancer patients by Wortman & Dunkel-Schetter, 1979).

Another consideration is that some problems, due to their exotic nature or complexity, offer little hope of resolution through lay consultation. The consultant may have something to offer for a persistant headache or a recommended liquid diet, but nonexpert information is probably less attractive and compelling in reference to pain produced by blinking or to a recommended chemoradiation treatment. It would seem that many problems would lead subjects to conclude that they have never heard of such a thing and that there is no reason to assume potential consultants to be any better informed. Consultants themselves should also be less willing or able to offer influential opinions when faced with very unusual or involved issues.

One final property of medical problems per se, which may mediate the frequency and impact of lay consultation, is the degree to which these difficulties interfere with normal activities. The discussion of illness roles by Parsons (1958) has as its basis the idea that people will engage in special role-prescribed sickness behaviors when their ability to execute their normal roles (e.g., worker, parent, etc.) is impaired. Because one of these sickness behaviors is to rely passively on others' guidance, I would expect lay consultation to increase in frequency and impact when medical uncertainties are related to the inability to perform normal functions. In another role-playing study, I again had subjects imagine they experienced a particular set of symptoms. A marked increase in their desire for comparison information from fellow students was produced by the addition of a phrase indicating that the symptoms interfered with taking notes in class. The idea of normal role disability may help to explain why: (1) Suchman (1965) found that for a general sample of symptoms, some involving impairment of normal functions, 74% of the respondents discussed their problems with others, and over 70% were influenced by the information they received; whereas (2) Miller (1973) found that for a sample of head and neck cancer symptoms, none of which involved normal role interference, only 62% engaged in lay consultation, and only 55% of these were influenced by the comparison information. Despite the apparent importance of role interference in mediating information discussions of medical problems, it should be noted that this factor may be culturally specific; Antonovsky (1972) reported high levels of lay consultation independent of role interference in an Israeli sample.

Personal characteristics of both subject and consultant are probably a third major governor of the lay conferral system. To begin with, certain personality variables should facilitate the relevant processes. Some people are more habitually self-evaluative than others (cf. Carver & Glass, 1976; Scheier, 1980). These self-evaluative types may be especially likely to be aware of and concerned by unusual symptoms and to clarify their self-evaluations via lay consultation. In contrast, those with little introspective tendency may continue to focus on external problems until the symptoms either disappear or worsen to the point where the need for professional attention is obvious. Mullen and Suls (1980) have obtained evidence suggesting that subjects high in self-awareness are more likely to engage in some form of stress-management tactic than subjects who rarely view themselves as objects of contemplation. This result may be due to the greater awareness possessed by self-evaluators in experiencing internal difficulties and in understanding the need to determine the precise nature of the problem and to embark on some remedial action. If this is the case, self-focused people should be particularly attracted to and influenced by the clarifying and action-facilitating properties of lay consultation.

A second relevant personality variable is the locus of control construct (Rotter, 1966) and, more specifically, the health locus of control orientation (Wallston, Wallston, Kaplan, & Maides, 1976). This variable refers to people's tendency to see self-relevant events such as illness and its treatment as being determined primarily by one's own efforts (internal locus of control) or by environmental forces beyond one's influence such as fate or powerful others (external locus of control). It would seem that people with a strong belief in the role of fate or luck would be unlikely to engage in lay consultation or to offer helpful advice because they would adopt a fatalistic attitude toward the difficulty in question and would assume that deliberate action was irrelevant to the eventual outcome. On the other hand, those who believe that events are determined primarily by one's own actions and/or those of powerful others would want to clarify the problem they were facing so that effective action could be taken; hence, they would be much more likely to seek and heed others' opinions and to offer action-oriented information.

Other individual differences that could directly influence lay consultation are:

1. Self-disclosure (Jourard, 1964). Some people find it easier to discuss intimate personal topics, whereas others feel either too vulnerable or intrusive when such issues are brought up. It is likely that someone who is comfortable in revealing weaknesses will be more likely to initiate and respond to lay consultation than someone who finds self-disclosure unpleasant. Similarly, those who feel at ease in discussing personal problems should be especially likely to listen carefully to others' complaints and confusion, thus drawing out the discussion and instilling an interest in and respect for their opinions.

2. Self-esteem. People with little respect for the validity of their opinions and the wisdom of their actions should be predisposed to initiate and respond to lay consultation; in contrast, those with high self-esteem should be most confident and persuasive in their analyses of others' problems.

3. Extraversion. Gregarious individuals will have developed a larger network of potential consultants than introverts and should feel easier in approaching others about their difficulties due to their greater social experience.

4. Dominance/submissiveness. Some people like to lead; others like to be led. It is clear that submissive types should find it easier to seek and heed others' opinions, whereas dominant types should be more compelling when offering opinions.

5. Trust. Again, it is true almost by definition that the greater one's belief in the capability and goodwill of others, the more likely one is to be a candidate for an influential lay consultation.

A somewhat different category of personal characteristics that probably exerts as much influence on lay consultation as personality variables is the individual's social standing. One prominent element of this category is socioeconomic status (SES). Miller (1973) reported that SES was inversely related to both the frequency and impact of lay consultation. That is, poorer people with less education are particularly likely to seek and respond positively to uninformed medical opinions. This tendency could be partly due to a greater prevalence of intuitive medical theories in lower-class areas, but is probably also the result of the fact that the higher one's SES, the more likely one is to number medical experts among personal acquaintances. Thus, members of the middle and upper classes are more likely to have the option of informal consultation with professionals to counter or obviate the impact of nonexpert information. Furthermore, one of the principal barriers to immediate professional consultation—financial cost—is of course more of a problem for low SES individuals.

Another aspect of social standing orthogonal to SES is one's depth and breadth of social and family interaction. The more people one encounters and/or the more intense one's relationships, the greater the probability that someone will be available who is similar to the subject, at ease with self-disclosures, or in possession of a compelling medical theory—in short, someone who inspires an influential lay consultation. Although no directly relevant data are available, several findings are consistent with the assumption that being married, having a strong family authority figure, and engaging in frequent superficial and/or intense relationships are all factors that increase the frequency and impact of lay consultation (e.g., Cobwin & Pope, 1974; Geertsen, Klauber, Rindflesh, Kane, & Gray, 1975; Hessler, Kubish, Kong-Ming, Ellison, & Taylor, 1971).

Although the preceding discussion of mediators of the lay conferral system's operation is by no means exhaustive, it should suffice to suggest the range of potential facilitating and inhibiting factors. The fact remains, however, that lay consultation is in general very common and influential, despite the numerous ways in which it might be short circuited. Thus, the basic pressures acting on people to participate in the lay conferral system, discussed in the previous section, must be quite strong indeed to be able to overcome so many potential sources of resistance.

Implications

Laypersons. People will often feel incapable of or uncomfortable about discussing medical problems with others due to considerations similar to those just reviewed. An alternative, and potentially dangerous, method of coping is to minimize the significance of the difficulties and try to ignore them. An awareness of the sources of resistance to lay consultation may help overcome them so that one can gain some degree of emotional clarity and initiate meaningful action. For example, it may be realized that a consultant's opinions do not seem helpful because he or she cannot be expected to share the subject's perspective (i.e., the consultant is a dissimilar other). If so, the subject has an idea of who to consult to obtain more useful information rather than continuing to feel that meaningful opinions simply are not available. A second implication of this section is that the urgency with which opinions are sought may not reflect the seriousness of the problem, but may instead be at least partly a function of medically irrelevant aspects of the interpersonal relationship, the nature of the problem, and the personal characteristics of the participants. Similarly, people should be aware that some opinions may seem more cogent than others not because they are more valid but, again, because of medically irrelevant factors such as those just reviewed.

Health Care Professionals. Particular attention should be devoted to providing information to patients who are unlikely to engage in lay consultation, as they would otherwise be trapped with their uncertainties and could become quite difficult to handle. On the other hand, patients who are especially susceptible to lay conferral should be asked about what they have heard so that serious misconceptions can be corrected. If it seems probable that the patient is consulting with particularly influential but nonexpert others (e.g., a similar, high self-esteem, authoritative family member), it may be advisable to co-opt such others into the medical team so that they can be used to reinforce the professional's viewpoint rather than be left free to subvert it.

POTENTIAL INFLUENCES OF SOCIAL COMPARISON

Thus far, we have been concerned with the general process of obtaining medical information from nonexperts. In the next two sections, attention is focused on the specific content of such information. The *possible* ways in which lay consultation may influence medically relevant behavior is discussed first; the determinants of the *actual* information obtained by social comparison are explored in the following section. In general, influence may be exerted at five different stages of health and illness: (1) behaviors that prevent or induce illness; (2) decisions about the meaning of symptoms; (3) decisions about the treatment of symptoms; (4) responses to professional care; and (5) recovery from illness. Each of these stages can be considered in turn.

1. Behaviors Relevant to the Onset of Illness. Although many medical problems may occur independently of consciously controlled behavior (e.g., congenital diseases), a great variety of difficulties can be forestalled or induced via particular activities. Such activities can range from the Type A workaholic syndrome that has been linked to coronary heart disease (cf. Friedman & Rosenman, 1974), through general exercise and dietetic patterns that can affect overall susceptibility to bodily malfunctions, to specific habits or acts linked to specific problems (e.g., smoking or taking birth control pills). Two forms of social comparison may influence the probability of an individual choosing to engage in or continue these behaviors. The first form is nonverbal and consists simply of comparing the frequency and intensity of one's own behaviors with those of salient others. This comparison will indicate the extent to which each behavior is normative or deviate within the reference sample. In turn, these estimates can encourage the individual to continue with or adopt behavior seen as normative, to abandon behavior seen as deviate, or to establish a sense of individuality by adopting, maintaining, or intensifying deviate behaviors and/or abandoning normative ones. The second form of social comparison influence is verbal, and this consists of individuals' clarifying ambivalent feelings toward a behavior by comparing their reactions with others' opinions. These ambivalences can involve decisions to adopt the behavior (temptations balanced against fears), to intensify the behavior (increased benefits balanced against unknown consequences or increased costs balanced against potential new benefits), or to abandon the behavior (reduced costs balanced against unknown consequences or reduced benefits in opposition to potential new benefits). Influence will be exerted by comparison sources adding more credence to one or the other set of conflicting beliefs and feelings through personal adherence to that set. Influence can also be exerted by *creating* ambivalence and setting the stage for behavioral change. This would occur via the expression of beliefs and feelings contrary to those held by the subject but previously not considered by him or her.

2. Decisions Relevant to the Meaning of Symptoms. When people become aware of some unusual bodily condition, they are usually interested in determining if this condition is symptomatic of some medical problem. Again, there are two forms of influence that can be exerted through social comparison. In the nonverbal form, one simply observes the frequency with which such bodily conditions (e.g., headache, shortness of breath) appear in others. On the one hand, a high frequency may suggest to the individual that the condition is a common, normal one, and nothing to cause alarm ("everybody gets headaches"). Alternatively, a high frequency may suggest the presence of some potent force to which both oneself and others have been exposed and therefore may favor the conclusion of some medical difficulty ("there's an epidemic"). The verbal form of comparison-based influence stems from discussions of possible antecedents of the condition in question. Attempts at clarification can focus on whether the antecedent was itself a medical problem; for instance, was a headache caused by too much time in the sun (not a medical problem per se) or by a flu virus (a problem in its own right)? Attempts can also focus on whether the antecedent is likely to produce additional symptoms; for instance, is the headache likely to be followed by a sore throat? In either case, the lay consultation is oriented at this stage toward determining if the symptoms can be safely ignored.

3. Decisions Relevant to the Treatment of Symptoms. If a person decides that it is not safe to ignore symptoms, the next stage of lay consultation is intended to provide some basis for action. Such action can take three basic forms. In symptom monitoring, the issues involve charting the time course of symptoms and/or being on the lookout for the appearance of additional symptoms. In addition, symptom monitoring may involve establishing criteria for determining whether danger has passed or intensified. Lay consultation can influence expectations about the symptom's time course and about potential new symptoms, and it can help establish criteria for further action as well as encourage the general monitoring approach. The second basic form of action at this stage involves pursuing some form of home remedy. These remedies can take the form of stopping behaviors suspected to have caused the symptoms, initiating behaviors thought to stimulate the appropriate bodily defenses, and/or taking some kind of nonprescription medical agent. Lay consultation can influence both the general and precise forms of home remedy to be adopted as well as support this overall course of action. The third basic action that can be taken if it is felt that symptoms are medically significant is to seek professional care. Aside from promoting this option, lay consultation can influence decisions involving the general kind of professional most likely to help (e.g., family doctor, emergency room, chiropractor, etc.); the choice of particular individuals on the basis of their interpersonal style, past success with certain symptoms, and so forth; and strategies of self-presentation when consulting professionals (e.g., exaggerate the difficulties so they will be taken seriously vs. act unconcerned so that unnecessary tests will not be hastily administered).

4. *Responses to Professional Care.* A large number of uncertainties can arise from professional care, and the manner in which these are resolved can have strong effects on the success or continuation of the professional/client relationship. The most common issues are probably: (1) the quality of the interaction—how much warmth, courtesy, and interest is the professional exhibiting, and are these levels typical? (2) the competence of the professional—are pet theories, prejudice, or ignorance interfering with the professional's ability to understand and treat the difficulty, and should additional expert opinion be sought? (3) the openness of the professional—is information being kept from the patient, and if so, what are the secrets, why are they being kept, and how can they be brought into the open? (4) the appropriateness of the patient's feelings, attitudes, and behavior—is too much being hoped for, will complaining do any good, should this cure-related side effect be mentioned, and so forth? (5) alternatives to current professional care—are there easier, cheaper, or more effective ways to deal with the difficulty than are currently being pursued, and if so, what are they and how can they be implemented? Furthermore, are there any drawbacks to discontinuing the current approach, and if so, what are they and how can they be avoided? Depending on the specific opinions given, lay consultation can either greatly facilitate or seriously interfere with the effectiveness of professional care.

5. *Recovery.* Social comparison can exert a variety of influences on a patient's recovery from illness, independent of resolving the uncertainties produced by professional care. In its simplest form, lay conferral consists of comparisons between one's own capacities and feelings and those of others who are either in good health or who are afflicted with similar or dissimilar problems (cf. the discussion of typical comparison strategies by Sanders & Kardinal, 1977). Being surrounded by others who are in better health than oneself can lead to subjective exaggeration of one's difficulties, whereas seeing that others are doing worse than oneself can lead to unrealistic optimism about future developments. On the other hand, comparing unfavorably with others could spur determination to improve, and favorable comparisons could lift flagging spirits. Aside from simply observing their relative standing, people can use social comparison with nonexperts to clarify many uncertainties unique to the recovery phase. Typical

problems that can be influenced by lay consultation include: the meaning of unanticipated side effects or of irregular periods of progress, backsliding, and status quo; the appropriate timing of the resumption of normal activity and/or termination of phases of treatment; and the chances of achieving certain results within a given interval. Answers to these problems can seriously affect the speed and completeness of recovery.

Although the preceding review of potential sources of social comparison influence is largely speculative and incomplete, it should serve to illustrate the central point of this section. And that point is that lay consultation is not only deep in terms of frequency and impact, but it is also broad in that it can, at least in principle, interact with and possibly affect in crucial ways virtually every aspect of every phase of the journey from health to illness and back again to health.

Implications

Laypersons. Decisions relevant to health care are not only affected by deliberate consultations with others but also by impressions of how often others perform particular behaviors, how many others possess certain bodily conditions, and how healthy others are relative to oneself. In turn, these impressions can influence the attractiveness and probability of health-relevant behavior patterns, the anxiety produced by the appearance of symptoms, and perceptions of and reactions to one's rate of recovery. Awareness that perceptions of health and illness are not strictly a function of one's actual health, nor even of one's conscious attempts to clarify feelings through lay or professional consultation, may help one achieve a more fully rational consideration of appropriate health behavior. It may also help one realize that the experience of illness can create a great amount of uncertainty along a large number of dimensions so that feelings of confusion and the inability to make independent decisions should not be viewed as an indication of personal inadequacy or of being at the mercy of unusually severe and debilitating problems. Those who serve as lay consultants may be impatient, overwhelmed, or flattered by the steady stream of issues they are asked to help resolve, but they should try to keep in mind that this can be a normal part of illness and does not necessarily reflect on either their own strengths or on the information-seeker's weaknesses.

Health Care Professionals. The provision of health care will almost certainly generate at least some uncertainty, and it would be desirable to anticipate the difficulties, bring them out into the open, and resolve them, rather than having them resolved by lay consultants or by having patients endure the stress of confusion. When making recommendations involving the adoption or termination of specific behaviors, some consideration should be given to the frequency of these behaviors in the patient's reference groups as well as to how the patient would react to performing normative or deviate acts. Attention should also be paid to whether the patient's recovery is being affected by favorable or unfavorable comparisons with the health or progress of others.

DETERMINANTS OF COMPARISON INFORMATION

Unfortunately, there are no relevant data that would enable us to specify the relative probability of each of the influences that have been reviewed. Without knowing how often lay consultants provide particular types of information, it is impossible to determine the overall harm or good produced by the medical opinions of nonexperts. As a first step in making such a determination, this section discusses various pressures acting on consultants to offer or withhold certain kinds of opinions. Some flavor of the total impact of lay consultation should emerge, but obviously this cannot substitute for empirical research into this central issue.

The concept of intuitive theories of illness was discussed earlier (e.g., the hot–cold theory), and these theories are probably a major determinant of the content of nonexpert opinions. Opinions resulting from intuitive systems are also likely to be particularly influential because the subject's problems are treated as exemplars of general and well-established rules, rather than as unique aberrations that require guesswork and trial-and-error solutions. It is therefore important to gain some empirical insight into the prevalence of such intuitive systems, their scope and depth in terms of the range of problems they typically address, and their general tendency to complement or interfere with professional treatment. One speculation can be hazarded at this point, however. The more coherent and comprehensive the theory and the more firmly embedded it is within a culture or community, the less likely it is to interfere seriously with the mantenance or restoration of good health. Such theories must have a considerable grounding in observation and experience and thus could not easily advocate policies with obviously undersirable consequences. If home remedies, for example, were markedly inferior to professional treatment, this difference would eventually be noticed and incorporated into the theory. From this viewpoint, it would appear that people are in greater danger of receiving harmful information when consulting about very unusual problems that cannot be placed in the domain of an established intuitive theory.

A related source of lay opinions is the set of attitudes specified by the Health Belief Model (cf. Becker, 1974). This set includes estimates of the susceptibility of various individuals to various problems, the severity of consequences produced by the problems, and the benefits and drawbacks of specific courses of action. The general effect of these attitudes is to tailor general theories to particular cases. Thus, it might be believed that in general sweating in a cold breeze will induce a fever, but that Joe or Betty will violate this rule owing to idiosyncratic characteristics, or that heat is a good cure for sore throats, but that Joe or Betty will experience dangerous side effects. These attitudes should serve to reduce the possibility of dangerous lay opinions further if it is assumed that, just as intuitive theories reflect general experience, health belief attitudes will usually be grounded in individual experience. However, as the individual yields a smaller number of observations than a collectivity, the possibility of erroneous conclusions is probably greater for specific health beliefs than for comprehensive general theories.

One final and even more specific source of nonexpert medical opinions is generalization from a single experience. For example, if a certain diet was followed by the disappearance of a stiff back, the same diet might be recommended for a stiff elbow; if a specialist was successful in controlling a migraine headache, a visit to that individual might be recommended for any complaint involving stress; if a broken toe heeled without a cast, someone with a broken arm might be dissuaded from following the doctor's recommendation of a cast; and so forth. Because such opinions are based on a single observation and because even slight changes in circumstances can seriously alter the impact of a given behavior, generalization probably represents the most potentially dangerous source of lay medical opinions.

There are a number of factors that may modify the tendency to express opinions solely on the basis of intuitive theories, health beliefs, and generalization. As discussed earlier, lay consultants are somewhat free of responsibility from the consequences of their information owing to the complexity of medical processes and the absence of control groups not exposed to their opinions. However, certain opinions are safer than others. This is particularly true of sentiments that professional advice should be sought or heeded. Even if negative consequences follow from seeing physicians and adhering to their prescriptions, the lay consultant who favored these actions can escape responsibility by placing it on the shoulders of the professionals. In contrast, if a suggested home remedy backfires or if advice to discontinue treatment results in a relapse, it is much more difficult for the consultant to avoid the feeling of contributing to those problems. Thus, rather than a random distribution of the contents of nonexpert information, a bias in favor of placing and maintaining people in the hands of professionals might be expected. Geertsen et al. (1975) found that the presence of a strong family authority figure or a network of close friends, both of which should increase the use and impact of lay consultation, has the effect of increasing an individual's use of professional health care facilities. This observation supports the idea that nonexpert opinions tend to be biased in favor of seeking and heeding professional advice. Similarly, Cobwin and Pope (1974) reported that the number and intensity of one's friendships were both positively related to the incidence of preventive vaccinations and medical and dental checkups. Furthermore, Davis and Eichorn (1963) found that 50% of those who indicated they were strongly influenced by lay consultation complied with a cardiac recovery regimen, whereas only 34% of those who rejected lay opinions complied with the regimen. Again, it seems that lay consultants tend to channel people into the formal medical system. In two more illustrations of this tendency, Suchman (1965) reported that 54% of the consultants presented with symptoms recommended seeing a doctor, and Apple (1960) found that if a nonexpert felt a person was ill, a doctor visit was urged in 81% of the cases. Interestingly, Apple also noted that professional care was suggested more often if the symptoms were unfamiliar to the lay consultant. Unfamiliar symptoms should reduce the applicability of intuitive theories, health beliefs, and generalization, and therefore should increase the pressure to avoid responsibility by advising doctor visits.

A rather different bias in the content of social comparison information is related to the concept of role interference, discussed earlier. At least in contemporary American culture, there seems to be a tendency to encourage action only when medical difficulties impair the performance of normal functions (i.e., if one cannot operate effectively in social or work roles because of the problem). Apple (1960) found that the tendency of symptoms to interfere with role behavior was the major determinant of whether the symptoms were viewed as constituting medical problems and that role-interference symptoms were 50% more likely to elicit the recommendation of some action from lay consultants. Additionally, Amarasingham (1980) observed that it is commonly believed that medicine should only be taken for as long as one feels sick, with sickness in turn determined largely by role interference. Friedson (1961) also concluded that nonexperts will tend to react to noninterfering complaints as part of one's normal ups and downs and discourage remedial action as well (see also Hartley, 1961, for a developmental perspective on this issue). Although more extensive data are needed, it may be tentatively concluded that lay consultants will tend to resolve medically related uncertainties by minimizing the need for concern or action if the subject is capable of pursuing normal activities. Furthermore, the results of Miller's (1973) study suggests that when action is recommended for noninterfering complaints, lay opinions are much more likely to favor home remedies and monitoring than the aforementioned tendency to channel people into the professional health care system.

Two more influences shaping the content of nonexpert opinions may be tentatively advanced. First, Twaddle (1969) noted that when people are formally, officially under the care of a professional, their reliance on lay consultants is markedly diminished. Similarly, observations by Skipper, Tagliacozzo, and Mauksch (1967) and by Wortman and Dunkel-Schetter (1979) indicate that hospitalized patients feel frustrated in attempts to clarify their situation through discussions with both experts and nonexperts. Although there are probably a number of valid explanations for this reduction, one likely possibility is that lay consultants feel uncomfortable about expressing their true opinions to people whose problems are sufficiently intense to require professional care. This discomfort, in turn, could arise from the ambivalence created by a confrontation with others' serious problems. On the one hand, there is a desire to offer sympathy and encouragement, which may be irrelevant to the patient's current concerns. At the same time, there is a tendency to avoid discussing clearly unpleasant topics, partly out of fear that they will aggravate the patient's condition and partly because they are depressing and upsetting to the consultants themselves. The result of this ambivalence would be a suppression of true feelings, mixed messages of encouragement and aversion to the patient, and/or a total avoidance of illness-related discussion (cf. Wortman & Dunkel-Schetter, 1979). None of these tendencies would provide the patient with very confident or useful opinions. In short, lay consultants may be willing to expound calmly and informatively on what a functioning colleague should do about unusual lumps or what a patient in remission should do to prevent a relapse, but when faced with the emotional concerns of people who are clearly suffering or frightened, half-hearted and ambiguous opinions are more likely to be the bill of fare.

A second and final speculation on the forces shaping nonexperts' opinions arises from a study by Campbell (1975). He found that mothers had a tendency to see symptoms as being more serious if they appeared in their children than if they were manifest in the mothers themselves. Again, there is a variety of plausible explanations for what Campbell termed an "attributional double standard," but one intriguing possibility is that subjects are motivated to suppress the threatening implications of their medical uncertainties, whereas observers/consultants are more likely to respond objectively. For example, unusual lumps may be discounted by a subject who is unconsciously fearful of cancer, whereas a lay consultant would feel remiss in not at least suggesting the possibility of malignancy; the difficulties of breaking off a long relationship and finding a new physician may lead a subject to accept the competence of professional advice, whereas a consultant would be more apt to raise questions; and a subject may try to avoid thinking of the pain involved in a treatment program, whereas the negative overtones likely to surface in a consultant's reactions may force a consideration of this factor. On an overall basis, then, the opinions of lay consultants may be likely to emphasize negative possibilities avoided by the subject because of the threat they pose to the self. Although this proposed tendency of lay consultants to emphasize the threatening aspects of medical uncertainty could have diverse effects, it would almost certainly help clarify the subject's feelings by bringing covert fears into the open where they can at least potentially be resolved.

In summary, the content of nonexperts' opinions is probably determined primarily by idiosyncratic, intuitive medical theories, health beliefs, and generalizations (which are probably least, more, and most potentially misleading, respectively). In addition, general pressures to place and maintain subjects in the professional health care system, to encourage action only when role interference occurs, to offer unsatisfactory information when faced with clearly serious and unpleasant problems, and to raise threatening possibilities may all interact with these idiosyncratic contents of comparison information in complex and unknown ways. To be sure, much of the discussion in this section has been speculative, and it is best viewed as a guide for empirical research rather than a definitive statement of the issues. However, two implications of this review seem basically sound. First, the number of forces shaping the content of lay opinions, as well as the diversity of these forces, is probably sufficiently large to insure that subjects stand a good chance or being exposed to a range of information reaching from greatly beneficial through innocuous to lethal. Second, the factors that have been reviewed do not point to the lay conferral system as a necessarily inept or undesirable institution but rather allow for the possibility that it does more good than harm. Given the frequency and impact of lay consultation, this is a comforting thought that invites an empirical test. On an even more global level, Hessler et al. (1971) found that a high level of social interaction, which could reflect a large amount of lay consultation, was negatively associated with both physical and psychological disorders. Of course, interpretation of these findings is impaired by the presence of many confounding factors and the use of a correlational design. However, such results encourage follow-up research using longitudinal methods and clear measures of the frequency and content of nonexpert information.

Implications

Laypersons. People should be careful, when giving or receiving comparison information, to avoid placing too much emphasis on the subject's ability or inability to perform normal functions. Although the origins of this role interference bias are open to speculation, it seems clear that there is no necessary relationship between the seriousness of medical problems and the extent to which they inhibit routine behaviors (e.g., the "innocuous" first signs of head and neck cancer). Similar caution should be exercised against the tendency to use generalization as a guide for action because superficially similar cases may differ in subtle but critical ways. Patients in serious or unpleasant conditions may benefit from knowing that their inability to obtain useful comparison information from lay consultants does not necessarily reflect on the poor quality of their relationships or on the hopelessness of their case; rather it is a common problem caused by ambivalent feelings on the part of the consultants. In turn, the consultants themselves would do well to realize that their reluctance to express their true opinions freely comes at a time when patients are most in need of discussion and clarification and that the patient's inability to have a meaningful exchange of opinions can be more stressful than anything the consultants might have to say.

Health Care Professionals. Lay consultation has the potential to reinforce and supplement the professional's concerns and goals beneficially. It would therefore be wise not to discourage the receipt of lay opinions automatically, but instead to determine the content of such opinions first to see if they are or can be helpful. Second, if it is known that some generalizations are particularly misleading (e.g., if treating a broken arm like a broken toe would be dangerous), special care should be taken to advise clients against such reasoning. Third, the tendency of lay consultants to discourage action if the subject is able to function in normal work and social roles requires special vigilance in administering preventative or recovery programs under these conditions. Finally, patients who are in serious condition and under the professional's direct care may be frustrated in their customary attempts to clarify their condition via lay consultation, so it is especially important for professionals to address and resolve uncertainties in these stages of illness.

IMPLICATIONS OF LAY CONSULTATION FOR HEALTH CARE MODIFICATION

Thus far, we have been exploring the issue of nonexpert medical information as a world unto itself, isolated from other pressures and concerns inherent in health care behavior. In this concluding section, attention is focused on some examples of how lay consultation might affect the success of deliberate attempts to improve people's health through prediction or modification of their behavior.

A good starting point for this discussion is provided by the Health Belief Model (HBM). As was mentioned in the preceding section, the HBM describes an interrelated set of beliefs about an individual's need for professional care together with the costs and benefits associated with such care. This model was formulated in order to facilitate predictions about the likelihood that a person will participate in preventive programs and/or adhere to professionals' suggestions. In turn, good predictive power would allow professionals to concentrate and expand their influence on those targets whose beliefs are likely to interfere with their health. Although the HBM has often successfully predicted relevant behavior, the overall associations are rather weak (correlations of less than .14 are typical), and there have been almost as many complete failures as successes (e.g., Haynes, Taylor, Snow, & Sackett, 1979, Table 5). Furthermore, in most cases of successful "prediction" the correlational methods have left open the possibility that the behavior caused the attitudes, not vice versa. Although there are many possible sources of the HBM's weakness (e.g., the generally unreliable casual link between attitudes and behavior, cf. Wicker, 1969), the influence of lay consultation is a likely contributor. The idea here is that health beliefs may predict relevant behavior, *but those beliefs are likely to change as a result of nonexpert comparison information.* That is, as the subject progresses through an illness experience, uncertainties may be resolved by lay consultation in such a way that the subject's original health beliefs are altered. Any attempt, then, to use the HBM as a predictive device should determine that the attitudes used to make the prediction are still held by the subject when the relevant behavior is measured. An illustration of this principle is provided by Taylor's study, described by Becker, Maiman, Kirscht, Haefner, Drachman, and Taylor (1979). He found that when beliefs about the seriousness of hypertension and the safety of combative drugs were measured prior to being diagnosed as hypertensive, these beliefs failed to predict pill-taking compliance. However, the same attitudes were successful predictors if they were measured 6 months after diagnosis. This clearly suggests that the experience of illness results in a modification of health beliefs. Lay consultants, in turn, are a probable source of such modification.

A second approach to controlling health behavior that should be affected by nonexpert information is the attempt to induce rational decisions by providing objective medical information. The highly publicized seven warning signs of cancer represent one such attempt to offer reliable information as a basis for health behavior. To the extent such information is seen as being an objective description (i.e., a true statement of reality), this approach should theoretically eliminate the influence of lay consultation. Festinger's theory of social comparison (1954) proposed that people would not use comparisons with others to clarify their uncertainties if an objective basis for evaluation was available (Hypothesis II and Corollary II B). This position implies that if people were given an objective basis for health care decisions, such as whether to see a doctor or whether to continue treatment, lay consultants would have relatively little input. However, the existence of substantial interference with the persuasive impact of objective information is indicated by the frequently observed failure of this approach to affect compliance with remedial or preventive regimens (e.g., Haynes et al., 1979, Table 5; Schmidt, 1977). That is, given clear and abundant information about the nature of their problems and the costs and benefits of compliance, patients are more likely than not to ignore or discount this objective knowledge. A possible explanation is that, despite Festinger's propositions, lay consultation continues to be influential when contrasted with objective information, and perhaps the former is even more influential than the latter.

As a preliminary exploration of this possibility, I had subjects role-play the development of symptoms and then gave them both objective and social comparison information relevant to the need to see a doctor (Sanders, in press). It was found that if the objective information suggested that a doctor should be consulted, the effect of comparison opinions to the contrary (i.e., not to go) was completely eliminated, as hypothesized by Festinger. On the other hand, if the objective information suggested there was no need for alarm, the effect of contrary comparison opinions (i.e., to see a doctor) remained at full strength. For whatever reasons, subjects were much more willing to believe that an objective test could "prove" that they were ill than that they were healthy, relying in the latter case on the opinions of nonexperts. In general terms, these results suggest that objective information does not automatically rule out the use and impact of lay consultation. Research into the conditions under which objective information is successful in overriding social comparison information should help to pinpoint areas where health education programs will be most effective.

One final example of the interaction of lay consultation with health modification efforts involves the use of social support groups to ease the burdens of chronic illness and to hasten recovery from acute episodes (cf. Kaplan, Cassel, & Gore, 1977, for background on the social support concept). The basic approach here is to enlist the involvement of family, friends, or other patients in the subject's problems and coping efforts. It is hoped that these support groups can offer numerous benefits to the subject, such as bringing disturbing fears into the open and dispelling or minimizing them, offering sympathy and encouragement, performing chores that are stressful or that interfere with treatment requirements, and serving as calm and effective models that generally set a good example for the subject to follow. Despite all these potential benefits, however, the one extensive attempt to improve health via support groups has yielded rather negative results (Caplan, Robinson, French, Caldwell, & Shinn, 1976). These investigators divided patients receiving hypertension medication into three groups: Control, in which normal therapist/patient relationships were unmodified; Lecture, in which patients attended four 1-hour presentations on the nature of high blood pressure and its treatment; and Social Support, in which the lectures were supplemented by the joint participation of family and friends of each patient and a group-dynamics expert was present to supervise various discussions and role-playing exercises designed to encourage the exchange of socioemotional support. It was found that both the Lecture and Social Support groups surpassed the Control group in both the motivation to adhere to regimens and in the actual adherence, as well as in subjects' satisfaction with efforts being made on their behalf. The surprising result was that the Social Support treatment not only failed to improve upon the gains made by the Lecture treatment, but it was actually somewhat, and on occasion significantly, less effective. For example, subjects felt that others' concern was less helpful, that they received less tangible support, and that their medical information was less adequate if they were in a Social Support group than if they just heard the lectures. Thus, the attempt to involve others actively in the patient's problems only served to disrupt the positive effect of objective information mildly. Several reasons for the failure of social support to be truly supportive are discussed by Wortman and Dunkel-Schetter (1979). All of these reasons basically specify ways in which unwanted and/or disturbing comparison information can be supplied by lay consultants. It seems clear that increasing social support will also increase the frequency and impact of nonexpert opinions. As discussed in an earlier section on the possible influences of such opinions, it is quite possible, though not necessary, for these opinions to counter or even reverse the beneficial aspects of social support. Therefore, it is important to determine what kind of comparison information is likely to result from the introduction of social support. For example, in the particular situation studied by Caplan et al. (1976), hypertension did not significantly interfere with normal functions. As discussed earlier, lay consultants are biased in the direction of recommending inaction in the absence of role interference. Thus, most patients may have been told by their social support groups that preventive efforts were not necessary, resulting in the failure of social support to improve adherence despite the groups' potential benefits.

These three examples should suffice to illustrate the general point that the operation of the lay conferral system can often interact with and impair the effectiveness of attempts to predict or modify health behavior. As further research clarifies the frequency, impact, and content of comparison information in various situations, it should be possible to design health care programs that either neutralize the influence of lay consultation or that use its influence to their own advantage.

SUMMARY

It is very common for people to seek and heed the opinions of nonexperts in clarifying uncertainties and taking actions relevant to health and illness. Although it is surprising that uninformed medical advice would be sought or offered, this practice has a solid basis in people's experiences, attitudes, and goals. Despite the overall frequency and impact of lay consultation, numerous sources of variation in its magnitude can be identified. The lay conferral system is likewise variable in terms of the types of influence it can exert as the subject moves from health to illness and back again to health. General sources of the content of nonexpert opinions can be specified, together with certain biases that help shape these opinions, but little is known about the relative or absolute frequency of specific types of information. Nonetheless, it seems clear that lay opinions *can* be beneficial despite their lack of expertise, and this may be the case more often than not. Finally, it is important for designers of health care modification programs to anticipate how lay consultation will interact with their efforts and, when possible, to incorporate it into their procedures.

REFERENCES

Amarasingham, L. R. Social and cultural perspectives on medication refusal. *American Journal of Psychiatry*, 1980, *137*, 353–358.

Antonovsky, A. A model to explain visits to the doctor: With special reference to the case of Israel. *Journal of Health and Social Behavior*, 1972, *13*, 446–454.

Apple, D. How laymen define illness. *Journal of Health and Human Behavior*, 1960, *1*, 219–228.

Becker, M. H. (Ed.). The health belief model and personal health behavior. *Health Education Monographs*, 1974, *2*, 324–473.

Becker, M. H., Maiman, L. A., Kirscht, J. P., Haefner, D. P., Drachman, R. H., & Taylor, D. W. Patient perceptions and compliance: Recent studies of the health belief model. In R. Haynes, D. Taylor, & D. Sackett, (Eds.), *Compliance in health care*. Baltimore, Md.: Johns Hopkins University Press, 1979.

Campbell, J. D. Attribution of illness: Another double standard. *Journal of Health and Social Behavior*, 1975, *16*, 114–126.

Caplan, R. D., Robinson, E. A., French, J. P., Caldwell, J. R., & Shinn, M. *Adhering to medical regimens: Pilot experiments in patient education and social support*. Ann Arbor, Mich.: Institute for Social Research, 1976.

Carver, C. S., & Glass, D. C. The self-consciousness scale: A discriminant validity study. *Journal of Personality Assessment*, 1976, *40*, 169–172.

Cobwin, D., & Pope, L. R. Socioeconomic status and preventive health behavior. *Journal of Health and Social Behavior*, 1974, *15*, 67–78.

Davis, M. S., & Eichorn, R. L. Compliance with medical regimens: A panel study. *Journal of Health and Human Behavior*, 1963, *4*, 240–249.

Elder, R. *Social class and illness behavior in response to symptoms of a common chronic disease, osteorarthritis*. Unpublished doctoral dissertation, Yale University, 1968.

Festinger, L. A theory of social comparison processes. *Human Relations*, 1954, *1*, 117–140.

Fillenbaum, G. G. Social context and self assessments of health among the elderly. *Journal of Health and Social Behavior*, 1979, *20*, 45–51.

Friedman, M., & Rosenman, R. H. *Type A behavior and your heart*. Greenwich, Conn.: Fawcett, 1974.

Friedson, E. *Patients' view of medical practice*. New York: Russell Sage Foundation, 1961.

Geertsen, R., Klauber, M. R., Rindflesh, M., Kane, R., & Gray, R. A re-examination of Suchman's views on social factors in health care utilization. *Journal of Health and Social Behavior*, 1975, *16*, 226–237.

Goethals, G. R., Darley, J. M. Social comparison theory: An attributional approach. In J. Suls, & R. Miller (Eds.), *Social comparison processes: Theoretical and empirical perspectives*. Washington, D.C.: Hemisphere, 1977.

Hartley, E. L. Determinants of health beliefs and behavior. *American Journal of Public Health*, 1961, *51*, 1541–1547.

Harwood, A. The hot–cold theory of disease: Implications for treatment of Puerto Rican patients. *Journal of the American Medical Association*, 1971, *216*, 1153–1158.

Haynes, R. B., Taylor, D. W., Snow, J. C., & Sackett, D. L. Annotated and indexed bibliography on compliance with therapeutic and preventive regimens. In R. Haynes, D. W. Taylor, & D. L. Sackett (Eds.), *Compliance in health care*. Baltimore, Md.: Johns Hopkins University Press, 1979.

Heinzelmann, F., & Bagley, R. Responses to physical activity programs and their effects on health behavior. *Public Health Reports*, 1970, *85*, 905–911.

Hessler, R. M., Kubish, P., Kong-Ming, N. P., Ellison, D. L., & Taylor, F. H. Demographic context, social interaction and perceived health status: Excedrin headache #1. *Journal of Health and Social Behavior*, 1971, *12*, 191–199.

Jourard, S. M. *The transparent self*. Princeton, N.J.: Van Nostrand Reinhold, 1964.

Kaplan, B. H., Cassel, J. C., & Gore, S. Social support and health. *Medical Care*, 1977, *15*, 47–64.

Miller, M. H. Seeking advice for cancer symptoms. *American Journal of Public Health*, 1973, *63*, 955–961.

Mullen, B., & Suls, S. *"Know thyself": Stressful life changes and the ameliorative effect of private self-consciousness*. Unpublished manuscript. SUNY/Albany, 1980.

Osterweis, M., Bush, P., & Zuckerman, A. Family context as a predictor of individual medicine use. *Social Science and Medicine: Medical Psychology and Medical Sociology*, 1979, *13A*, 287–291.

Parsons, T. Definitions of health and illness in light of American values and social structure. In E. G. Jaco, (Ed.), *Patients, physicians and illness*. New York: Free Press, 1958.

Rotter, J. B. Generalized expectancies for internal versus external control of reinforcement. *Psychological Monographs*, 1966, *80*, (Whole no. 609).

Sanders, G. S. *Social comparison with similar others as an influence on health care decisions*. Unpublished manuscript. SUNY/Albany, 1980.

Sanders, G. S. The interactive effect of social comparison and objective information on the decision to see a doctor. *Journal of Applied Social Psychology*, in press.

Sanders, J. B., & Kardinal, C. G. Adaptive coping mechanisms in adult acute leukemia patients in remission. *Journal of the American Medical Association*, 1977, *238*, 952–954.

Scheier, M. F. The effects of public and private self-consciousness on the public expression of personal beliefs. *Journal of Personality and Social Psychology*, 1980, *39*, 514–521.

Schmidt, D. D. Patient compliance: The effect of the doctor as a therapeutic agent. *Journal of Family Practice*, 1977, *4*, 853–856.

Skipper, J., Tagliacozzo, D. M., & Mauksch, H. D. Some possible consequences of limited communication between patients and hospital functionaries. *Journal of Health and Social Behavior*, 1967, *8*, 33–44.

Suchman, E. A. Stages of illness and medical care. *Journal of Health and Social Behavior*, *10*, 105–114.

Suls, J., & Miller, R. (Eds.). *Social comparison processes: Theoretical and empirical perspectives*. Washington, D.C.: Hemisphere, 1977.

Tesser, A., & Rosen, S. The reluctance to transmit bad news. In L. Berkowitz (Ed.), *Advances in experimental social psychology* (Vol. 8). New York: Academic Press, 1975.

Twaddle, A. C. Health decisions and sick role variations: An exploration. *Journal of Health and Social Behavior*, 1969, *10*, 105–114.

Wallston, B. S., Wallston, K. A., Kaplan, G., & Maides, S. Development and validation of the health related locus of control (HLC) scale. *Journal of Consulting and Clinical Psychology*, 1976, *44*, 580–585.

Wicker, A. W. Attitudes versus actions: The relationship of verbal and overt behavioral responses to attitude objects. *Journal of Social Issues*, 1969, *25*, 41–78.

Wortman, C. B., & Dunkel-Schetter, C. Interpersonal relationships and cancer: A theoretical analysis. *Journal of Social Issues*, 1979, *35*, 120–154.

Zola, I. Pathways to the doctor: From person to patient. *Social Science and Medicine*, 1973, *7*, 677–689.

III PROFESSIONAL/CLIENT INTERACTION

6 The Doctor and the Patient: A Psychological Perspective

Steven J. Mentzer
Brigham & Women's Hospital, Boston

Melvin L. Snyder
Dartmouth College

THE CASE PRESENTATION

Imagine that you are a young physician, having just completed a training program in primary care medicine. You have taken a position in a city clinic, and this is your first week on the job. Awaiting your next patient, you sit in a small examining room consisting of a chair, a stool, an examining table, and an instrument table. Remember that there are 1304 formal disease entities noted in a standard compilation (Berkowitz, 1967). Your challenge is to decide whether the incoming patient has one or more of these diseases or no medical problem whatsoever. You have 20 minutes.

The door opens letting in the nervous chatter of the waiting room. In walks Emil Rucker. He is a tall, well-nourished man in his mid-30s. His sleeves are rolled up revealing bronzed muscular arms. A package of cigarettes in his shirt pocket partially obscures the inscription *Bell Telephone Company*. Emil does not look up as he turns to close the door. You stand and shake hands and introduce yourself. Mr. Rucker sits in the chair next to the examining table. He rubs his palms together and fidgets uncomfortably in his chair. His gaze is fixed on the corner of the room. You comment on what a cold day it is and ask him where he lives in town. You ask his age. His answers are short; his gaze unchanged. You begin: "What brings you here today?" (concerned)

"Well Doc, I just don't have any pep anymore."

"Tell me more."

"I'm feeling kind of tired all the time. I don't even play with the kids much anymore; everytime I start to play ball with the boys, I get really fatigued."

"Do you have any guesses as to why you are so fatigued?"

"I haven't been able to figure it out, Doc." (frown)

"When is the fatigue a problem? Early in the morning? At the end of the day?"

"Anytime that I am active."

"How much does it limit you? For example, how many blocks can you walk before you get tired?"

"About three or four blocks."

"Did you have any problem 6 months ago, say at Christmas time?"

"Maybe a little; I don't remember very well. It's gotten much worse the past month or 2."

"What helps the fatigue go away?"

"Just rest."

"Are you taking any medicine?"

"No."

"Have there been any big changes in your life lately? At home? At work?"

"No."

"Are you working at the same job? Same number of hours?"

"Yes."

"Have you ever had any problems with anemia? Does the word sound familiar?"

"No."

"Do you have any problems with swelling in your ankles? Shortness of breath? Chest pain?"

"No, I can't say that I have."

"Any dizziness?"

"I get dizzy when I get up too fast. I think it may be getting a little worse."

"How long have you been smoking?"

"About two packs a day for maybe 15 to 20 years."

"Do you have a cough?"

(frown) "Oh, once in a while."

"Do you ever cough anything up?"

"No."

"Do you ever have any chest pain?"

"No."

"Do you think your weight has changed?"

"I've probably lost a few pounds the past couple of months."

"Is that due to any change in appetite?"

"My appetite probably isn't what it was 6 months ago."

"Have you had any fever? Or chills? Nightsweats?"

"No."

"When you are in a room with other people, are you generally warmer or colder than most?"

"I haven't noticed."

"Are you constipated?"

"No."

"Do you have dry skin?"

"I've got terribly dry skin. But I shower a lot—and in the wintertime—well you know."

"Have you been feeling down lately?"

"Not really down, Doc, actually . . . well . . . I think I've been pretty irritable lately."

"Irritable?"

"Yes. I'm usually pretty low-key, but the last several weeks things have been getting on my nerves."

"What kind of things?"

"Little things—you know."

"Any person in particular?"

"Nobody in particular."

"Do you have any guesses why you are irritable?"

"Not that I can focus on."

"What kind of personal or financial problems are there at home?"

"None."

". . . at work?"

"None."

"Do you have any significant health problems?"

"No."

"Have you ever had any surgery? Have you ever been hospitalized before?"

"No."

"Tell me about your family."

"Well, I've got a wonderful wife and three strong boys." (smile)

"How is their health?"

"Fine."

"Do you have any brothers or sisters?"

"One older brother—he's healthy as a horse."

"Are your parents still living?"

"My father died of lung cancer 3 years ago. My mother has some problems with her blood pressure, but she is doing well."

"Any history of heart disease in your family? Depression? Anemia? Thyroid disease? Diabetes? Any disease that seems to run in the family?"

"No . . . not that I know of."

"You mentioned that you have a wife and three boys. What is it like living at home?"

"Pretty hectic sometimes . . . you know, three boys get pretty active sometimes." (smile)

"What do you do for fun?"

"Play ball with the boys. I like fishing and hunting, too."

"Now, I'm going to ask you a little checklist of questions . . . take you from head to toe . . . to see if we missed anything and see if I can jog your memory."

The questioning reveals only that the patient has had some nausea in the past 6 weeks; it is seemingly unrelated to meals, time of day, or activity. The physical examination reveals a dark skinned young man with a blood pressure of 110/80, pulse 90, temperature 99. There were no additional physical findings.

You talk with Mr. Rucker and explain that you do not know what is causing his tiredness. You do think, however, that some blood tests are indicated. You explain that these may give some additional clues. It will take several days for the tests to come back; therefore, he should schedule an appointment for 1 week, and you can go over the tests results together at that time.

THE CASE IN PSYCHOLOGICAL CONTEXT

With each new patient that enters the clinic, the primary care physician is confronted with an enormous diagnostic challenge. The physician must be prepared to make the diagnosis of one or more of hundreds of diseases and medical conditions. Moreover, many of these people, probably most, will come to the clinic with complaints that do not represent any medical problem. The task is highly complex; the physician must cope with a high degree of uncertainty.

The physician attempts to reduce the uncertainty by undertaking a formalized evaluation process. The typical *work-up* involves three parts: the history, the physical examination, and laboratory studies. The history, or medical interview, tries to identify the patient's problem. The problem is then further defined along several dimensions. Useful information about symptoms includes their location, their time course, their quantity or quality, and factors that exacerbate or attenuate them such as time of day, meals, or specific places and activities. The history is then followed by the physical examination. In most cases, this examination involves a thorough search for the physical manifestations of disease. The emphasis of this examination is often determined by the findings in the history. Finally, the clues obtained in the history and physical examination are followed up with laboratory studies. The modern laboratory offers wide variety of X-ray, chemical, and physical tests.

Many physicians would argue that, of these three parts, the medical history is the most important element of the diagnostic process. A figure often quoted is that 75% of any physician's diagnosis are made on the basis of history alone (Leitzell, 1977). Because of its importance in everyday practice, we have chosen the medical interview to illustrate several psychological issues in the doctor–patient interaction.

Self-Disclosure and Rapport

The physician's primary objective is to help the patient with his or her problem. To achieve this goal, the physician needs to identify what is *the most significant problem to the patient.* For example, Mr. Rucker may complain of not being able to play with the kids; perhaps he is not having fun on the job. Continued questioning clarifies the complaint. The primary problem appears to be fatigue and tiredness. This refined version of the patient's problem is called the *chief complaint.* The importance of this self-disclosure is emphasized in major textbooks on medical interviews (Froelich & Bishop, 1972; Prior & Silberstein, 1977). Medical educators preach during medical training about its importance (*Introduction to Clinical Medicine,* 1978). Everyone argues it is important; but what role does the chief complaint play in the doctor–patient interview?

One answer lies in information theory. Identification of the chief complaint constitutes a huge gain in information. Consider that there are 1304 possible diagnoses, and you have 20 minutes to diagnose Mr. Rucker. The physician cannot ask questions about 1304 possibilities. He or she must quickly focus on a handful of disease states. This is possible if the patient can reliably disclose the most significant problem. In Mr. Rucker's case, fatigue and tiredness are associated with 13 common disease states (Hart, 1973). After a positive statement of the primary problem, the number of possibilities has been narrowed from 1304 to 13. Conversely, a negative response to the direct question "Do you have any problems with fatigue or tiredness?" eliminates only 13 problems. The physician is still faced with 1291 possibilities. Little information has been gained because the number of possibilities has hardly been narrowed at all.

As Blois (1980) notes in an informative review on diagnostic strategies, the "diagnostic" or "selective" power of a positive response can be more than 100 times greater than a negative response. The implications for developing an efficient interview strategy are clear. As patients nearly always volunteer positive statements, instead of asking a set of specific questions the physician should encourage the patient to state his or her own case. The patient's spontaneous disclosure efficiently selects the handful of diagnostic possibilities. The physician's uncertainty is markedly decreased, and attention is directed toward the 13 causes of fatigue and tiredness. He or she then structures the remaining interview to sort out these possibilities. In contrast, a failure to obtain reliable self-disclosure maintains a high degree of uncertainty and leaves the physician's thinking unfocused.

Having identified the chief complaint, the physician then begins to consider what its origins might be. We presented the initial portion of the Rucker interview—in which the chief complaint of fatigue is revealed—to a sample of physicians in a variety of specialties. We then asked them to list the diagnostic possibilities they would choose to pursue in the remainder of the interview. The number of possibilities volunteered ranged from four to six. Diagnoses commonly considered were anemia, infection, heart disease, depression, thyroid disease, and cancer. The number of hypotheses generated by our sample of physicians was consistent with recommendations that have been made by other researchers. According to Elstein and his co-workers (Elstein, 1976; Elstein, Shulman, & Sprafka, 1978), two to six is an effective range of tentative hypotheses. More than six or seven hypotheses result in cognitive overload and an inability to manipulate and compare them.

Precisely because the chief complaint controls the physician's thinking, its premature identification is a potential source of error. Consider the possibility that fatigue was important to Mr. Rucker, but perhaps it was secondary to concerns he was hesitant to reveal. For example, patients are often hesitant to reveal problems related to sexual dysfunction or concerns about a recent death. The physician who does not recognize this reticence could naively pursue fatigue and tiredness through the entire differential diagnosis of organic diseases. The cost in time, energy, and money can be substantial.

Several strategies are available to the physician who wishes to elicit accurate self-disclosure from the patient. For one, there is evidence that people are more self-revealing in cozy surroundings than in harshly lit, bare-walled rooms (Chaikin, Derlega, & Miller, 1976). Another approach is simply increasing exposure to the patient. In general, we expect that communication improves with time. But, of course, more than simple exposure is involved in the doctor–patient relationship. We suspect that accurate self-disclosure is promoted by the same variables that enhance patient compliance with doctor's recommendations. For example, patient cooperation is correlated with the quality of the doctor–patient relationship. In a study of pediatricians, Francis, Korsch, and Morris (1969) found than when the mother believed: 1) the doctor did not understand her concerns; or 2) the doctor was "businesslike," there was a significant lack of cooperation (manifest by the patient's failure to cooperate with the physician's advice). On the other hand, cooperation was the highest with high patient satisfaction. Alpert (1964) studied patients who failed to keep doctors' appointments and found that only 63% of these patients felt they had a doctor with whom they could talk. This compares with 79% of the patient group who did not fail to keep their appointments. Davis (1968), using tape-recorded interviews and multiple follow-up interviews, found that the doctor–patient relationship suffered when physicians sought information without providing feedback.

The quality of a doctor–patient relationship and the doctor's ability to communicate appear to have an intimate association. Of the 800 patients in the Korsch, Bozzi, and Francis (1968) sample, 244 patients spontaneously signaled out the doctor's communication skills as being worthy of note. In this study there was a dramatic difference in satisfaction between those who commented favorably (86% satisfied) and those who commented unfavorably (25% satisfied) on the doctors communication skills.

Korsch et al. (1968) identified several specific characteristics that appear to be important in the development of doctor–patient rapport: 1) warmth and friendliness; 2) clear-cut explanations regarding diagnosis and illness; 3) recognition of patient concerns and expectations. These results may be best summarized by Friedson (1961) who suggested that physicians look at the patient as a person. Given the association between rapport, cooperation, and communication in the doctor–patient relationship, we find it plausible that the quality of the relationship affects the reliability of self-disclosures. Evidence bearing on this conjecture would be most welcome. If the physician makes a sincere investment in patient rapport, we predict that he or she will more likely be rewarded with reliable, informative disclosures. Thus, the nurturing of rapport, in addition to its inherent value, may advance not only the patient's compliance but an accurate diagnosis as well.

Limits on Communication with Words and the Use of Nonverbal Cues

The patient's verbal disclosures may also be limited by his or her perception of the role of the "good patient." Taylor (1979) suggests that the social prestige of the doctor and the traditional power the doctor has over our bodies is intimidating. The patient may be concerned about bothering the doctor (i.e., taking up too much time). As a consequence, the patient may fail to ask questions or volunteer relevant disclosures. This may extend to the stoic patient who is reluctant to disclose discomfort or pain. Limited by his perception of proper behavior, he may try to be the "good patient" to the detriment of effective self-disclosures.

There is a different way that the patient may respond to the exalted image of the physician. The patient may make the tacit assumption that self-disclosure is unnecessary, that all the doctor needs to do is examine the body as a mechanic might inspect a piece of machinery. Talk is seen as irrelevant and improper. This view may be more frequent among lower-class individuals (Leigh & Reiser, 1980). Even if the patient does appreciate the importance of verbal disclosure, often he or she may fail to recognize the relevance of a particular symptom. For example, the patient may have heart pain but perceive it as indigestion and simply not bother to mention it. Unusual symptoms probably are perceived as relevant, but at the same time their very unfamiliarity may mean the patient is at a loss as to how to describe them (Friedman, 1979). When the task is difficult, it is well known that high anxiety interferes with performance (Spence & Spence, 1966). And there is little doubt that a visit to the hospital or clinic commonly produces anxiety. Elevated blood pressure and heart rate are common in the visitor to the health care setting (Sackett, Haynes, Gibson, Taylor, & Roberts, 1977). In addition to psychological barriers to communication, there may be physical limitations. These range from a Parkinsonian patient with slurred speech to a patient with an endotracheal tube, completely unable to talk.

Irrespective of the reason, there are many potential limitations to verbal self-disclosure. To an extent the physician can compensate for such limitations by learning to be sensitive to nonverbal cues. Enelow and Wexler (1966) argue for the utility of making explicit what has been learned verbally and what has been learned nonverbally. For instance, in the Rucker interview, the patient verbalized his fatigue, his smoking habit, his father's death from lung cancer, and his mother's state of health. But simply by observing him, we learned that he was a working man. And from his avoidance of eye contact, his facial expression, and fidgety posture we inferred a level of anxiety beyond what might be expected during an office visit.

The validity of this sort of interpretation has been borne out in studies of nonverbal behavior. Argyle (1975), Ekman, Friesen, and Ellsworth (1972), and others have demonstrated that emotions are most clearly revealed in the face. Facial expressions may accurately reflect—and be used to grade the severity of—the impact of something as practical as the pain of a medical procedure. Leventhal and Sharp (1965), for example, have pointed out the usefulness of the face in assessing the pain of a woman in labor. Facial expressions may also convey more complicated emotions and motivational states. Indeed they may also be used to analyze interpersonal attitudes.

Ekman and Friesen (1974) provide evidence that when people are motivated to hide their feelings the true emotion is somewhat easier to detect by attending to the rest of the body. For example, Mr. Rucker's fidgety posture shows him to be more anxious than his face reveals. Detecting this anxiety is important. His discomfort with the topic of lung cancer suggests that he might minimize his symptoms. Realizing this, the physician must gently probe deeper, if for no other reason than to be able to provide reassurance if cancer turns out not to be the problem.

In the medical interview, as in other areas of communication, it is rarely the isolated nonverbal cue that is helpful. It is the combination of verbal and nonverbal elements that produces the unmistakable meaning (De Paulo, Rosenthal, Eisenstadt, Rogers, & Finkelstein, 1978). If Mr. Rucker had been talkative and outgoing, the physician might interpret his facial expression or posture differently. Conversely, if Mr. Rucker had presented himself with a calm and confident posture, it would change the interpretation of his reticence. In fact, it is the combination of his nonverbal behavior and his reticence that suggests Mr. Rucker's fear of cancer. Goffman (1967) suggests that it is this complex of verbal and nonverbal signals that allows us to understand what would otherwise remain hidden. In an experimental study, Friedman (1979) has explored the effect of combined verbal and nonverbal communication. He has found evidence that facial expressions may be necessary to impart meanings that words alone cannot convey.

Thus, for the physician, using all the senses (i.e., synthesizing diverse relevant cues) may be essential for arriving at an accurate diagnosis. Often the cues are very subtle. For example, certain patients may make glaring errors in speech. They may talk about "driving a catalog" or use the word "presidium" instead of "president." Upon initial examination, such mistakes may be interpreted as global confusion for which a common diagnosis is dementia. In one case after such a label was pinned on the patient, an astute physician noted that the patient's nonverbal behavior was appropriate. This observation led to the correct diagnosis: functional impairment of speech due to a stroke. Needless to say, treatment for the latter and for dementia differ substantially, and the timely treatment of the stroke victim can be important.

Assuaging Versus Creating Anxiety

Mr. Rucker's sensitivity to the issue of cancer illustrates a dilemma that plagues all practitioners. Physicians and patients alike are sensitive to and self-conscious about symbolic issues such as sexual function or feelings about death. When the diagnostic process infringes on these subjects, it is common for both the doctor and the patient to be uncomfortable. The interview may purposefully drift away from these threatening topics. The consequence of this avoidance may not even be addressed consciously (Raimbault, Cachin, Limal, Eliacheff, & Rappaport, 1975).

The anxiety in these situations can be understood in terms of the theory of self-awareness (Wicklund, 1975). The theory suggests that an analysis of symptoms and bodily sensations will promote self-consciousness—generally an unpleasant state in which discrepancies between real self (e.g., sick) and ideal self (e.g., healthy) loom larger. Self-criticism can occur on a variety of dimensions besides health (e.g., physical appearance, intelligence, personality). The consequence is a general reduction in feelings of well-being. When we feel that we are the object of another's gaze, the result may be this aversive sort of self-awareness.

There are two ways to assuage the anxiety of self-awareness. One is simply to avoid thinking about oneself either in general or in terms of a specific problem. Mr. Rucker's confession that his father died of lung cancer, but his mother is doing well is an example. Mr. Rucker clearly does not want to talk about his father's lung cancer.

A more complex coping device is described as *discrepancy reduction.* This means that the individual tries to eliminate any discrepancies or any variety of within-self contradiction. A first step is to recognize the problem. For Mr. Rucker, this may entail accepting that smoking causes lung cancer. Once he acknowledges that he is at risk, a more reliable history and a more thorough evaluation can be obtained, and efforts at discrepancy reduction—a cure—can begin.

Whether to push the patient toward self-consciousness is a choice often made by the physician. At times, when diagnostic uncertainty is high, it may be necessary to discuss sensitive issues. At other times, the odds for discovering valuable information may be very small. The vigilant pursuit of the issue would only translate into wasted time and enhanced patient anxiety. In a study of the management of renal transplant patients, Whittaker, Vieth, Soberman, Lalezori, Tellis, and Freed (1973) argue that there can be serious consequences to the zealous pursuit of information. They illustrate these dangers of what they call the *black snake phenomenon:*

> This phenomenon derives from the story of the two campers who, arriving at their weekend camp site, divide the chores. One stays in camp and pitches the tent. The other sets out to gather wood and obtain water. A while later, the seeker of the water and wood returns to camp battered and bruised. He is limping, bleeding, and disheveled. He states that he has been attacked by a blacksnake. His companion, who remained at the camp site, chides him by saying, "Don't you know a blacksnake isn't poisonous?"
>
> "He doesn't have to be if he causes you to jump off a 50 foot cliff," is the reply. [p. 919]

In the Rucker case, is the allusion to cancer contributing to the diagnostic process? Or is the pursuit of such personal and sensitive information needlessly precipitating self-consciousness and anxiety? The diagnostic uncertainty surrounding this case suggests that all relevant questions should be asked; nonetheless, the physician must be aware that even the diagnostic interview may have a significant psychological and physiological impact.

Bad News and Good

It is apparent from Mr. Rucker's nonverbal and verbal responses that the topic of cancer was a sensitive issue. The physician in the case, however, does not address this issue directly. He is clearly reluctant to inform the patient that cancer may be at the root of the fatigue.

The physician's reluctance to talk to Mr. Rucker about cancer can be seen in the context of a more general phenomenon—a reluctance to deliver bad news. Tesser and Rosen (1975), working in the psychology laboratory, found that several factors contribute to this reluctance. In one study, they manipulated the perceived emotionalism of the recipient of bad news. They found that the communicator was much more reluctant to relay bad news if the recipient was perceived as emotional. This could explain the physician's reluctance to discuss the topic of cancer. Whereas Mr. Rucker would not ordinarily be perceived as emotional, the topic of cancer has clearly disturbed him. The physician could easily have mislabeled Mr. Rucker as exceptionally prone to anxiety (Snyder & Frankel, 1976). There is a general tendency for observers who view another's behavior to underestimate the current situation's contribution to it; rather they infer that it stems from a corresponding characteristic of the actor (e.g., emotional behavior is seen as stemming from a disposition to be emotional) (Jones & Nisbett, 1971).

Rosen, Johnson, Johnson, and Tesser (1973) considered other explanations for the reluctance to transmit bad news. Possibly, the communicator feels guilt or fears a negative evaluation. Whether influenced by guilt or a negative evaluation, one is led to predict less communication the more attractive the recipient. Guilt should be greater and so should concern about the recipient's reaction. In one study, attractiveness of the recipient was varied by describing her as similar in attitudes and pleasant or as just the opposite. Results showed that communicators more readily transmitted bad news if the recipient was attractive rather than unattractive. The suggestion that a physician would hesitate to communicate bad news because of fear of negative evaluation or guilt is weakened by these data.

Tesser and Conlee (1973) also found support for the view that people are reluctant to deliver bad news because the communicator must adopt an appropriate bad mood. This study presents evidence that the communicator's mood fluctuates or "shifts" in the direction that was consistent with the affective nature of the message. When the communicators were already in an unpleasant mood, they tended to communicate bad news more spontaneously than communicators in a pleasant mood. The implication of these data for the practicing clinician relate directly to the psychological costs of adopting the appropriate mood. Physicians, like other people, may be reluctant to shift mood in the course of a day at a busy clinic—sensitive, perhaps unconsciously, to its attendant costs. These costs may be reflected not only in how they feel but also in their impact on others and in their general efficiency. We believe, however, that the cost to the patient of not being informed is even greater.

Many physicians explain their reluctance to communicate bad news by claiming that patients do not really want to know. Oken (1961) found that physicians who remain silent about issues such as cancer often claim that: "Patients really do not want to know regardless of what people say [p. 1123]." Such a belief may have a very memorable origin. The physician may have told a patient bad news. The patient may then have gotten upset, or the physician may have surmised that the patient was upset (cf. Snyder & Frankel, 1976). The physician may have concluded that it is better not to tell. Tesser, Rosen, and Waranch (1973) and Tesser and Rosen (1975) suggest that this conclusion mistakes the patient's desire to avoid having the disease for the desire to avoid hearing about it. No one wants to have a life-threatening disease; yet it may be more distressing to suspect it and remain uncertain than to know. A variety of laboratory studies have shown that people often prefer to be informed about uncertain outcomes—both positive and negative (e.g., Lanzetta & Driscoll, 1966).

The evidence in the studies by Korsch et al., (1968) Davis, (1968), Alpert (1964), Argyle (1975), and Friedson (1961) shows that patients want clear-cut information about their diagnosis and illness. The patient expects the physician to address their concerns. Even when the issue is life-threatening, surveys reveal that about 80% of the public would want to know their diagnosis (Blumenfield, Levy, & Kaufman, 1978, 1979; Cappon, 1962; Kelly & Friesen, 1950). Surveys of this type may have had an impact on physician behavior. Whereas 20 years ago physicians were often reluctant to disclose a diagnosis of cancer (Fitts & Ravdin, 1953; Oken, 1961), patients are routinely informed of their diagnosis in most centers today (Mount, Jones, & Patterson, 1974; Noyes & Travis, 1973; Travis, Noyes, & Brightwell, 1974). The reason for this shift may be that because of these and similar studies physicians are now aware of patient desires. The studies of Conlee and Tesser (1973) suggest that patient desires could significantly influence the transmission of information. Working in the psychology laboratory, they found greater news transmission—both good and bad—to recipients who were perceived as having a high desire to hear it.

Keeping patients informed has a variety of beneficial effects. Work by Bertakis (1977) confirmed that outpatients are more satisfied with their physician the better they understand their illness. Moreover, Svarstad (1976) found that the physician's efforts to instruct and motivate the patient had a positive correlation with the patient's evaluation of the treatment plan. Information and instructions have a distinct impact on patient satisfaction.

Ley (1977) reviewed 13 studies that demonstrated the usefulness of providing patients, prior to surgery, with information about what to expect (e.g., how they will feel or what to do, breathing techniques, exercises). For example, Egbert, Batitt, Welch, and Bartlett (1964) examined the impact of instruction on 97 patients hospitalized with intra-abdominal operations. Unknown to the attending surgeons or nursing staff, the anesthesiologist provided pre- and postoperative information and encouragement to half of the patients. In these brief visits, the anesthesiologist would teach the patients how to manage their abdominal incision pain; that is, they were taught how to breathe and move without aggravating their abdominal incision discomfort. On an average, these patients required half the narcotics and were discharged 2.7 days sooner than their uninstructed counterparts.

Across a variety of such studies, patients given information required, in general, fewer analgesics and had shorter hospital stays by an average of anywhere from 1 to nearly 3 days. A contributing psychological factor might be the sense of control that Seligman (1975) discusses or perhaps what Antonovsky (1979) calls the sense of coherence. As Ley points out, even if these findings turn out to be due to the placebo effect, they are important not only for improving patient care but also for reducing health care expenses.

To Explain Is to Believe

Suppose that Mr. Rucker's physician has decided to consider the hypothesis of Addison's disease. Once such a cognitive commitment is made, Nisbett and Ross (1980) suggest that the hypothesis might not be easily discarded. They argue that, for most people, to generate an explanation promotes belief in it. This phenomenon is well-known in medical training centers. Medical students in particular have a predilection for this error. When presented with a patient or a case history, students typically have naive confidence in the first plausible diagnosis that comes to mind.

The classic example is the case of a 60-year-old man with back pain, which was being presented to faculty, house staff (residents), and students in a major medical center's "grand rounds." Weeks of diagnostic efforts were explained to the distinguished group; all of the available results were presented. At the end of the presentation, the group was posed with the question: What proved to be the cause of the back pain?

A lone hand was raised, and a medical student was called upon to make the diagnosis. "Retroperitoneal fibrosis," replied the student.

The moderator appeared shaken. "That's fantastic," she said, "it took us months to establish that diagnosis. How did you know it was retroperitoneal fibrosis?"

The student's response: "What else causes back pain?"

In contrast to the naive medical student, the experienced clinician knows that most of the time there are a number of potential causes for each clinical picture. Only occasionally is there a pathognomic symptom or finding, that is, a single sign uniquely associated with a disease. When these do occur, great reliance is placed upon them. But the experienced clinician knows that typically just having a given etiologic hypothesis be consistent with the available data is not adequate. What is required are those findings that discriminate among all plausible hypotheses.

The Primacy Effect: One Explanation (the First) Is Enough

A related pitfall is the tendency for first impressions to have a disproportionate influence. If the physician's initial diagnosis had been Addison's disease, laboratory evidence suggests that this diagnosis would be more difficult to relinquish. The phenomenon, in a more general context, is called *the primacy effect*.

One factor is that the initial diagnosis has the physician's greatest attention (Jones, 1977). With each succeeding diagnostic possibility, there is a decrement in attention and gradual increments of fatigue. The result is that the initial hypothesis receives a disproportionate amount of energy. In Mr. Rucker's interview, the physician's initial hypotheses were systematically pursued with a variety of direct questions. It is doubtful that any subsequent hypotheses would be considered as carefully. The result may be a diagnostic work-up that Schiffman, Cohen, Nowik, and Selinger (1978) describe as "systematically distorted to support prior decision." Barrows and Bennett (1972) add further support to this conclusion. After studying the diagnostic processes of clinical neurologists, they concluded that physicians actively search to confirm hypotheses and slight data that support other interpretations.

Testing the Explanation: The Easy Leap from Evidence to Conclusion

Mr. Rucker's initial medical interview revealed a muscular 35-year-old man with bronzed skin who complained of fatigue, dizziness, weight loss, decreased appetite, irritability, and nausea. These symptoms do not immediately suggest a common symptom constellation. At a minimum, they do not support the hypotheses suggested by our sample of physicians who were provided only with the chief complaint. Given this uncertainty, Prior and Silberstein (1977) state that the role of the physician is to: "sort out, to weigh, and to differentiate minutiae from the more significant aspects of the narrative history [p. 3]." Physicians must ask themselves a number of questions. Is the decreased appetite significant or is it a consequence of the inactivity? Is the irritability reported by Mr. Rucker a diagnostic point or is it the result of his fatigue or inactivity? Does Mr. Rucker simply have a "touch of flu"—the importance of which has grown with continued awareness? Is the dark skin color important or is it just a variation of normal?

A critical assessment of each clue is important to avoid what might be called a *relevance error*. The fundamental relevance error can be observed in everyday life and has recently been characterized in the psychological laboratory (Nisbett & Ross, 1980). It is the error that people commit when they treat evidence as more supportive of their hypothesis than it really is.

This error can be illustrated with the case of Mr. Rucker. Suppose the physician was considering the diagnosis of Addison's disease or Endocrine flu. Addison's disease is characterized by a number of Mr. Rucker's symptoms: nausea, myalgia, and fatigue. Dark or bronzed skin is also a sign of Addison's disease. For the physician trying to make a diagnosis, the flu symptoms might suggest Addison's disease. In such a case, Mr. Rucker's bronzed skin might be viewed as confirmatory. But should it be? In a 100 cases with the particular pattern of flulike symptoms reported by Mr. Rucker, only a small number, say 5, are likely to have Addison's disease. For the sake of argument, let us assume that all cases of the disease show the finding of bronzed skin. So for all 5 cases of Addison's, all 5 display the symptom. Next, we need to ask how common bronzed skin is in the other 95 cases. If we are in Minnesota during the winter, bronzed skin is unusual, occurring in perhaps only 15 of the 95 remaining cases. The association of bronzed skin with the disease is unmistakable. But consider that 20 of the 100 cases (5 with and 15 without the disease) have bronzed skin, but only 5 have the disease. Even if the finding appears in every instance of Addison's disease, it can be possible that only 25% of those with the finding have the disease. The presence of the finding sharply increases the probability of the disease, from 5% to 25%, yet the chance is still well under 50% and nowhere near the certainty subjectively felt by the diagnostician. If we fail to consider the base rate of the symptom (i.e., its frequency in cases without the disease), we may jump to an erroneous conclusion (Nisbett & Ross, 1980). We note, in passing, that a Bayesian approach handles this sort of problem rather well (e.g., Gorry, Parker, & Schwartz, 1978; McNeil, Keeler, & Adelstein, 1975).

The Law of Small Numbers

The formulation of a diagnostic work-up for Mr. Rucker raises several practical issues. In weighing the findings, the physician must first decide if the constellation of complaints in this interview really constitutes a disease state. A new patient is at a disadvantage. Doctor–patient rapport has only begun to be established, and patient reliability is unknown. Moreover, a symptom complex that defies ready categorization does not lend itself to laboratory study. Considering the high degree of uncertainty, how should the physician allocate time, energy, and money? Does the problem warrant vigorous diagnostic efforts? Which direction or hypothesis should be pursued? Should only one hypothesis be pursued or should a "shotgun" approach be taken?

To address these questions, we asked our sample of physicians to examine the entire case and then make recommendations for laboratory work. These recommendations, not surprisingly, were quite varied. The laboratory requests ranged from a hemoglobin level ($5) to several laboratory tests including serum cortisol levels ($15) and chest X-ray ($50).

The disagreements in the management of this case highlight the ambiguity in many clinical situations. Whereas we expect experts to agree more often than not (Einhorn, 1962, 1974), disagreements are not unusual in patient management. Lasagna (1976) reports disagreements among experts in a survey of recommendations for use of various treatment regimens and suggests two reasons for disagreement. First, physicians make different value judgments. He illustrates these value differences using the risk–benefit dimension. Coronary artery bypass surgery has a mortality rate of 5%. Some physicians advise against it on this basis; others feel the benefit is worth the risk. Second, physicians have different data bases. Some are more experienced with relevant cases.

There is yet another reason for the differences we observe in our physician sample (Snyder & Mentzer, 1978). Even if their values were identical and even if they had equal exposure to relevant cases, the data experts possess can vary simply according to the laws of chance. Consider a disease state for which there is no established treatment: 50% of the patients die; 50% recover. If an experimental treatment works once or twice, few would conclude it was effective. Alternatively, if the treatment is tried in six cases and saves all but one, most people would feel they were on to something. With only six cases, however, an 83% success rate could easily occur by chance. Yet, we suspect that most of us would begin to feel confident about the efficacy of the treatment.

This phenomenon, which Tversky and Kahneman (1971) have called a *belief in the law of small numbers,* is a widespread bias. When a group of mathematical psychologists were tested, they also showed this bias. Tversky and Kahneman concluded that: "Apparently an acquaintanceship with formal logic and with probability theory does not extinguish erroneous intuitions [p. 109]." They suggest that people believe that random samples, regardless of their size, must be representative of the sample from which they are drawn. If there are five positive results in six attempts, the law of small numbers erroneously predicts that the finding will be unchanged whether the sample is 60, 600, or 6000. Detmer, Fryback, and Gassner (1978) have also documented this insensitivity to sample size in a survey of university physicians.

Tversky and Kahneman (1974) use the concept of psychological availability to explain unwarranted extrapolation from small samples. This idea is based on the tendency of people to judge the probability of an event by the ease with which it comes to mind (i.e., how psychologically available it is). With five positive cases and one negative case, a positive case is more likely to come to mind first. There are several ways for a memory to be salient. For the physician, the reasons that a case might be memorable are many (e.g., the patient may not have done well, perhaps the patient died). The physician may have been embarrassed by the failure of a therapy, or alternatively the physician may have been proud of an unexpected success. The case may be memorable because it refuted an old theory or fit a new one. All of these factors may affect the assessment of clinical judgment.

One might expect these erroneous conclusions to be corrected as more data are available. The evidence suggests, however, that this might not always be true. If one initially has five positive results and one negative result, and then has a run of only two positive results in four attempts, it is easy to think of a reason for this change of events. The motivation to find such a reason may be high if one has treated many patients, told colleagues, or published the theory. The well-known process of dissonance reduction—justification of one's behavior—may provide much of the incentive. Alternatively, the physician's prejudiced views may create a "self-fulfilling prophecy" (Jones 1977), an expectancy that leads to its own confirmation. A physician who evaluates only one therapeutic protocol has little basis for claiming its benefits over rival regimens.

THE CASE IN MEDICAL CONTEXT

There are many social and psychological variables that influence the effectiveness of the doctor–patient interaction. Adverse psychological responses in Mr. Rucker's case were characterized by his anxiety and unfamiliarity with the sick role. The newness of this role may have led to a limited ability to express his symptoms. The intimidating social context may have also contributed to this limitation. Many of these adverse reactions could be offset by a doctor–patient relationship predicated on communication, warmth, and friendliness. Studies indicate that the physician who provides information, instruction, and motivation to the patient significantly contributes to the overall adjustment to the health care setting.

This case also illustrated practical concerns involved in the diagnostic interview. Clearly, self-disclosures are important in providing a basis for diagnostic strategies. Contributing to these strategies are reliable patient cues—both verbal and nonverbal. There are also pitfalls in diagnosis. Many of these pitfalls are a consequence of physicians being subject to common psychological processes. Everyone has a desire to avoid an uncomfortable confrontation or a depressive affect. The price, however, is unusually high in the practice of medicine. A vital patient disclosure may be overlooked or an important point might be left unspoken. Premature fixation on a single hypothesis and the tendency to see supporting data as conclusive also assume much greater significance in the health care setting.

Many of these issues complicate the diagnosis of Emil Rucker; nonetheless, all of the important historical information was available to the diagnostician. What was your diagnosis?

The decision that determined whether or not the diagnosis could be confirmed was the choice of laboratory studies. The hormone level that is diagnostic for Addison's disease was not obtained because of its cost and the rather low likelihood that Mr. Rucker had the disease. Six days later, the patient was involved in a motor vehicle accident. The stress of the accident put Mr. Rucker into an *adrenal crisis.* A crisis is a life-threatening event and is a direct consequence of Addison's disease. If you were the physician, would this experience alter your tolerance of diagnostic uncertainty? How would you interpret the bronzed skin of the next patient with flulike symptoms? Before ordering the expensive lab test, would you recall the base rates of Addison's disease or would you remember the near fatal consequences for Emil Rucker?

EPILOGUE

In writing about the psychology of the physician, we have no doubt committed a variety of sins, but we will confess to only one. We have noted the human tendency to adopt a simplified view of reality, to be content with the first explanation for the patient's symptoms that comes to mind, to favor evidence that supports it, and to fail to generate or assess adequately other accounts. But we have been guilty of a comparable preference for simplification in our discussion of the chief complaint. Implicit in our remarks is that the patient is entitled to only a single problem. For example, in Rucker's case we focused on fatigue rather than irritability. This sort of thinking is part of what Antonovsky (1979) calls *the magic bullet approach,* which holds that not only is the patient entitled to but one disease, but also that the disease is presumed to have only a single cure.

The magic bullet approach grows out of the emphasis on pathogenesis. Its presumptions are that people are healthy until a specific element, the pathogen, comes along and raises havoc. The job of medicine is seen to be the identification of specific pathogens—germs, viruses, foods, chemicals—associated with specific diseases and to develop specific counterattacks (e.g., antibiotics). Antonovsky (1979) acknowledges the important role of the pathogenic approach in the recent history of medicine. Indeed it has had a critical role in providing a scientific base for the practice of medicine. Although it will continue to make a contribution, it can be argued that we have reached the point where returns are beginning to diminish and where a fresh perspective is needed to complement the traditional point of view.

Antonovsky (1979) provides us with one: *salutogenesis.* Salutogenesis asks what the general causes of health are. The salutogenetic approach argues that pathogens (both physical and psychological) are ubiquitous, that health and illness should be viewed as a continuum not as a dichotomy, that most people fall somewhere in the middle of this continuum, that health problems of varying degrees of severity are common, and finally that the real mystery is how any of us manage to stay as healthy as we do in a world full of germs, stress, carcinogens, and so on. The answer is that there are a number of factors that contribute to health, and their relevance is general—not specific—to a particular disease. Antonovsky calls these *generalized resistance resources,* and they include such factors as physical condition, money, identity, knowledge, intelligence, social support, and cultural coherence.

We have taken the time to sketch the salutogenetic approach because we view it as truer to the complex realities of health and illness, because it recognizes and begins to organize the many levels of factors that influence health, and because it thereby serves as one sort of cure for the singlemindedness against which we have railed.

REFERENCES

Alpert, J. J. Broken appointments. *Pediatrics,* 1964, *34,* 127–132.

Antonovsky, A. *Health, stress and coping.* San Francisco: Jossey-Boss, 1979.

Argyle, M. *Bodily communications.* New York: International Universities Press, 1975.

Barrows, H. S., & Bennett K. The diagnostic (problem solving) skill of the neurologist. *Archives of Neurology,* 1972, *26,* 273–277.

Berkowitz, S. B. *Differential diagnosis.* Springfield, Ill.: Thomas, 1967.

Bertakis, K. D. The communication of information from physician to patient: A method for increasing patient retention and satisfaction. *The Journal of Family Practice,* 1977, *5,* 212–222.

Blois, M. S. Clinical judgments and computers. *New England Journal of Medicine,* 1980, *303,* 192–197.

Blumenfield, M., Levy N. B., & Kaufman D. Do patients want to be told? *New England Journal of Medicine,* 1978, *299*:1138.

Blumenfield M., Levy N. B., & Kaufman D. The wish to be informed of a fatal illness. *Omega,* 1979, *9,* 323–326.

Cappon, D. Attitudes of a physician towards the dying. *Canadian Medical Journal,* 1962, *87,* 693–700.

Chaikin, A. L., Derlega, V. J., & Miller, S. J. Effects of room environment on self-disclosure in a counseling analogue. *Journal of Counseling Psychology,* 1976, *23,* 479–481.

Conlee, M. C., & Tesser, A. The effects of recipient desire to hear on news transmission. *Sociometry,* 1973, *36,* 588–599.

Davis, M. S. Variations in patients' compliance with doctors' advice: An empiric analysis of patterns of communication. *American Journal of Public Health,* 1968, *58,* 274–288.

DePaulo, B. M., Rosenthal R., Eisenstadt R. A., Rogers P. L., & Finkelstein, S. Decoding discrepant nonverbal cues. *Journal of Personality and Social Psychology,* 1978, *36,* 313–323.

Detmer, D. E., Fryback, G., Gassner, K. Heuristics and biases in medical decision-making. *Journal of Medical Education,* 1978, *53,* 682–683.

Egbert, L. D., Batitt G. E., Welch, C. E., & Bartlett, M. K. Reduction of post-op pain by encouragement and instruction of patients: A study of doctor–patient rapport. *New England Journal of Medicine,* 1964, *270,* 825–827.

Einhorn, H. J. Expert measurement and mechanical combination. *Organizational Behavior and Human Performance,* 1962, *7,* 86–106.

Einhorn, H. J. Expert judgment: Some necessary conditions and an example. *Journal of Applied Psychology,* 1974, *59,* 562–571.

Ekman, P., & Friesen, W. V. Detecting deception from the body or face. *Journal of Personality and Social Psychology,* 1974, *29,* 288–298.

Ekman, P., Friesen, W., & Ellsworth, P. *Emotion in the human face.* New York: Pergamon Press, 1972.

Elstein, A. S. Clinical judgment: Psychological research and medical practice. *Science,* 1976, *194,* 696–700.

Elstein, A. S., Shulman, L. S., & Sprafka, S. A. *Medical problem solving: An analysis of medical reasoning.* Cambridge, Mass.: Harvard University Press, 1978.

Enelow, A. J., & Wexler, M. *Psychiatry in the practice of medicine.* New York: Oxford University Press, 1966.

Fitts, W. T., & Ravdin, I. S. What Philadelphia physicians tell patients with cancer. *Journal of the American Medical Association,* 1953, *153,* 901–904.

Francis, V., Korsch, B. M., & Morris, M. J. Gaps in doctor–patient communications: Patients' response to medical advice. *New England Journal of Medicine,* 1969, *280,* 535–540.

Friedman, H. S. The interactive effects of facial expressions of emotion and verbal messages on perception of affective meaning. *Journal of Experimental Social Psychology,* 1979, *15,* 453–469.

Friedson, E. *Patient views of medical Practice.* New York: Russell Sage Foundation, 1961.

Froelich, R. E., & Bishop, F. M. *Medical interviewing.* St. Louis, Mo.: Mosby, 1972.

Goffman, E. *Interaction ritual.* Chicago: Aldine, 1967.

Gorry, G. A., Parker, S. G., & Schwartz, W. B. The diagnostic importance of the normal finding. *New England Journal of Medicine,* 1978, *298,* 486–489.

Hart, F. D. (Ed.). *French's index of differential diagnosis.* Baltimore, Md.: Williams & Watkins, 1973.

Introduction to clinical medicine. University of Minnesota Medical School, 1978.

Jones, E. E., & Nisbett, R. E. *The actor and the observer: Divergent perceptions of the causes of behavior.* In E. E. Jones, D. E. Kanouse, H. K. Kelley, R. E. Nisbett, S. Valins, & B. Weiner (Eds.), *Attribution: Perceiving the causes of behavior.* Morristown, N.J.: General Learning Press, 1971.

Jones, R. A. *Self-fulfilling prophecies: Social, psychological and physiological effects of expectancies.* Hillsdale, N.J.: Lawrence Erlbaum Associates, 1977.

Kelly, W. D., & Friesen, S. R. Do cancer patients want to be told? *Surgery,* 1950, *27,* 822–826.

Korsch, B. M., Bozzi, E. K., & Francis, V. Gaps in doctor–patient communication. 1. Doctor–patient interaction and patient satisfaction. *Pediatrics,* 1968, *42,* 855–871.

Lanzetta, J. T., & Driscoll, M. J. Preference for information about an uncertain but unavoidable outcome. *Journal of Personality and Social Psychology,* 1966, *3,* 96–102.

Lasagna, L. Consensus among experts: The unholy grail. *Perspectives on Biology and Medicine,* 1976, *19,* 537–548.

Leigh, H., & Reiser, M. F. *The patient.* New York: Plenum, 1980.

Leitzell, J. D. Patient and physician: Is either objective? *New England Journal of Medicine,* 1977, *296,* 1070.

Leventhal, H., & Sharp, E. Facial expressions as indicators of distress. In E. E. Tompkins & C. E. Izard (Eds.), *Affect, cognition and personality: Empirical studies.* New York: Spring, 1965.

Ley, P. Psychological studies of doctor–patient communication. In S. Rachman (Ed.), *Contributions to medical psychology (Vol. 1).* New York: Pergamon Press, 1977.

McNeil, B. J., Keeler, E., & Adelstein, S. J. Primer on certain elements of medicine decision making. *New England Journal of Medicine,* 1975, *293,* 211–215.

Mount, B. M., Jones, A., & Patterson, A. Death and dying—Attitudes in a teaching hospital. *Urology,* 1974, *4,* 741–748.

Nisbett, R., & Ross, L. *Human inference: Strategies and shortcomings of social judgment.* Englewood Cliffs, N.J.: Prentice-Hall, 1980.

Noyes, R. J., & Travis, T. A. The care of terminal patients. *Archives of Institutional Medicine,* 1973, *132,* 607–611.

Oken, D. What to tell cancer patients. *Journal of the American Medical Association,* 1961, *175,* 1120–1128.

Prior, J. A., & Silberstein, J. S. *Physical diagnosis: The history and examination of the patient.* St. Louis, Mo.: Mosby, 1977.

Raimbault, G., Cachin, O., Limal, J. M., Eliacheff, C., & Rappaport, R. Aspects of communication between patients and doctors. An analysis of discourse in medical interviews. *Pediatrics,* 1975, *55,* 401–405.

Rosen, S., Johnson, R. D., Johnson, M. J., & Tesser, A. Interactive effects of news values and attraction on communicator behavior. *Journal of Personality and Social Psychology,* 1973, *28,* 298–300. Sackett, D. L., Haynes, R. B., Gibson, E. S., Taylor, D. W., Roberts, R. S., & Johnson, A. L. Hypertension control, compliance and science. *American Heart Journal,* 1977, *94,* 666–667.

Sackett, D. L., Hayes, R. B., Gibson, E. S., Taylor, D. W., Roberts, R. S., & Johnson, A. L. Hypertension control, compliance, and science. *American Heart Journal,* 1977, *94,* 666–667.

Schiffman, A., Cohen, S., Nowik, R., & Selinger, D. Initial diagnostic hypotheses: Factors which may distort physicians' judgment. *Organizational Behavior and Human Performance,* 1978, *21,* 305–315.

Seligman, M. E. P. *Helplessness.* San Francisco: Freeman, 1975.

Snyder, M. L., & Frankel, A. Observer bias: A stringent test of behavior engulfing the field. *Journal of Personality and Social Psychology,* 1976, *34,* 857–864.

Snyder, M. L., & Mentzer, S. Social psychological perspectives on the physician's feelings and behavior. *Personality and Social Psychology Bulletin,* 1978, *4,* 541–547.

Spence, J. T., & Spence, K. W. The motivational components of manifest anxiety: Drive and drive stimuli. In C. D. Spielberger (Ed.), *Anxiety and behavior*. New York: Academic Press, 1966.

Svarstad, B. Physician–patient communication and patient conformity with medical advice. In D. Mechanic (Ed.), *The growth of bureaucratic medicine*. New York: Wiley, 1976.

Taylor, S. E. Hospital patient behavior: Reactance, helplessness, or control? *Journal of Social Issues*, 1979, *35*, 156–184.

Tesser, A., & Conlee, M. C. Recipient emotionality as a determinant of the transmission of bad news. *Proceedings, 81st Annual Convention, American Psychological Association*, 247–248, 1973.

Tesser, A., & Rosen, S. The reluctance to transmit bad news. In L. Berkowitz (Ed.), *Advances in experimental social psychology* (Vol. 8). New York: Academic Press, 1975.

Tesser, A., Rosen, S., & Waranch, E. Communicator mood and the reluctance to transmit undesirable messages (the MUM effect). *Journal of Communication*, 1973, *23*, 266–283.

Travis, T., Noyes, R., & Brightwell, D. The attitudes of physicians towards prolonging life. *International Journal of Psychiatry in Medicine*, 1974, *5*, 17–26.

Tversky, A., & Kahneman, D. Belief in the law of small numbers. *Psychological Bulletin*, 1971, *76*, 105–110.

Tversky, A., & Kahneman, D. Availability: A heuristic for judging frequency and probability. *Cognitive Psychology*, 1973, *5*, 207–232.

Tversky, A., & Kahneman D. Judgment under uncertainty: Heuristics and biases. *Science*, 1974, *185*, 1124–1131.

Whittaker, J. R., Vieth, F. J., Soberman, R., Lalezori, P., Tellis, I., & Freed, S. Z., Glied-man, M. L. The fate of the renal transplant with delayed function. *Surgery, Gynecology and Obstetrics*, 1973, *136*, 919-922.

Wicklund, R. A. Objective self-awareness. In L. Berkowitz (Ed.), *Advances in experimental social psychology* (Vol. 8). New York: Academic Press, 1975.

7 Social Psychology and Prevention

Howard Leventhal
Robert S. Hirschman
University of Wisconsin—Madison

The words *prevention, health promotion,* and *holistic health* (e.g., Ardell, 1979; Hastings, Fadiman, & Gordon, 1980; LaLonde, 1975; Pelletier, 1979) raise hopes for a longer, healthier life and present an attractive arena for applied social psychological research. Have we at last found the magical world where social science can do well by doing good? In our judgment, research in prevention will be of mutual benefit to social psychology and to public health. The applied setting provides a forum for generating substantive theory and specifying contextual factors that moderate relationships among theoretical variables (Deitz, 1978; Garner, 1972; Leventhal, 1980). This is a recent development, as social psychology has traditionally relied on laboratory research to generate theory. In our view, laboratory studies are most appropriate for testing and rejecting single hypotheses. Although field studies can also be designed to test and reject single hypotheses (Ellsworth, 1977), this use appears inefficient when compared with their value in generating comprehensive models of behavior.

Public health is benefited on three levels. First, on the sociocultural level, we can examine how the activities of governmental, legal and financial structures shape social values and control behavior. These institutions can influence the risk of industrial accidents, environmental pollution, the sale of risk-promoting foods and drugs, and the fostering of norms for risky and dangerous behavior. Second, on the health care institutional level, we can investigate failure to seek care when needed (Safer, Tharps, Jackson, & Leventhal, 1979), failure to comply with medical regimens (Haynes, Taylor, & Sackett, 1979), improve physician–patient communication (Ley, 1977; Svarstad, 1976), and how individuals structure and appraise their own coping regimens (Leventhal, Meyer, & Nerenz, 1980). Third, on the personal level, we can study individual choice and life-style patterns involving diet, exercise, smoking, substance use, hygiene, and so on. Research in this area focuses on factors motivating change in risk behavior patterns, commitment to change, action planning, and maintaining long-term change (Hirschman & Leventhal, in press; Lando & McCullough, 1978; Leventhal & Cleary, 1979; Pechacek & Danaher, 1979).

The risk for social psychology is that it can be constrained by the parochial perspective and needs of medical practice. If our efforts yield nothing more than a collection of techniques to solve specific problems and if they ignore explanatory mechanisms, we will fail to contribute both to science and to the development of an effective problem-solving technology. There is also the risk that the desire to enhance social welfare may encourage the undertaking of large-scale intervention projects, which as yet are premature. Such projects may better follow smaller scale field or laboratory study. Their cost, in time and money, demands that they be carefully conceptualized, designed, executed, and evaluated (Leventhal, Safer, Cleary, & Gutmann, 1980).

The overall objective of this chapter is to take a step toward the development of a comprehensive framework for social psychological research on prevention. Because the problem of prevention is multidimensional, research may develop along a variety of unrelated avenues, which in the absence of an integrative framework may reduce its cumulative impact. We hope this chapter takes one step toward the formulation of a framework that can help to integrate these separate lines of investigation and that it stimulates others to contribute to this development.

The chapter is divided into three sections. The first presents the biomedical view of prevention and identifies areas for prevention research specified by medicine. We review some of the positive features of this perspective and also spell out its limitations. In the second section, we review studies in an attempt to identify the underlying themes of prevention research and specify various problems this research has yet to resolve. As is shown, much prevention research has been conducted from a biomedical perspective. This research has generally failed to focus on behavioral processes and measures. Research conducted from a behavioral perspective has corrected this omission, but only recently has it begun to study the factors critical for long-term maintenance of preventive behaviors. Finally, in the third section, we emphasize principles of self-regulation in coping with health threats as one possible frame of reference for prevention research. This section aims to be integrative and suggestive of factors relevant to long-term health promotion.

THE BIOMEDICAL VIEW OF PREVENTION

The Biomedical Definition of Prevention

The biomedical model focuses on three types of preventive action: primary, secondary, and tertiary. Primary prevention encompasses all actions and technology to prevent disease prior to its occurrence. Secondary prevention is concerned with the detection of early signs of the disease, hopefully prior to the establishment of the disease proper, and the elimination of the disease process. Tertiary prevention involves treating and halting the development of disease so as to limit damage and restore normal functioning.

Biomedicine encourages a particular approach to each of the three problems. It searches for a specific preventive, looks for the impact of the preventive on specific outcome measures, and focuses on disease avoidance within an expert model of the practitioner–patient relationship. We discuss these features of the biomedical model later and examine the prevention research it has generated to see if it has achieved the objective of all prevention research: the creation of lasting barriers to illness.

A Model for Disease Causation and Treatment

In the 19th century, Pasteur and Koch firmly established the germ theory of disease, positing the existence of microorganisms and a specific cause for every illness. These ideas were implicit in the biblical practice of isolating people with contagious disease, and they were made explicit in 1546 by Frascatoro in his theory of contagion by miniscule animals (Lilienfeld & Lilienfeld, 1980). These early statements of the germ theory were used to justify quarantines of cattle and humans during the epidemics of the 17th and 18th centuries (Dubos, 1959; Lilienfeld & Lilienfeld, 1980; Rosen, 1975).

It is only during the past 50 years that the germ theory of disease has impacted medical practice with its technical contributions to primary, secondary, and tertiary prevention. For example, inoculations (primary prevention) and screening for early detection (secondary prevention) seem able to prevent most major infectious diseases such as tuberculosis, scarlet fever, influenza, pneumonia, diptheria, whooping cough, small pox, and typhoid fever. However, the extent of these contributions to prevention can be questioned, as the rates of every one of these diseases had been reduced to very low levels *prior* to the introduction of the biomedical technology (McKeown, 1976; McKinlay & McKinlay, 1981). These ills were eradicated primarily by socioeconomic advances, which improved community-wide sanitation and individual diets. It is the environmental and behavioral interventions ignored by biomedicine that have played the critical role in prevention.

It is ironic that biomedicine, which grew out of environmental practices to isolate people from disease agents, has chosen to ignore environmental interventions in favor of more technical solutions. Despite impressive advances, it has yet to be demonstrated that medical technology can achieve the reduction in disease rates in large populations that has been attained with environmental and behavioral change. Nonetheless, the biomedical model provides the primary frame of reference for the evaluation of preventive methods. For this reason, it is important to be aware of its assumptions and examine how they have guided prevention research.

The biomedical view of the pathway from agent to disease and the mechanisms for intervention and prevention are depicted in Fig. 7.1. The basic assumptions of the biomedical model include: (1) positing a separate agent for each illness; (2) specifying a physiological and biochemical process underlying normal structure and function, which is upset in a particular way by the disease agents; and (3) specifying a technical procedure for defeating the agent or blocking disease vectors (e.g., Winkelstein, 1975). To insist that we use only those preventive measures that modify specific physiological processes and destroy specific antecedent agents requires that we ignore much of what has been and yet remains to be done for effective disease prevention (Breslow, 1977). For example, biomedical investigators will ignore preventive and health promotive behaviors, as these appear nonspecific and inadequate when evaluated from the biomedical paradigm (Bennett, 1977; Thomas, 1977). We now review biomedicine's focus on specific preventive measures, specific and limited outcome criteria, and the expert model of communication.

The Search for the Specific Preventive

Immunization is the paramount example of a specific technological solution to prevention. Individuals are injected with a substance that stimulates an immune response that makes them invulnerable to the disease agent (Mortimer, 1978; Saward & Sorenson, 1978). The elusive, and possibly nonexistent, "safe cigarette" would be another technical solution (Gori, 1976), as would the long sought for chemical cure for addiction (Brecher, 1972).

There are several possible reasons why medical researchers and practitioners focus exclusively on medical technology, and ignore behavioral change as a technique for prevention. First, behaviors lack a specific one-to-one causal relationship with disease processes. Most risk behaviors have multiple consequences (e.g., smoking increases the incidence of many different cancers along with diseases of the heart, vasculature, and lungs). Because there is insufficient evidence on how the risk behavior leads to a specific pathological process, the causal relation between the behavior in question and illness is suspect. For example, behaviors such as eating fatty foods or not exercising may be given insufficient emphasis because the physiological processes by which they increase risk of coronary disease are poorly understood (Ahrens, 1976). Second, behavioral interventions are more complex than typical medical interventions. Compare the single act of injection with the ongoing, multifaceted actions required to implement and maintain a weight control program. This discourages their use by the practitioner.

Third, the biomedical model provides no technology for the manipulation of behavior and leaves the practitioner without guides for preventive intervention. For example, even immunization is losing its value as a preventive measure as large numbers of people are not going in for their shots, resulting in a steady

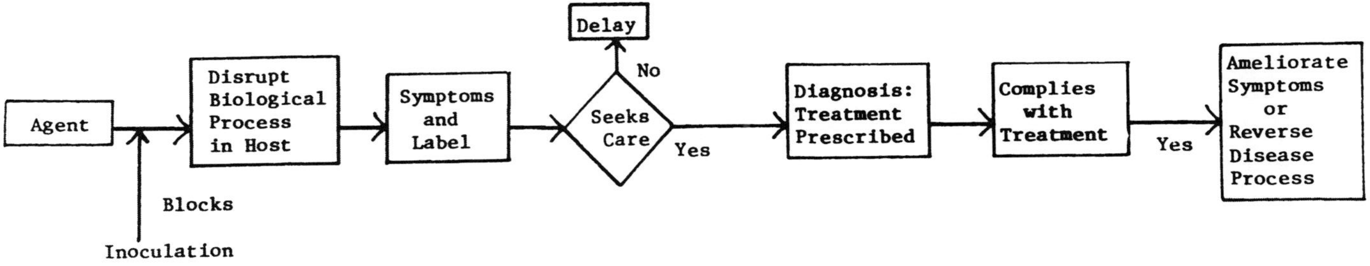

FIG. 7.1 The biomedical model of prevention.

decline of the proportion of the population that is protected against infectious diseases (Mortimer, 1978). Failure to address behavior can undercut our most advanced biomedical technology (Engel, 1977).

The Search for the Specific Outcome

The biomedical model focuses on reductions of morbidity and mortality. Amelioration of pain and suffering is considered a halfway measure (Bennett, 1977; Thomas, 1977). It is inappropriate to use morbidity and mortality as the only criteria evaluating behavioral risk reduction programs because these factors do not tell us the degree to which we have succeeded in changing behavior. Moreover, they do not show which techniques for altering behavior were responsible for the change in morbidity and mortality or whether any of a variety of nonspecific factors such as structure, self-selection, commitment, or change in social environment induced the changes (Green, Levine, & Deeds, 1975).

In designing and evaluating prevention programs, it would be more appropriate to consider a sequence of outcome criteria and measures such as the following. First, the targeted population should be adequately defined. For example, the effectiveness of a smoking control program in reducing morbidity and mortality depends on who is exposed to the program (how many smokers, light vs. heavy smokers, members of the same family, etc.). Second, behavior should be measured to see if the program succeeded in changing behavior. In our smoking control program, we may want to measure type and amount of change as well as the duration of the change. Third, specific factors of the behavioral change process should be measured and analyzed. Process measures will help us extract some principles of change that can be readily applied to new settings. Fourth, we should examine how behavioral change affects morbidity and mortality. For example, in assessing the effectiveness of our smoking control program on reducing morbidity and mortality, we need to be aware of limitations in the effects because the link between smoking and disease is not perfect, nor is the reversibility of the disease process (Rogot & Murray, 1980). Finally, evaluations should measure outcomes related to an individual's quality of life (Andrews & Withey, 1976; Kaplan, Bush, & Berry, 1976) and his or her self-assessed health status (Hunt, McKenna, McEwen, Backett, Williams, & Papp, 1980), as these tend to reflect and influence individuals' physical and mental health status.

Focus on Disease Avoidance and the Expert Model of Communication

Because biomedicine views prevention as the avoidance of specific diseases or a return to adequate functioning after exposure to a disease agent, it encourages us to view prevention within a disease avoidant framework. Disease avoidance is a particular type of negative motivation most likely to be called into play when people are symptomatic (Mechanic & Volkart, 1961; Meyer, Leventhal, & Gutmann, in press; Safer et al., 1979). Symptoms lead individuals to define themselves as ill and seek help for their illness. Disease avoidance is likely to be a less potent motive when people are well and when other motives such as work achievement, economic gain, and social success are salient.

Health can also be viewed as a positive goal and growth process, rather than simply as a matter of avoiding disease (Ardell, 1979; Bradburn, 1969). Steuart (1975) differentiates between health-directed goals, which operate primarily when symptoms are present, and health-related goals in which individuals strive to maintain or improve their health as part of their everyday activities. Unfortunately, the biomedical model does not address the issue of positive health motivation. Its focus has been to provide an accurate characterization of the relationship between the individual and the disease agent and to identify specific changes to block the agent. In practice, this has meant communicating the expert's view of the problem to the public and insisting on public adoption of preventive practices.

The expert perspective of health practitioners leads them to attribute an individual's failure to use technology to a dispositional, noncompliant trait. Clearly, biomedical prescriptions do not always lead to compliant action (Engel, 1977). As we have indicated, immunization levels for polio are dangerously low (Mortimer, 1978). Water fluoridation is hotly debated. Announcements about carcinogenic risk in widely used substances are met with ridicule. Problems in the use of technology exist at every level of social organization. Labeling the foregoing problems as issues of noncompliance reflects a bias referred to as the fundamental attribution error (Kelley, 1967), which places all moral and causal accountability for the occurrence or nonoccurrence of actions on the individual (Kelley, 1971; Lerner & Matthews, 1967). As Knowles (1977) states, each person has: "an individual moral obligation to preserve one's own health—a public duty if you will [p. 59]." This perspective ignores the important role played in preventive behavior by situational factors and the individual's understanding of both the risk and the prevention technology.

The expert model of communication also discourages active participation with the recipient and leaves the practitioner with little understanding of what the recipient is actually thinking and doing. The status and information differential in the practitioner (expert) and patient (layperson) relationship are barriers to the mutual understanding needed to displace trait inferences.

Finally, the biomedical perspective makes no suggestions about how to maintain long-term change. Once an attribution or inference is made, the individual is presumed to be always compliant or noncompliant. However, even compliant people frequently fail to remain compliant, as demonstrated by the consistent relapse curves for alcohol and smoking cessation (Hunt, Barnett, & Branch, 1971; Hunt & Matarazzo, 1973). The expert orientation of biomedicine may be responsible for the focus of past evaluations of medical practice on how well the expert (practitioner) performed the technical procedure, instead of examining the long-term behavioral consequences of these procedures.

In sum, the biomedical model is an incomplete guide for preventive practice. The focus on specific interventions and outcomes ignores the importance of complex intermediary steps and positive motivation in initiating and maintaining long-term changes in everyday behavior. The expert model of communication and its emphasis on compliance limit two-way interaction and participation. These limitations lead to unproductive trait attributions of noncompliance on the individual level and public rancor and ridicule of prevention policies. The question is, what needs to be changed and added to guide more adequate preventive health practices and policies? This question should be kept in mind when reviewing the prevention research literature.

PREVENTION RESEARCH

So far, we have articulated the basic concepts of the biomedical model and its approach to prevention. Although we have criticized this model for ignoring important behavioral and environmental factors (see also Engel, 1977), it has been the predominant guide to prevention research. In the first part of this section, we discuss investigations conducted from the biomedical frame of reference. We explore the biomedical emphasis on compliance problems and the focus on characteristics of patients related to following doctors' orders. The second part of this section reviews research conducted from behavioral and social psychological perspectives. These studies focus more on situational factors affecting performance of preventive actions, both in the laboratory and in the community.

The behavioral studies have added to our understanding of the determinants of behavior, which the biomedical investigations have largely ignored. However, both types of research have failed to resolve the same critical problem: What are the essential steps needed to achieve long-term adherence to recommendations for preventive health behavior? The most recent behavioral studies have begun to address this issue seriously. Cognitive notions of self-regulation have been incorporated into the behavioristic framework. These models overlap with the control or feedback theory that we elaborate in the final section of this chapter. In our view, control theory offers the most powerful heuristic for analyzing the problem of achieving continued performance of behaviors that do not ameliorate any current malady or symptomatic experience.

Compliance Research

Medical researchers who have studied individual's compliance with preventive and therapeutic recommendations have made several important contributions. First, this research has helped to identify behaviors that pose risk for the individual. Knowing which behaviors to change is an essential ingredient for any prevention program. Second, compliance research has linked alteration of risk behaviors with reductions in morbidity and mortality. This helps establish whether it pays to modify a given behavior and also specifies whether the risk reduction is of clinical value. For example, a reduction in blood pressure of 5 mm/hg may not be of clinical value, whereas one of 20 mm/hg may be of clinical significance for a hypertensive patient. In evaluating the impact of a change in behavior on morbidity and mortality, we must consider the effect size and the clinical significance of the effect, not just its statistical significance. The third contribution of compliance research has been to provide means of detecting populations who are at risk so that we can focus our efforts on changing risk behaviors in these populations. Methods of early detection include Pap smears, breast self-examinations, testing for blood in the stool, glucose tolerance tests, and blood pressure readings. In many instances, early detection has paid off in decreased mortality for screened populations as compared with unscreened controls (Sackett, 1975; Shapiro, 1975). However, there are problems with screening as it is now conducted. For example, some programs screen when there is no treatment or remedy available, or they ignore the everyday health habits of the participant during the screening process (Haynes, Taylor, & Sackett, 1979; White, 1973).

A fourth important contribution of this research has been to document the extent of the noncompliance problem. Clearly, identifying and asking people to alter risk behaviors is of little use if individuals do not adhere to these recommendations. Yet, a large number of studies have shown consistently high rates of noncompliance (Haynes et al., 1979; Ley, 1977). For example, Elling, Whittemore, and Green (1960) found that 30% of the mothers in a pediatric clinic failed to follow the prescribed regimen for penicillin in treating their children for rheumatic fever, and Becker, Drachman, and Kirscht (1972) report that 51% of the mothers failed to follow recommended medication schedules in treating their children for middle ear infections.

Noncompliance rates occasionally reach 80–90% in adult populations. The most prominent example is that of hypertension. The National High Blood Pressure Education Program (1973) and Schoenberger, Stamler, Shekelle, and Shekelle (1972) found that a ½ rule applies to the control of hypertension: ½ of those detected fail to appear for a second confirmatory reading, ½ of those who are confirmed drop out or fail to enter treatment, and ½ of those who enter treatment are not adequately controlled. Thus, 87.5% of known hypertensives are not adequately controlled. More recent figures suggest a ⅓ rule, or about 70% are not adequately controlled (Ward, 1977). In some cases, however, the noncompliance problem may be getting worse. In surveys conducted in England and Wales in 1969 and 1977, Anderson (1980) finds indications that a growing proportion of the population may not be taking their medications as instructed.

Although compliance investigators have made important contributions in identifying risk factors and documenting the noncompliance problem, they have been less successful in explaining and altering noncompliant behavior. At first, these investigators looked at age, education, sex, personality, and other patient characteristics thought to be related to noncompliance. In most instances they found no relationship (Marston, 1970). Svarstad (1976) suggests that traits of noncompliance cannot be found because the correlations among compliance behaviors as well as other preventive behaviors are themselves low (Langlie, 1979). Additionally, little would be gained even if we could identify a noncompliant type, as many of these variables are fixed and not subject to manipulation (Rogers, 1968).

Medical practitioners and investigators became more appreciative of the environmental factors that posed barriers to compliance as they learned more about patients and their situations. For example, Finnerty and Mattie (1973) found that their hypertension clinic patients waited about 2 hours to see their physician and another 2 hours to fill their prescriptions from the hospital pharmacist. Providing specific appointments for each patient produced a dramatic increase in compliance, both for keeping appointments and using medication. Haynes (1979) reviewed the factors affecting compliance in the medical setting and found higher levels of compliance when waiting time in the clinic is reduced, when time between making the appointment and the visit is reduced, and when regimens of brief duration and low complexity are used (see also Kasl, 1978).

It is interesting to view the progression of compliance research just discussed in terms of attribution theory. As expert observers, compliance investigators are likely to make the fundamental attribution error and see actors as the cause of their noncompliant behaviors. This seems particularly likely when: (1) the practitioner comes from an upper socioeconomic background and is unfamiliar with many of the environmental factors impinging on his or her patient; (2) the practitioner is overly familiar with his or her paradigm and its associated procedures and, therefore, views them as obvious and simple to execute (Langer, Blank, & Chanowitz, 1978); (3) the conceptual framework of practice calls for diagnostic labeling of the patient's disease state, which is but a small step from labeling patients in order to account for their noncompliant behavior; and (4) the prescribed regimen is for the patient's benefit, making noncompliance a self-destructive and highly deviant action that encourages labeling.

As practitioners learned more about their patients, they became better able to appreciate the situational constraints their patients confronted and subsequently removed situational barriers to compliance. However, these studies have contributed relatively little to our understanding of compliant and noncompliant behavior, particularly why removing situational constraints sometimes fails to improve compliance (Leventhal, Meyer, & Gutmann, 1980). Therefore, we have little insight into the following questions: (1) Why do some people comply even when it is inconvenient to do so? (2) Why do some people fail to comply even when it is convenient? (3) Why do some people who are initially compliant become noncompliant?

Even where compliance research has contributed to our ability to improve compliance, the effects are generally short lived. None of the studies that we are aware of have reported sustained behavioral change at a long-term follow-up. One possible reason for this inability to sustain compliance is that the compliance framework interprets less than total adherence to a prescription as failure. The motto is: "Once a smoker, always a smoker" or "Once an alcoholic, always an alcoholic." Apart from the discrepancy between this view and data that many exalcoholics succeed in controlling drinking despite some social drinking, this view may well be the basis for many harmful self-attributions made when a person fails to adhere to a rigid abstinence program (Marlatt & Gordon, 1980). Health providers could facilitate a more productive set that would view risk reduction as a process of experimentation using a number of techniques. Partial successes would be acknowledged and attributed to the individual's ability to implement the program, and lapses would be attributed to the inadequacy of the techniques themselves. If one technique is faulty, the individual can actively experiment with another (Hirschman & Leventhal, in press; Kopel & Arkowitz, 1975).

In sum, biomedical research has done well in identifying risk behaviors and populations at risk, but it has done poorly in understanding and resolving behavioral compliance problems. Defining prevention as a problem of compliance has led to the focus on the patient rather than the practitioner as a cause of failures to follow recommendations (Stimson, 1974). This perspective has also focused research on long-term consequences of risk behaviors (e.g., lung cancer after 20 years of smoking) instead of on the immediate rewards of the action itself (e.g., being able to handle the stresses of social and work situations). The individual has not been viewed as an active health agent whose perceptions and interpretations of health threats and actions guide his or her behavior. These factors may be very important in motivating and effecting behavioral change and maintaining such change over the long term (Hirschman & Leventhal, in press; Leventhal, Zimmerman, & Gutmann, in press; Marlatt & Gordon, 1980).

Noting the failure to resolve these behavioral issues, investigators began to study motivation and to focus their tests of educational materials on behavioral criteria. Behaviorally oriented studies have been conducted in the laboratory, the clinic, the community, and the schools, and a review follows.

Behavioral and Social Psychological Research

Whereas biomedical research has targeted risk behaviors to be changed, behavioral investigations have looked at determinants of behavior and mechanisms of behavioral change. These investigations have been independently pursued along a number of pathways including cognitive attitude change, fear induced motivation, operant behavior change, problem-solving strategies, and so forth. Although each line of research uses a different strategy to pursue a specific question, they all have one feature in common: They all specify rules for communicating with individuals. Therefore, we first lay out a model describing the steps in the communication process. We then use this step model to describe and critique the behavioral research in each of four settings: laboratory, clinic, community, and school.

A Step Model of Communication. As we have stated, the mechanisms leading to behavioral change can be viewed from a communications framework. In all of the settings, a message with some specified content (cognitive, emotional, etc.) is constructed and sent from a source to a recipient (individuals or groups of varying types and degrees of risk) via specific channels (face-to-face, media, etc.). We propose using a variation of McGuire's (1969) "step" model of communication to describe this process and to understand how the different types of investigation have contributed to our understanding of behavioral change (see Fig. 7.2). Our step model of communication is as follows: (1) a message is constructed and sent by a source; (2) the message is attended to and received by the target; (3) the target comprehends the text of the message and interprets its meaning in relationship to previously held conceptions; (4) the recipient retains the message in memory; (5) the individual personally accepts the message and changes his or her attitudes if required; (6) the person changes his or her behavior.

Studies of the Individual in the Laboratory. Early investigations focused on inducing motivation to change behavior. Operationalization of the Freudian concepts of fear dynamics (Dollard & Miller, 1950; Taylor, 1953) led to studies of the effects of fear on motivating escape and avoidance behavior (Janis & Feshbach, 1953). The overall empirical picture generated by a large number of investigations was that higher levels of fear lead to more attitude change and slightly more behavioral change over a wide range of health issues, including

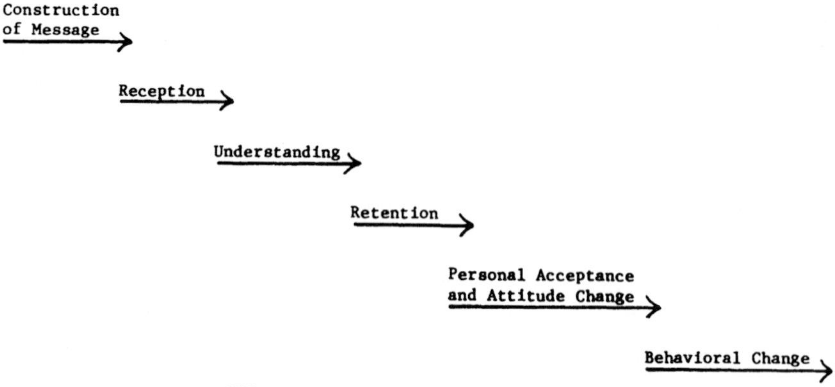

FIG. 7.2 A step model of communication.

dental hygiene, use of seat belts, taking tetanus inoculations, and reducing or quitting cigarette smoking (see Leventhal, 1970; Rogers & Mewborn, 1976; Sternthal & Craig, 1974, for reviews).

At first, these studies mainly manipulated the amount of fear arousal in order to specify the optimal level. This emphasis on the main effect ignored numerous and important interactions between fear motivation and moderating variables. The subsequent study of these moderating factors produced a number of key findings that still pose challenges for theory and research. These findings include:

1. The effects of fear tend to be short-lived, with enhanced motivation, attitude change, and behavioral change dissipating within a week (Kornzweig, 1967; Leventhal & Niles, 1964; Leventhal, Watts, & Pagano, 1967).

2. If threat is to lead to change in behavior in addition to change in attitude, one must add specific action instructions to the threat message (e.g., Dabbs & Leventhal, 1966; Leventhal, Singer, & Jones, 1965). Although these action-instruction packages contain many of the ingredients used by more recent skills training approaches (Meichenbaum, 1974), their major goal was to encourage people to identify specific places in their ongoing, daily routines where recommended health practices could be easily inserted. Identifying specific cues and rehearsing specific responses (e.g., refusing a cigarette at a party or buying magazines instead of cigarettes) appeared to be critical for moving from attitude to action.

3. Individual differences such as self-esteem (Kornzweig, 1967) and feelings of vulnerability (Leventhal & Niles, 1964) played a significant role in response to fear messages. People low in self-esteem or high in perceived vulnerability respond as though they lack the ability or psychological strength to perform recommended protective actions (Bandura, 1977; Rosen, Terry, & Leventhal, in press).

Overall, the fear studies have contributed to our understanding of what types of messages can motivate adoption of protective measures. Both fear and action instructions appear to be important components in mediating attitude and behavior change. However, these studies have failed to address many of the processes in the previously described step model. For example, factors affecting attention to and reception of the message are largely ignored. Outside the laboratory, such factors may be highly variable and critical for even the best of messages to have its desired effect. Individuals at high risk may be particularly resistant to exposing themselves to mass media messages about the risk (Weinstein, 1978). These problems of external validity of the laboratory findings may be substantial (Campbell & Stanley, 1966).

We should also recognize that these studies rely primarily on a negative or disease avoidance motivation. However, positive health motivations may be just as effective in producing change. For example, Becker et al., (1972) found that mothers who complied with treatment regimens for their children were more likely than noncompliers to want their children to be socially mobile and to give the children special foods and vitamins.

Another important omission is the failure to study how subjects understand the message and relate it to their own understanding of the health threat. Investigators tend to construct fear messages based on what they think will produce an effect instead of on how subjects understand the threat and its potential effects on them. Even the highly differentiated health belief model (Becker, 1974), which addresses an individual's readiness to receive and accept the message, cost–benefit factors for alternative behaviors, and availability of cues to action, overlooks the importance of the recipient's understanding of the threat.

Studies of the Individual in the Clinic. Studies in the clinic go a long way toward correcting the problems of external validity found in laboratory studies. In particular, the physician's office provides an appropriate setting for motivating and helping to implement protective health action. Individuals will visit their physicians with moderate frequency and regularity (Hershey, Luft, & Gianaris, 1975). Further, the physician represents a credible and authoritative source of information about health threats. For example, Russell, Wilson, Taylor, and Baker (1979) have found significant smoking reduction among patients whose doctors delivered a simple, brief antismoking recommendation. Although the percentage compliant with these recommendations may be small, the overall effect could be substantial if all physicians advised their smoking patients to quit.

The first step in transmitting a health message is to set the context and construct the message. Although the office itself may set an atmosphere conducive to preventive messages, the physician's rapport with patients, or "bedside manner," may be a large influence. A number of studies have shown that physician's warmth and empathy increased patients' satisfaction with the encounter. Ware and Snyder (1975) found that patients judge interpersonal effectiveness as an indicator of the physician's competence. Affective components of messages have been found to determine both the patient's assessment of the quality of the treatment and his or her satisfaction (Ben-Sira, 1980). Ratings of physicians' friendliness and warmth were also found to be related to patients' satisfaction (Francis, Korsch, & Morris, 1969; Korsch & Negrete, 1972). A study by Hall, Roter, and Rand (1981) shows that patients' contentment with medical visits is positively related to the physician's use of sympathetic words as well as to his or her responding in a negative or angry tone. Clearly, physician expressiveness is an important area deserving of further study. As Capella (1981) has persuasively argued, expressive behavior plays a crucial role in the communication and mutual influence process.

There is reason to believe that training physicians to be aware of the verbal and nonverbal communication they transmit as well as receive will enhance patients' contentment (DiMatteo, Taranta, Friedman, & Prince, 1980). However, it is open to question whether enhancing patients' contentment will improve their adherence to health recommendations. For example, Ley (1977) found that variables correlated with satisfaction are not necessarily correlated with compliance.

Practitioners' expectations about their patients' receptiveness and ability to change behavior may also influence the context and transmission of information. Therapists have failed in efforts to achieve smoking cessation in their patient in cases when the patient's spouse smoked owing to the belief that patients could not stop smoking under such conditions. This outcome did not hold for patients if their therapist did not hold that belief (Schwartz & Dubitzky, 1968). Further, doctors who are nonsmokers or who have successfully quit are better able to influence their patients to reduce or quit smoking (Burnum, 1974; Leventhal & Cleary, 1980). Clearly, the context for communication and how messages are transmitted are important determinants of behavioral change in the clinical setting.

The second step in the communication process is the reception of the message. Clearly, preventive recommendations will not be acted on if they are not received. Investigators assumed that reception was not a problem in the clinic, as it is a face-to-face setting that should insure exposure to the information (e.g., Hovland, 1959). Svarstad (1976) has documented the discrepancy between what physicians think they transmitted and what patients actually received. For example, about 63% of the physicians' communications to patients exhibited low use of clear, specific, and consistent instructional techniques. Practitioners frequently failed to specify precise regimens, relying instead on a few compact words that subsumed a host of actions, which the patient was expected to infer. Further, the practitioner may present information in ways that minimize attention to it. For example, a patient may not attend to the details of a recommended coping regimen if it is presented right after the diagnosis of a serious or traumatic illness. The practitioner may also assume that the patient does not want or care about information or that someone else has told him or her what to do (Ley & Spelman, 1967). Clearly, behavioral investigators need to explore how the message is sent and received before they can effectively study how message content affects the recipient's beliefs and behavior.

Comprehension is the third stage in the communication process. A message that is received but not understood will probably have little impact on attitudes and behavior. Ley (1977) has shown that, contrary to practitioners' beliefs, patients want intelligible information (see also Cartwright, 1967). Yet, much of what is communicated to the patient is incomprehensible. Ley (1977) has carefully documented three areas that lead to this lack of understanding: "(1) material presented to patients is often too difficult for them to comprehend; (2) patients often lack elementary technical medical knowledge; (3) patients often have active misconceptions which militate against proper understanding . . . [p.

19].'' The excessive difficulty of the material was documented by scoring the reading level of booklets commonly used in primary care settings. The reading level of these booklets was found to be several grade levels above the population being served.

The use of technical medical terms that are poorly understood may stem from a number of factors. The practitioner, who is overly familiar with these terms, may expect their meaning to be obvious to the recipient. Alternatively, the provider may perceive the patient as ignorant and incapable of understanding even when the terms are explained. The provider avoids elaborate discussion, thereby discouraging patient questions and reinforcing his or her view of the patient as ignorant (McKinlay, 1975; Pratt, Seligman, & Reader, 1957). Similarly, behavioral change clinics will run into problems if psychological jargon is used, tasks such as monitoring or reinforcement are inadequately laid out, or the target behaviors are only vaguely defined or illustrated.

Another source of misunderstanding is the misconceptions held by the patient about the body and illness threats. Boyle (1970) found that roughly half of a sample of laypeople did not know the location of the heart, lungs, stomach, and kidneys. Spelman and Ley (1966) found that nearly a third of a sample of laypeople thought that lung cancer was not very serious and easily curable. Pervasive misconceptions about the nature and control of hypertension have also been documented (Meyer et al., in press). For example, individuals told that they have hypertension may erroneously interpret this as nervous tension and reduce their stresses at work without seeking or implementing any treatment (Meyer, 1981).

Ley (1977) summarizes a number of studies showing that improving comprehension will enhance patient satisfaction and increase the likelihood of behavioral change. For example, Ley (1976) found that improved comprehension aided compliance to a dietary regimen and increased weight loss. This is a surprising finding given that weight loss is very difficult to achieve and is assumed to require strong motivational appeals and intensive skill training (Leon, 1979).

Issues of sending and receiving messages are important not only in the physician's office but in other types of clinics as well. For example, individuals with a high blood pressure reading may not be told the importance of a follow-up reading or when it should be taken. Similar issues hold in screening for cancer (Cole & Morrison, 1978) as well as in health hazard appraisal or screening for behavioral risk factors (Hall & Zwemer, 1979). For example, presenting someone with a multiple risk logistic score or relative risk probability ratio may have little influence because it is not likely to be understood by most laypeople.

Message retention is a fourth important issue. Ley (1977) reports that general practice patients had forgotten 50% of the statements made to them by their doctor within 5 minutes. Further, patients were particularly prone to forget advice and instructions. Part of the failure to implement preventive action regimens is due to poor methods of presenting messages that minimize long-term retention. Improvements in retention can be accomplished by having physicians present instructions and advice at the beginning of the message, giving information in explicit categories, and repeating and stressing the importance of the key instructions. Relating instructions to the goals that the instructions are supposed to help the patient accomplish may also improve retention (Hoffman, Mischel, & Mazze, 1981).

Whether a message is personally accepted or produces attitude change may be an important mediator of behavioral change (Bentler & Speckart, 1981). Presumably, information that is personally relevant should be most salient and therefore most likely to be used by an individual making a decision to take action (Bower & Gilligan, 1979; Carver, 1979; Taylor, Crocker, Fiske, Sprinzen, & Winkler, 1979). For example, individuals who are self-conscious may be particularly likely to notice and cope with body stresses (Mullen & Suls, in press).

The health belief model (Becker, 1974) specifies attitudes about personal vulnerability and the severity of health threats as important in guiding behavior. Yet, individuals who see themselves at risk are no more likely to seek information about the threat or to take preventive action than are those who do not perceive themselves at risk (Harris & Guten, 1979; Weinstein, 1978; White & Albanese, 1981). This may be due to the low self-esteem of people who see themselves as vulnerable to illness, as low-esteem individuals show difficulty acting in response to threatening circumstances (Brockner, 1979; Leventhal, 1970; Rosen et al., in press). Information needs to be directed to specific behaviors. Fishbein and Ajzen (1975; see also Jaccard, 1975) are able to make relatively accurate predictions of behavior based on the individual's attitude toward the behavior, his or her perception of community norms supportive of the behavior, and his or her intentions to behave. However, it is questionable that we greatly advance our understanding and ability to influence behavior by concentrating on the measurement of factors so proximate to action that we are practically using measures of the beginning of the act to predict the action itself.

Behavioral change is the bottom line of preventive efforts in the clinic. It is clear that physicians have not lived up to their potential as behavioral change agents, as visits to physicians are not correlated with other preventive behaviors (White & Albanese, 1981; Williams & Wechsler, 1972). Innovations in medical education are being designed to encourage physicians to develop effective preventive interventions (Love & Stone, 1978; Segall, Barker, Cobb, Jackson, & Carey, 1981), although it is still too early to tell whether these can be effective or not. We anticipate that many medical schools and practitioners will resist the incorporation of preventive behavioral training as an integral part of the physician's role.

Those health professionals who do wish to encourage preventive behaviors have a substantial body of literature to draw upon. Behavioral scientists have made innovations in controlling diet (Mahoney & Mahoney, 1976; Stunkard,

1979), smoking (Danaher & Lichtenstein, 1978; Leventhal & Cleary, 1980), stress (Benson, 1975; Schwartz & Beatty, 1977), and alcohol use (Baker & Cannon, 1979; Nathan & Goldman, 1979). Some of these techniques are used in health clinics. There is a potential for greater and more effective use if the principles underlying these therapies are used to develop new approaches to fit specific settings and specific patients with particular problems (Kanfer, 1975; Leventhal & Cleary, 1979).

Attempting to maintain behavioral change over the long term remains the largest problem of behavioral change efforts in clinic settings. Many investigators assume that adherence to behavioral regimens can be achieved for the long term, indeed for a lifetime, simply by adding factors to the initial intervention package (Marlatt & Gordon, 1980). However, all the data on risk reduction point to one salient fact: No matter what the behavior—smoking, alcohol use, drug abuse, compliance to antihypertension medication, weight loss, etc.—about two thirds of the participants have returned to the pretreatment base line within 90 days of leaving treatment (Hunt et al., 1971; Hunt & Bespalec, 1974; Stunkard, 1977). Procedures to prevent relapse are essential!

A number of studies on preventing relapse are beginning to appear, but their results have been mixed. For example, Hamilton and Bornstein (1979) found that adding social support and paraprofessional training to a treatment package consisting of aversive conditioning and self-control helped reduce relapse of smoking at 3 months after the therapy, but not at 6 months.

Self-control techniques offer one promising path for maintenance of new behaviors (Tomarken & Kirschenbaum, in press). There is some encouraging news in studies that examine differences between individuals who are successful at self-control and those who are not. According to Perri, Richards, and Schultheis (1977), individuals successfully reducing smoking for at least 4 months were generally more motivated; used a greater number of techniques; applied the techniques more frequently, consistently, and over a longer period of time; received more positive feedback; and used more self-reinforcement techniques than individuals who tried but failed. Self-control failures tended to be more habitual smokers and less committed to change.

It is possible that we can use these and similar findings to develop self-control procedures that can produce lasting effects. Communicating the risk clearly so that it is understood, remembered, and personally accepted could solidify motivation to change. Commitment to change can be enhanced by increasing the individual's sense of free choice, facilitating decisions to take the first step or to make a personal obligation, and embedding the desired change in other attitudes and behaviors of the individual (Burger & Petty, 1981; Freedman & Fraser, 1966; Freedman & Steinbruner, 1964). Explicit commitments to immediate, midterm, and long-term goals may also help the individual cope with pressures to slide back at these various points (Hirschman & Leventhal, in press). Practicing relapse in "dangerous" situations may also help reduce the changes of more dramatic relapse (Marlatt & Gordon, 1980). How some of these ideas can be incorporated within a self-regulatory model of preventive behavior are discussed in the final section of the chapter.

In sum, many of the studies of individuals in clinical settings tend to overlook various aspects of the communication process. Taken together, we can begin to examine how information is sent, received, understood, remembered, accepted, and related to behavioral change. In particular, we can begin to specify how failures at any of these steps may hinder preventive efforts. We have also become aware of an enormous problem in terms of maintaining change. Although efforts are being made to deal with this problem, it is open to question whether any clinic intervention that ignores the individual's environmental context can produce stable change. We now turn to studies in community and school settings to review how they have contributed to promoting stable, preventive behaviors, and where they have fallen short in doing so.

Studies in the Community. The substantial cost of therapeutic approaches and the difficulties faced in maintaining behavioral changes led to the initiation of large-scale community studies using mass media interventions. The idea that environmental factors can promote maintenance of behavioral change is held for a number of reasons. First, studies of the environmental effects on behavior indicate that both the immediate and remote features of the environment can have substantial effects (Craik, 1973; Proshansky, Ittelson, & Rivlin, 1970). Second, the effects of the environment tend to multiply as changes in one person's behavior influences that of others (McClure, Cannon, Allen, Belton, Connor, D'Ascoli, Stone, Sullivan, & McClure, 1980). Third, long-term environmental shifts can lead to a change in the social climate that can alter the norms or goals around which individuals regulate their behavior (Insel & Moos, 1974).

These findings have many implications for preventive health. First, simply regulating the availability of substances such as liquor, cigarettes, candy, salt, and high cholesterol foods will affect the ease and frequency with which people adopt harmful as opposed to healthy habits. Second, the environment can reinforce the individual's self-image as someone active in prevention. For example, a section in the supermarket for saltfree foods can remind hypertensives that they are regulating their diets to prevent heart disease. Similarly, nonsmoking areas in restaurants can serve as a reminder that the individual has decided to quit and should resist temptations to smoke. Third, changes in the cultural climate can have powerful effects. For example, Warner's (1977) analysis suggests that the 1964 Surgeon General's report and various antismoking ads held cigarette smoking to a level 30% below its projected growth. This decade-long effect is twice that reported in studies of therapeutic measures conducted on volunteer samples during that same period of time.

Investigators have undertaken large-scale community prevention programs with much enthusiasm. Unfortunately, very few of these have been systematically evaluated, and those that have tell us less about the communication and change process than do the clinical studies reviewed earlier. One reason is that they fail to control adequately for various threats to internal validity including placebo, Hawthorne, and social desirability effects (Campbell, 1969; Green, 1977). A second reason is that they often fail to conceptualize and use the measures needed to assess communication and behavioral change processes.

One of the first needs of a community program is to define its intended targets. If participation is voluntary, the investigators need to ascertain who actually participated and how they arrived at the decision to do so or to abstain. For example, members of some community group may experience more pressure to participate than do nonmembers. Furthermore, those who choose not to participate may still receive the message and may affect the people who do agree to participate and be measured.

A second need of community programs is to determine how their message is understood. As we stated earlier, people's common-sense ideas as to how the body and how behavioral change is related to physiological change will strongly influence how they interpret program information (Leventhal, Nerenz, & Straus, 1980). Beliefs about trade-offs form one such set of beliefs. For example, people may expect increased exercise to balance the risks involved in continuing to smoke. They may be willing to make changes in some areas but not others, and their common-sense views of disease causation may guide their justifications of these decisions. Additionally, common-sense beliefs involving the misperception of consequences may lead people to select inappropriate criteria for assessing risk reduction (Herzlich, 1973; Leventhal, Meyer, & Nerenz, 1980). A dramatic example is the person who persists in smoking because it is seen as relaxing or reducing stress and, therefore, beneficial in reducing the risk of coronary disease. Another misperception has to do with the common expectation that coping behavior will have immediate, observable effects. For example, people may expect their bronchial symptoms to disappear as soon as they quit smoking, but actually they may worsen at first as sensation begin to return to the injured lungs. Similarly, cardiac patients may unrealistically expect to lose 15 pounds and to show extensive rehabilitation only 1 week after instituting a diet and exercise program. Clearly, inappropriate criteria and unrealistic time lines can have disastrous consequences for continued adherence to preventive programs (Leventhal & Nerenz, in press). Therefore, community programs need to study how common-sense notions affect comprehension of messages sent through the media.

A third need of community programs is to document attitude and behavioral change. Medically oriented investigators have tended to focus on measures of physiological state to the exclusion of behavioral measures. Whether programs change behavior is the critical question. A program to change behavior must be evaluated by its success in that area. Whether behavioral changes lead to physiological changes, and whether these in turn lead to changes in disease rates, are important but separate questions. The importance of multiple measures in evaluating community programs is well stated by Cowen (1978): "Because programs have multivariate, differential, and changing outcomes, multiple criteria, including behavioral ones wherever possible, should be used to evaluate them [p. 800]."

A final need of community programs is to assess the stability of change. Behavioral changes that were artifacts of momentary pressures and behaviors that fail to meet ongoing individual or group demands and are not supported by the postprogram environmental context will probably revert to preprogram base lines on follow-up (Cowen, 1978). Community investigators need to document whether or not these effects occur and which features of the environment act to maintain behavior change.

The most recent and complete community-wide experiment is the Stanford three community study (Meyer, Nash, McAlister, Maccoby, & Farquhar, 1980). The Stanford investigators obtained measures of knowledge, dietary practices, smoking, exercise, blood pressure, and blood lipids at four points in time: base line, and 1, 2, and 3 years after the start of an intensive mass media campaign. There was a control community, a media-only community, and a combined program community including the media package and face-to-face therapy for a sample of persons at high risk for coronary heart disease. Two years after the end of the therapy treatment, the percentage of high risk people quitting smoking was substantially greater among those participating in the combined program community than in the media-only or control communities. Changes in knowledge and reported diet were also greater in both media communities than in the control community.

But do the Stanford results truly support the notion that community change provides an ideal way of influencing preventive practices for the long term? There are a number of reasons for caution in answering "yes" (Kasl, 1980; Leventhal, Safer, Cleary, & Gutmann, 1980). First, the study failed to provide a picture of community process or how messages were transmitted and received. For example, the fact that the investigation team and not community members solicited participation, developed media materials, and provided therapeutic services may have been important factors in the program's success. Many communities may lack such expert help. Further, we do not know if the people who participated were more likely to belong to health-oriented groups (e.g., sports clubs) rather than other formal (e.g., religious and civic organizations) and informal groups (e.g., bridge clubs). Such groups may have important effects both on who is exposed to the community program and on how the program affects receipt of information and attitude and behavioral change (Heller & Monahan, 1977). We also do not know if exposure to the media programs played a direct or indirect role in the change process. For change to occur, it is unclear whether it was necessary for the individual to be exposed to the media, as opposed to having the media affect a community leader or change agent who then influenced the individual (Katz & Lazarsfeld, 1955; Weiss, 1969).

A second shortcoming of the Stanford study was the use of inadequate measures of change. The investigators followed a standard epidemiological approach and computed a multiple risk logistic equation that combined variables such as smoking, blood pressure, and blood lipids to measure pre- through postprogram changes. This obscures whether or not behavioral and medical variables were correlated with each other and whether changes in behavior attributable to the program were actually responsible for changes in physiological indicators.

These omissions undoubtably reflect realistic limits as to what can be accomplished in a single study. However, they leave us without a clear view as to what features of the environment were crucial both for initiating and for maintaining behavioral change. Issues of how community process affected transmission and reception of information, how common-sense notions affected comprehension and interpretation of messages, and how behavioral change was initiated, maintained, and interacted with physiological change needed further exploration. This is true for community programs directed to mental health as well as physical health (Kirschenbaum & Ordman, 1981).

Studies in Schools. Throughout our history, we Americans have looked toward our schools as vehicles for solving social problems. It should not be surprising that schools are now seen as a major target for public health efforts at primary prevention. Given that certain risk behaviors such as smoking are so resistant to change in adults (Gritz & Siegel, 1979), it is sensible to try to prevent individuals from developing unhealthy habits. We focus on school programs to prevent the uptake of cigarette smoking because smoking increases the risk of more illnesses by greater amounts than any other risk behavior. There is also extensive literature on school programs to prevent smoking.

Some of the better school programs reduce the number of children attracted to smoking by roughly half the amount in control groups (e.g., Piper, Jones, & Mathews, 1974). Unfortunately, these effects tend to be short lived as the proportion of new and current smokers in the experimental schools returns to levels in the control schools 1 to 2 years after program termination (Monk, Tayback, & Gordon, 1965). Reports such as this led Thompson (1978) to label as failures all of the school studies conducted between 1960 and 1976 that she reviewed. As Leventhal (1973) had suggested, it is probably unreasonable to expect health education efforts with children to create enduring resistance to risk behaviors unless they are supported by later individual, social, and cultural changes.

In this section, we suggest some reasons why school programs have such short-lived effects. First, many of the school programs studied usually focus on one specific behavior such as tooth brushing (Kegeles, 1963) instead of a cluster of preventive behaviors. Second, school programs have tried to create barriers to external pressures (e.g., the peer group) to adopt injurious behaviors such as smoking, and have not dealt with the development of such behaviors. Third, most studies have not used an adequate conceptualization of the communication process. In particular, the school studies have not addressed issues of what types of information to transmit, to which youngsters the information should be transmitted, and what types of effects are desireable and expected. We can discuss three areas in which school programs may be improved by more adequate conceptualization of these issues: (1) the context for communication including the complexity of the individual's link to his or her social environment; (2) making use of knowledge about the development of health and risk actions to target specific interventions to appropriate youngsters; and (3) solidifying attitudinal and behavioral change by linking specific actions to the young person's self-system.

1. The Context for Communication. School studies clearly recognize the importance of combating peer pressure (Botvin, Eng, & Williams, 1980; Evans, Rozelle, Mittelmark, Hansen, Bane, & Havis, 1978; McAlister, Perry, & Maccoby, 1979). Antismoking messages have been constructed to develop skills and to encourage youngsters to cope with social pressures in the hope that this will prevent them from trying cigarettes. This view of individual-environment interaction ignores whether some social environments increase the individual's susceptibility to smoking pressures and help to maintain the behavior once it occurs. For example, Shuval (1970) observes that a breakdown in social identification due to migration to a new culture increases suseptibility to mass media and to nontraditional pressures. Perhaps the youngster's changes in school or residence, or living in transient neighborhoods increases his or her susceptibility both to media models of smoking and to peer pressures.

In a similar vein, chronic feelings of failure, rejection by parents, and random schedules in securing tokens of adult and parental esteem may generate a state of deprivation and dysphoria that stimulates and sustains heavy use of cigarettes, alcohol, drugs, and a variety of deviant behaviors. These displacement or adjunctive behaviors may disappear once the contextual stressors are removed (Falk, 1971). Therefore, teaching youngsters to resist peer pressures may be ineffective in the context of a turbulent environment. Helping children anticipate the impact of this turbulence and teaching them to cope with it may be an important way to improve program impact.

2. The Development of Health and Risk Behaviors. The smoking interventions studied to date have conceived the development of smoking as an all-or-none process. They assume that once children smoke, they are hooked. Therefore, they try to inoculate young people against ever trying a cigarette and ignore the fact that nearly 90% of youngsters will try a cigarette by the end of high school (Johnston, Bachman, & O'Malley, 1977).

It is clear that risk behaviors such as smoking do not suddenly develop. Indeed, peer pressure is not the earliest of the factors to predict smoking. Many children expect to try cigarettes before peer pressures stimulate experimental tries (Newman, Martin, & Petersen, 1978). Becoming a smoker may begin before the act of trying one's first cigarette! Furthermore, the developmental pattern of moving from the first cigarette to regular smoking is quite variable. Although 80% of those who try four cigarettes become regular smokers at some point in their lives (McKennell & Thomas, 1969), an average of 2 and as many as 20 years may pass as a person moves from occasional to regular smoking (Cartwright, Martin, & Thomson, 1959; Salber, Goldman, Buka, & Welsh, 1961).

Once we recognize that smoking or any risk behavior has a developmental history, we can begin to describe it, to conceptualize its determinants, and to develop effective interventions. The goal is to pinpoint the kinds of interventions that are most effective at each stage of becoming a smoker and those that are also most likely to have additive effects across stages.

The development of cigarette smoking can be readily divided into four stages (Leventhal & Cleary, 1980). In the first, preparatory stage, nearly all children voice negative attitudes against smoking and think of it as harmful. Yet many anticipate trying cigarettes, if not becoming smokers. It may be that the models who smoke among family and older peers cause the child's antismoking attitudes to erode. Exposing children to ambient smoke may also lead them to adapt to the aversive properties of their initial cigarette. Further, the child who observes others who smoke and do not get sick may be unable to appreciate the hidden, deteriorative impact of smoking on health. The dangers posed by smoking cigarettes are not immediately salient. On the antismoking side, it is possible that early exposure to models who are made ill by cigarettes or who struggle with withdrawal symptoms will convince the child that smoking is hazardous (Allegrante, O'Rourke, & Tuncalp, 1977).

Another fascinating possibility is that some children acquire ''addictive schemata'' in the preparatory stage well before they experiment with cigarettes. In our studies, children report using candy, soda, and over-the-counter medicines to cope with distress. Smoking a cigarette may be one of a sequence of age-related responses that comes into play to regulate dysphoria. Other substances such as alcohol and illegal drugs also may be used to cope with dysphoria. This may partially explain why cigarette smoking is linked to actions that pose health risks (Block & Goodman, 1978; Greene, 1980; Jessor & Jessor, 1977; Kandel, Kessler, & Margulies, 1978).

Experimentation, the second stage in the development of the smoking habit, can be divided into initial and subsequent tries. A child's initial cigarette may be either aversive or pleasant (Gilbert, 1979; Gorsuch & Butler, 1976). Because slightly less than half of those who try a cigarette try more or become regular smokers, we might suspect that the cigarette is more aversive for those who do not experiment further. These youngsters may develop a conditioned taste aversion to cigarettes (Garcia et al., 1974; Silverstein, Feld, & Kozlowski, 1980). Youngsters who continue to experiment may do so not only because of severe social pressure but also because they believe they are immune to harm as they adapt to the noxious taste and burning of the cigarette.

Regular and then heavy use, the third and fourth stages, may involve entirely new determinants. Regulation of dysphoria may be a factor in regular use, and craving and dependence may be factors in heavy use. But the notion of stages is more important than the listing of factors that we believe may play key roles at each stage. A developmental view of this risk behavior raises a range of questions that are largely ignored when one views smoking as a simple behavior, which once begun leads to dependence. The links from stage to stage and the possibilities of innovative stage-relevant interventions are all part of this more differentiated perspective.

3. Self-System and Health Action. A final area that may be important for the stability of attitude and behavioral changes is the link between the individual's self-concept and specific health or risk behaviors. As has already been discussed, the child's lack of feelings of self-worth may create dysphoric affects that lead to displacement activities ranging from substance use to aggressive and other deviant behaviors. Alternatively, people with a positive sense of self are likely to look ahead and be concerned with building and preserving their future welfare (Cottle, Howard, & Pleck, 1979; McClelland, 1978) as well as asserting their sense of personal autonomy.

The belief that one has the capacity to manage environments and perform specific actions is a self-attribute that may be critical for resisting pressures to adopt risk behaviors. Bandura (1977) suggests that self-efficacy expectations can be strengthened by a number of methods including actual performance, observing models, and communications from teachers, parents, and peers reinforcing the view of individual competence. For example, Rosen et al., (in press) found that giving someone feedback that he or she was competent improved smoking cessation particularly in low self-esteem subjects. These subjects reduced smoking for 3 months after seeing an antismoking film only when their sense of self-competence was bolstered.

A note of caution should be sounded as relatively weak relationships have been reported between personality measures and smoking (Wingard, Huba, & Bentler, 1979). We believe this reflects at least three factors. First, investigators have ignored the specific beliefs that connect personality characteristics or aspects of the self-schema to smoking. Second, different personality characteristics may account for more or less variance at different stages of the developmental history of becoming a smoker. Third, aspects of the self-schema may be particularly important for facilitating or inhibiting smoking for selected subgroups of smokers (see Bem & Allen, 1974, for a parallel example).

Much work needs to be done to document how aspects of the self-system can serve to stabilize attitudinal and behavioral resistance to risk behaviors. The following points and directions for research should be emphasized:

1. Self-directed behavior depends on a clear representation of a problem, including a set of differentiated goals and a range of available actions.
2. The problem-solving process includes self-monitoring and reappraisal in relation to one's goals.
3. If self-directed behaviors are to be durable, it would seem wise to strengthen the potentially stable features of the self-concept such as future orientation and sense of self-efficacy. Further, these self-attributes should be linked to specific actions.

It is our belief that an adequate conceptualization of the communication process must attend to the context in which the communication occurs, the targeting of different messages to different subgroups of potential smokers depending on their developmental stage of becoming a smoker, and the linking of health attitudes and behavior to aspects of the self-system. Doing this should greatly improve primary prevention investigations in schools and allow us to move toward programs capable of producing long-term preventive action.

In sum, we have reviewed attempts to modify risk behaviors and attempts to prevent them from occurring. We have pointed out their weaknesses, particularly in their failures to characterize the communication process, and have made suggestions as to where further research may be beneficial. A model of prevention would clearly help to organize and guide such research.

SELF-REGULATION AND COPING WITH HEALTH THREATS

Perhaps the single greatest error of biomedically oriented compliance research was its treatment of people as inert entities to be prodded and trained before they would take steps to protect their health. This compliance orientation ignores the vast amount of evidence showing that people are indeed motivated to protect their health. In large numbers, individuals shifted from nonfilter to filter cigarettes in the 1960s and to low tar, low nicotine cigarettes in the 1970s. Millions are eating less or are cutting down on salt, red meats, fats, and so on. Jogging and exercise have led to the vast growth of athletic clubs and sporting supplies. Classes and institutes abound for meditation, assertiveness training, self-control, and strategies for stress reduction. If you doubt that health is an important motive, search the 600 plus recent titles on self-care (Rosenzweig, 1978) in the large health section of several book stores and reacquaint yourself with medical articles in *Redbook* and with Joe's Thymus in *Reader's Digest*.

We believe it a grave error for prevention research to ignore everyday health promotion activities. In our judgment, an integrative theory of preventive behavior requires that we understand the actor's view of health threats and the beliefs, knowledge, and skills that affect the actions taken to reduce illness risks (Chrisman, 1977). The actor's perspective provides the starting point for a more comprehensive model of prevention. We now discuss the features of the actor's perspective we think important and then explore how they might relate to risk-avoidant and health-promotive models of prevention.

From a control systems perspective, the human brain is a marvelous integrator of information and regulator of behavior. It interacts with chemical regulatory processes at the cellular level and maintains an overall homeostasis without demands on our attention or conscious awareness (Cannon, 1936; Schwartz, 1979). It integrates information from the outer environment so we can act to regulate our relationship to it and balance our internal system as well. Maintaining our external balance makes demands on processes both outside and within awareness. In short, the individual has enormous capability for self-regulation and self-protection.

The problem from the viewpoint of health professionals is that the self-protective health actions selected by the individual may be dangerous or of little objective value. The rationality of these coping responses resides in their fit with the individual's own perceptions and interpretations of his or her health risks. It is a psychological consistency based on information of doubtful validity with respect to objective health dangers. A primary implication is that we must understand these perceptions and interpretations so that we can communicate effectively to stimulate and maintain meaningful health practices.

Common Sense of Illness Behavior and Care Seeking

Many of the health-oriented actions taken by most people are focused on illness. Individuals tend to think about illness only when they experience symptoms. When symptomatic, they seek a label for their illness, request a prescription to cope with it, expect the illness and symptoms to disappear with treatment, and believe this to be a sufficient involvement for health maintenance.

The data are clear that symptoms play an important role in motivating people to seek medical care. When individuals appear at a clinic, they are likely to have symptomatic complaints (Safer et al., 1979; Suchman, 1965; Zola, 1963). But the presence of a symptom is not usually sufficient to bring a person to seek care: 63% of the people use only self-care to treat symptoms, 12% use both self-care and a visit to a doctor, 8% use only a visit to a doctor, and 16% do nothing (Williamson & Danaher, 1978). What we see at a medical catchment is clearly not representative of the population at large.

One of the other factors that appears to enhance help seeking is life stress (Mechanic & Volkart, 1961). It should come as no surprise that emotional arousal exaggerates symptom-based help seeking. The human brain integrates internal symptomatic information with emotions aroused from external sources (MacLean, 1970). Emotion plays a critical role in the pain response, and the habituation and inhibition of emotional responding plays an important role in pain control (Leventhal & Everhart, 1979; Melzack, 1973).

It is also clear that social factors play a major role in seeking care. Sharing symptom experiences with a family member is likely to lead to delay in seeking professional help. Extensive discussion or reading about symptoms also encourages delay (Safer et al., 1979). On the other hand, there are occasions when social consensus is needed to legitimize help seeking before people seek needed health care (Zola, 1966; cf. Sanders, Chapter 5, this volume).

Social factors can also affect the kinds of attributions people make about the causes of illness, and these can lead to substantial delays in seeking care. This appears most likely with symptoms that are familiar and of mild severity. Strange or severe symptoms appear to lead to immediate help seeking (Safer et al., 1979; Suchman, 1965). Noticing that a symptom is common to all members of a household or is a normally expected part of the individual's role (e.g., tiredness in the wage earner of a blue collar family) leads to benign, nonillness interpretations and failure to seek care (Robinson, 1971). Gutmann, Pollock, Schmidt, and Dudek (1981) have found an average delay of 2 years in seeking medical care among a sample of coronary bypass patients who interpreted their physical symptoms as signs of gastric upset. People who suspected cardiovascular illness delayed an average of 2 weeks. Only when a symptom is regarded as a sign of a definite problem is the individual likely to seek diagnosis and treatment.

Labels and symptoms define bodily states. The appearance of symptoms causes individuals to search for explanations or labels to define their bodily states. Hence, bodily sensations play a central role in help seeking behavior. This should not be surprising because symptoms are continually available, one need not use special instructions to be aware of them, and they are linked to expectations of weakness and illness throughout an individual's life history.

The need to label symptoms, however, is only half the picture; the other half is the need to find symptoms for labels (Leventhal, Meyer, & Nerenz, 1980). In an extensive investigation of the treatment of hypertension, Meyer (1981) found that approximately 90% of hypertensives believed they could tell when their blood pressure was elevated. Of patients just entering treatment, 71% believed they could tell when their blood pressure was elevated; 6 months later 90% thought they could. Yet hypertension is presumably asymptomatic. Not one of these patients had definite evidence that his or her blood pressure was high when they were symptomatic and low when they were asymptomatic, and people with symptoms did not have higher blood pressure than those without symptoms. Furthermore, 80% of the respondents believed that other people could not detect blood pressure changes.

This symmetrical relationship between symptoms and illness labels is based on the individual's illness history. Typically, diagnoses of illness have followed the detection of symptoms. Further, if a person is diagnosed or labeled as hypertensive, the threat to one's sense of control may generate emotional distress and more symptoms (see Skelton & Pennebaker, Chapter 4, this volume).

There is more to the representation of an illness than the linking of symptoms to labels. People's representations also appear to include notions of cause and the time needed for the illness to be cured. In many instances, these notions of cause, symptoms, labels, and time to cure form implicit, comprehensive models of illness. These models or schematic frameworks bias the individual's information processing and leads him or her to ask certain types of attributional questions along various dimensions (Leventhal, Nerenz, & Straus, 1980; Wong & Weiner, 1981). The most common of these is the "acute disease" model. This schematic framework suggests that illness is present when one is symptomatic, and treatment is expected to alleviate the symptoms. Meyer (1981) found that newly treated hypertensive expect their treatment to be brief. When their symptoms disappear, they drop out of treatment. If they remain in treatment, they use medications when symptoms are present and ignore medication when symptoms are absent. Even chemotherapy patients suffering from lymphatic cancer expect a cure (i.e., a finite treatment will produce a definitive removal of the illness). Hence, when their symptoms disappear, they are distressed by continued treatment (Nerenz, 1980). Similarly, breast cancer patients who do not have a metastatic disease are more distressed by the symptoms of chemotherapy treatment to prevent disease recurrence than are breast cancer patients with metastatic disease. Patients often view the removal of symptoms as equivalent to the removal of the disease. If the cancer has been surgically removed (they are asymptomatic), why should they suffer the illness (severe side effects) of chemotherapy (Ringler, 1981)?

Illness is a state of the body, a state of mind, and a state of behavioral readiness. When the state disappears, thoughts and behaviors turn to other directions. When measured against the schema of acute illness, wellness is the absence of disease. When we are well, we have the illusion of permanent life (Masserman, 1957), and we overestimate our ability to control and solve problems (Alloy & Abramson, 1979) as well as underestimate the occurrence of illness. Hence, if health behavior is linked exclusively with illness thinking and acute representations of health problems, prevention could well be a lost cause.

Models of Thought for Prevention

We need to develop and teach a model for prevention if we expect people to initiate and sustain complex sets of healthy behaviors and if we expect them to be supported in this activity by their social environments. This model must be both abstract to be able to tie together various risks and actions, and concrete to permit the development of automatic, salient perceptions of risk and related preventive behaviors. If we are to teach people or have people teach themselves the art of prevention or how to regulate their behavior toward optimal health goals, we must be able to articulate what these goal states are, specify action sequences that can be used to achieve these goals, and provide abstract labels or justifications for this process. We are assuming that we can achieve long-term self-regulation by putting into place each of the components (representations, coping skills, and criteria for evaluation) of the self-regulation process.

Coping behavior is structured by the individual's common-sense representations of illness threats and causation. These representations and concomitant coping behavior are resistant to change. The stability of inappropriate representations (e.g., the acute disease model) may partly account for the long-term failures of therapies for smoking cessation, weight control, and withdrawal from alcohol and drugs. This points to a need to study further the stable representations held by people who maintain long-term patterns of preventive action. Apart from illness thinking, we discuss two other areas where representations and their related preventive strategies can be investigated: (1) risk avoidance; (2) health promotion.

Risk Avoidance. Patients with chronic diseases frequently adopt health measures not prescribed by their physicians. These additions to their regimens are designed to minimize the presumed impact of factors that initiate and sustain the disease process. Hayes-Bautista (1976) reported that many additive procedures, such as exercise and diet or vitamin enrichment, were adopted by his hypertensive patients. Nerenz (1980) and Ringler (1981) found that similar additive measures were undertaken in their cancer cases. All three investigators also reported subtractive changes such as reduced work schedules to control stress and to minimize disease. Patients often view these strategies as strengthening and helping the healthy parts of their bodies to resist penetration by disease agents and as reducing the impact of external causes such as stress and poor diet. Actions to avoid or prevent disease onset are also taken when the condition is in remission or under control. Individuals appear to select these behaviors based on their common-sense notions as to what caused their own or another person's symptoms or illness.

We suspect that much avoidance action is a generalization of actions taken during past illness episodes. Coping responses that were associated with symptom reduction and give the impression of controlling one's own body signals seem likely candidates (Geer, Davison, & Gatchel, 1970). This hypothesis seems reasonable given the potential of nearly all coping behaviors to reduce emotional distress and minimize symptom experiences. Emotional and illness representations share many properties (Leventhal, in press). They both integrate bodily sensations or symptoms, affective feeling tone, and labels. They also both arise under definable external conditions and share common coping patterns (Folkman & Lazarus, 1980). One can also acquire affective reactions and coping responses through modeling (Bandura, Blanchard, & Ritter, 1969; Minuchin, Rosman, & Baker, 1978), although little data exist on the role of parental, peer, and expert models (e.g., taking vitamin C because Linus Pauling does) on the development of disease avoidant health behaviors.

Both Gutmann et al. (1981), in a series of interviews with coronary bypass patients, and Nerenz (1980), in his study of lymphoma patients, have observed that some people act to avoid risk, not just to cure chronic illness. At first, they work to reduce symptoms. When they succeed in doing so, they convert symptom absence into a sign for continuing preventive action. Why they do this rather than simply stop, the more common response, is not clear. Perhaps they have actively coped with cycles where symptoms have disappeared, reappeared, and disappeared again, and they have become convinced of the need to remain active for symptom avoidance. Therefore, a long-term pattern of active coping to reduce risk is acquired. Why relatively few chronic illness patients learn this pattern, and how individuals who are relatively well can learn to regulate continually to avoid risk, are areas greatly in need of further exploration.

Health Promotion. There may be substantial differences between the health behavior of people who consider themselves well and that of people who consider themselves in the early stage of disease (Baric, 1969; Kasl & Cobb, 1966). Well people need have no particular illness-avoidance goal in mind when engaging in health promotive behaviors such as exercise, following a sound diet, getting adequate rest, and so on (see Belloc & Breslow, 1972). Both the holistic health movement (Ardell, 1979; Gordon, 1980; Pelletier, 1979) and the self-care movements (Ferguson, 1979; Gartner & Riessman, 1977; Sehnert & Eisenberg, 1975) emphasize positive health seeking. For example, Dunn (1961) maintains that nurturing the body's own restorative capacities and integrating body, mind, and spirit for the individual, family, and community can produce full and effective living.

In general, we find that these writings lack clear conceptualizations and guides for developing a self-regulative process. They may make good choices with respect to the selection of health promotive behaviors on the basis of sound biomedical and epidemiological investigation, although these latter studies have little to do with the conceptual base of health promotion rhetoric. When they make recommendations as to how one might carry out these behaviors, they often suggest interventions typical of cult and faddist movements and add little to our understanding of how to introduce and sustain people's involvement in health promotion activities.

Despite these weaknesses, the health promotion literature does point to a number of factors to which social psychologists could direct their attention. First, we can examine the role of cultural and group processes in health promotion. For example, it would be interesting to identify when and why people (both practitioners and users) are attracted to such movements. An examination of the social support networks that keep people involved in health activities (Salloway & Dillon, 1973) could also provide insights into maintaining behavioral change. We might ask whether different networks are used to maintain different activities such as diet, exercise, and so on. It would be interesting to know how the subcultures and groups involved in various aspects of the health promotion movement interrelate to each other and to the culture at large. How ideas are transmitted from the health promotion movement to the culture at large and vice versa would be a reasonable starting point for investigation (Katz & Lazarsfeld, 1955). Because individuals' attitudes and values are their representations of group or cultural norms (Thomas & Znaniecki, 1918), health research could help us understand how ideologies spread through a population.

Prevention research can make a special contribution by exploring how group norms and values are validated in personal experience. Festinger (1954) pointed out that we seek social validation for ideas that cannot be validated in physical reality. People also seek to validate social norms in physical, concrete experience (Leventhal, Meyer, & Nerenz, 1980). We all experience symptoms and dysphoric moods a good deal of the time, which can be exaggerated when they are attended to and given threatening interpretations. Do health promotion groups and norms serve to direct individual attention so as to sustain positive beliefs and actions? That is, do they focus attention on positive body sensations (e.g., ease of movement, muscle relaxation) and positive affect (e.g., feelings of vigor following exercise, feelings of health and lightness after weight loss) and provide individuals with self-confirming information to support their behavior? Perhaps linking these positive affective experiences with abstract goals or wellness labels encourages individuals to form stable, long-term patterns of self-regulation for health promotion.

There are two other ways in which health promotion research could add to social psychological theory. First, it offers a conceptual challenge similar to that found in the investigation of social motives such as need achievement (McClelland, Atkinson, Clark, & Lowell, 1953). Thus, prevention is an area in which we could elaborate the structure and function of a motive for maintaining and promoting one's health. For example, we could first specify the goals of health promotion and explore their time dependent nature (e.g., jogging 1 mile today, jogging 5 miles a day by next year, and still jogging when I'm 80 years old). We could then elaborate environmental supports and barriers, the specific actions needed to advance health promotion goals, the affects associated with performance and goal attainment, and so forth. Storytelling could be used to see if people generate these themes and to see if they are susceptible to situational influence. We could identify aspects of them that are more permanent, develop training programs for generating health promotion imagery, and embed these in the individual's daily environment.

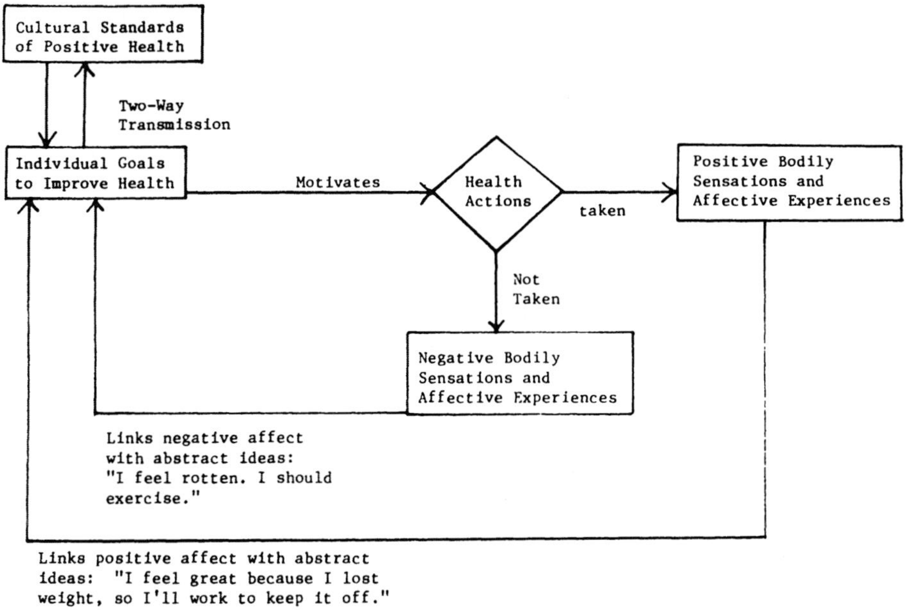

FIG. 7.3 Self-regulation of health promotion.

Second, the maintenance of health promotive activity could be approached in the same way that psychologists have approached the maintenance of addictive behaviors. For example, we might explore how the conditioning of contrasting or opponent emotions operate in health promotive activities. Behaviors such as running may initially generate noxious affective experiences, leading to a sequence of positive experiences immediately after running, and an opponent negative emotional state when running stops for a long period of time. This negative reaction can be eliminated only by reinstating the initial, running behavior (Solomon & Corbit, 1974). For many, running is indeed an addiction. If barred from it, they become sullen, depressed, and morose. Running brings on the high that eliminates the craving to run. Perhaps similar affective regulatory patterns could be facilitated for other health promotive activities.

The notions implicitly suggested by the health promotion movement and articulated here are summarized in Fig. 7.3. Positive health goals motivate health actions, which result in positive emotional experiences. These emotions become linked with these goals and increase their power to motivate health action. Once this pattern is firmly established, the cessation of health action will generate a negative emotional experience, which will motivate the individual to resume action to remove the dysphoria. Once these patterns are acquired by enough individuals, they can reinforce cultural norms of positive health, which in turn can provide a climate conducive to sustaining and helping more individuals acquire such self-regulatory patterns.

Clearly, much work needs to be done to specify how these self-regulatory mechanisms actually work and how they can be extended to a number of specific health protective actions if not to whole life styles (Haggerty, 1977; McCamy & Presley, 1975). Changes in the cultural climate will help expose more individuals to health protection messages. However, these messages could be more effective if they were constructed so they would teach about both the concrete and abstract features of health promotion goals, themes, actions, and affects, and what it means to self-regulate toward optimal health on a long-term basis.

CONCLUSION

Prevention research has much to offer to social psychology and social psychology has much to offer to prevention research. But the situation is not without risk. A narrow and naive view of biomedicine has encouraged excessive preoccupation with the question of compliance and has directed attention away from people's everyday self-protective activities. The seduction to a biomedical framework is not simply the fault of medical institutions; social psychologists, public health practitioners, and the lay public all share a naive, dogmatic view of illness and disease causation. Good biomedicine is multivariate and process oriented because it allows for differences in individual vulnerabilities as well as disease agents. It posits interaction between mental and physical systems because both operate on a common biochemical base (Ganong, 1980). It recognizes the hierarchical structuring of systems from the cellular to the cultural and sees malfunction at any one level as a potential source of perturbation at others (Weiner, 1972). Hence, it recognizes the need for considering all levels in the maintenance of health. There is no reason for discarding good biomedicine.

We also wish to make clear that we are not advocating that investigators ignore the sound compliance, social psychological, and behavioral research that has already been done. However, we believe it necessary to view this work in a broader context. This context should include a coherent characterization of the communication process, a focus on existant perceptions of health risks and existant strategies for illness avoidance and health promotion, and a conception of the relationship between the active self-regulator and the subgroups and norms of his or her community.

Each of these areas poses great challenges. Can we determine the conditions that lead some people but not others to perceive themselves as at risk and to adopt illness avoidance strategies? Can we tease out the interrelationship between social process and awareness of bodily change that reinforces health promotion? Can we define the role played by emotions in altering attention to the body, encouraging action, and leading to the conviction that one holds a shared and correct view of prevention? These are challenging questions. Hopefully, research during this decade will provide new insights and a set of new questions for the decade following.

ACKNOWLEDGMENTS

Preparation of this chapter was supported in part by grant DA02336 from the National Institute on Drug Abuse, and grant HL24543 from the National Heart, Lung, and Blood Institute. Both authors contributed equally and the order of the names is random. We would like to thank Marty Safer, Peter Mosbach, Jerry Suls, and Glenn Sanders for their comments on an earlier draft of this chapter.

REFERENCES

Ahrens, E. H. The management of hyperlipidemia: Whether, rather than how. *Annals of Internal Medicine*, 1976, *85*, 87–93.

Allegrante, J. P., O'Rourke, T. W., & Tuncalp, S. A multivariate analysis of selected psychosocial variables on the development of subsequent youth smoking behavior. *Journal of Drug Education*, 1977, *7*, 237–246.

Alloy, L. B., & Abramson, L. Y. Judgment of contingency in depressed and nondepressed students: Sadder but wiser? *Journal of Experimental Psychology: General*, 1979, *108*, 441–485.

Anderson, R. Prescribed medicines: Who takes what? *Journal of Epidemiology and Community Health*, 1980, *34*, 299–304.

Andrews, F. M., & Withey, S. B. *Social indicators of well being*. New York: Plenum Press, 1976.

Ardell, D. B. *High level wellness*. New York: Bantam Books, 1979.

Baker, T., & Cannon, D. S. Taste aversion therapy with alcoholics: Techniques and evidence of a conditioned response. *Behavior Research and Therapy*, 1979, *17*, 229–242.

Bandura, A. Self efficacy: Toward a unifying theory of behavioral change. *Psychological Review*, 1977, *84*, 191–215.

Bandura, A. A., Blanchard, E. B., & Ritter, B. Relative efficacy of desensitization and modeling approaches for inducing behavioral, affective, and attitudinal changes. *Journal of Personality and Social Psychology*, 1969, *13*, 173–199.

Baric, L. Recognition of the "at-risk" role: A means to influence health behavior. *International Journal of Health Education*, 1969, *12*, 24–34.

Becker, M. H. (Ed.). The health belief model and personal health behavior. *Health Education Monographs*, 1974, *2*, 324–508.

Becker, M. H., Drachman, R. H., & Kirscht, J. P. Predicting mothers' compliance with pediatric medical regimens. *The Journal of Pediatrics*, 1972, *81*, 843–854.

Belloc, N. B., & Breslow, L. Relationship of physical health status and health practices. *Preventive Medicine*, 1972, *1*, 409–421.

Bem, D. J., & Allen, A. On predicting some of the people some of the time: The search for cross-situational consistencies in behavior. *Psychological Review*, 1974, *81*, 506–520.

Ben-Sira, Z. Affective and instrumental components in the physician–patient relationship: An additional dimension of interaction theory. *Journal of Health and Social Behavior*, 1980, *21*, 170–180.

Bennett, I. L. Jr. Technology as a shaping force. In J. H. Knowles (ed.) *Doing better and feeling worse: Health in the United States*. New York: Norton, 1977.

Benson, H. *The relaxation response.* New York: Morrow, 1975.

Bentler, P. M., & Speckart, G. Attitudes "cause" behaviors: A structural equation analysis. *Journal of Personality and Social Psychology,* 1981, *40,* 226–238.

Block, J. R., & Goodman, N. Illicit drug use and consumption of alcohol, tobacco, and over the counter medicine among adolescents. *International Journal of the Addictions,* 1978, *13,* 933–946.

Botvin, G. J., Eng, A., & Williams, C. L. Preventing the onset of cigarette smoking through life skills training. *Preventive Medicine,* 1980, *9,* 135–143.

Bower, G. H., & Gilligan, S. G. Remembering information related to one's self. *Journal of Research in Personality,* 1979, *13,* 420–432.

Boyle, C. M. Differences between doctors' and patients' interpretations of some common medical terms. *British Medical Journal,* 1970, *2,* 286–289.

Bradburn, N. M. *The structure of psychological well-being.* Chicago: Aldine, 1969.

Brecher, E. M. *Licit and illicit drugs.* Boston: Little, Brown, 1972.

Breslow, L. A policy assessment of preventive health practice. *Preventive Medicine,* 1977, *6,* 242–251.

Brockner, J. Self-esteem, self-consciousness, and task performance: Replications, extensions, and possible explanations. *Journal of Personality and Social Psychology,* 1979, *37,* 447–461.

Burger, J. M., & Petty, R. E. The low-ball compliance technique: Task or person commitment? *Journal of Personality and Social Psychology,* 1981, *40,* 492–500.

Burnum, J. F. Outlook for treating patients with self-destructive habits. *Annals of Internal Medicine,* 1974, *81,* 387–393.

Campbell, D. T. Reforms as experiments. *American Psychologist,* 1969, *24,* 409–429.

Campbell, D. T., & Stanley, J. C. *Experimental and quasi-experimental designs for research.* Chicago: Rand McNally, 1966.

Cannon, W. B. *Bodily changes in pain, hunger, fear, and rage* (2nd ed.). New York: Appleton-Century-Crofts, 1936.

Capella, J. N. Mutual influence in expressive behavior: Adult-adult and infant-adult dyadic interaction. *Psychological Bulletin,* 1981, *89,* 101–132.

Cartwright, A. *Patients and their doctors.* London: Routledge & Kegan Paul, 1967.

Cartwright, A., Martin, F. M., & Thomson, J. G. Distribution and development of smoking habits. *Lancet,* 1959, *31,* 725–727.

Carver, C. S. A cybernetic model of self-attention processes. *Journal of Personality and Social Psychology,* 1979, *37,* 1251–1281.

Chrisman, N. J. The health seeking process: An approach to the natural history of illness. *Culture, Medicine and Psychiatry,* 1977, *1,* 351–377.

Cole, P., & Morrison, A. B. Basic issues in cancer screening. In A. B. Miller (Ed.), *Screening in cancer.* Geneva: International Union Against Cancer, 1978.

Cottle, T. J., Howard, P., & Pleck, J. Adolescent perceptions of time: The effects of age, sex, and social class. *Journal of Personality,* 1969, *37,* 636–650.

Cowen, E. L. Some problems in community program evaluation research. *Journal of Consulting and Clinical Psychology,* 1978, *46,* 792–805.

Craik, K. H. Environmental psychology. *Annual Review of Psychology,* 1973, *24,* 403–422.

Dabbs, J., & Leventhal, H. Effects of varying the recommendations in a fear-arousing communication. *Journal of Personality and Social Psychology,* 1966, *4,* 525–531.

Danaher, B., & Lichtenstein, E. *Become an ex-smoker.* Englewood Cliffs, N.J.: Prentice-Hall, 1978.

Deitz, D. M. Current status of applied behavior analysis: Science versus technology. *American Psychologist,* 1978, *33,* 805–814.

DiMatteo, M. R., Taranta, A., Friedman, H. S., & Prince, L. M. Predicting satisfaction from physicians' nonverbal communication skills. *Medical Care,* 1980, *18,* 376–387.

Dollard, J., & Miller, N. E. *Personality and psychotherapy.* New York: McGraw-Hill, 1950.

Dubos, R. *Mirage of health: Utopias, progress, and biological change.* New York: Harper, 1959.

Dunn, H. L. *High level wellness.* Arlington, Va.: R. W. Beatty, 1961.

Elling, R., Whittemore, R., & Green, M. Patient participation in a pediatric program. *Journal of Health and Human Behavior,* 1960, *1,* 183–191.

Ellsworth, P. C. From abstract ideas to concrete instances: Some guidelines for choosing natural research settings. *American Psychologist,* 1977, *32,* 604–615.

Engel, G. L. The need for a new medical model: A challenge for biomedicine. *Science,* 1977, *196,* 129–136.

Evans, R. I., Rozelle, R. M., Mittelmark, M. D., Hansen, W. B., Bane, A. L., & Havis, J. Deterring the onset of smoking in children: Knowledge of immediate physiological effects and coping with peer pressure, media pressure, and parent modeling. *Journal of Applied Social Psychology,* 1978, *8,* 126–135.

Falk, J. L. The nature and determinants of adjunctive behavior. *Physiology and Behavior,* 1971, *6,* 577–588.

Ferguson, T. *Medical self-care: Access to medical tools.* New York: Summit Books, 1979.

Festinger, L. A theory of social comparison processes. *Human Relations,* 1954, *7,* 117–140.

Finnerty, F., & Mattie, E. Hypertension in the inner city. *Circulation,* 1973, *47,* 73–78.

Fishbein, M., & Ajzen, I. *Belief, attitude, intention and behavior: An introduction to theory and research.* Reading, Mass.: Addison-Wesley, 1975.

Folkman, S., & Lazarus, R. S. An analysis of coping in a middle-aged community sample. *Journal of Health and Social Behavior,* 1980, *21,* 219–239.

Francis, V., Korsch, B. M., & Morris, M. J. Gaps in doctor–patient communication: Patients' response to medical advice. *New England Journal of Medicine,* 1969, *280,* 535–540.

Freedman, J. L., & Fraser, S. C. Complicance without pressure: The foot-in-the-door technique. *Journal of Personality and Social Psychology,* 1966, *4,* 195–202.

Freedman, J. L., & Steinbruner, J. D. Perceived choice and resistance to persuasion. *Journal of Abnormal and Social Psychology,* 1964, *68,* 678–681.

Ganong, W. *Fundamental physiological mechanisms of neuroendocrine function.* Paper presented at the annual meeting of the Academy of Behavioral Medicine Research, June, 1980, Charlottesville, Va.

Garcia, J., Hankins, W. G., & Rusiniak, K. W. Behavioral regulation of the mileau interne in man and rat. *Science,* 1974, *185,* 824–831.

Garner, W. R. The acquisition and application of knowledge: A symbiotic relation. *American Psychologist,* 1972, *27,* 941–946.

Gartner, A., & Riessman, F. *Self help in the human services.* San Francisco: Jossey-Bass, 1977.

Geer, J. H., Davison, G. C., & Gatchel, R. I. Reduction of stress in humans through nonveridical perceived control of aversive stimulation. *Journal of Personality and Social Psychology,* 1970, *16,* 731–738.

Gilbert, D. G. Paradoxical tranquilizing and emotion-reducing effects of nicotine. *Psychological Bulletin,* 1979, *86,* 643–661.

Gordon, J. S. The paradigm of holistic medicine. In A. C. Hastings, J. Fadiman, & J. S. Gordon (Eds.), *Health for the whole person.* Boulder, Colo.: Westview Press, 1980.

Gori, G. B. Low risk cigarettes: A prescription. *Science,* 1976, *194,* 1243–1246.

Gorsuch, R. L., & Butler, M. C. Initial drug abuse: A review of predisposing social psychological factors. *Psychological Bulletin,* 1976, *83,* 120–137.

Green, L. W. Evaluation and measurement: Some dilemmas for health education. *American Journal of Public Health,* 1977, *67,* 155–161.

Green, L. W., Levine, D. M., & Deeds, S. Clinical trials of health education for hypertensive outpatients: Design and baseline data. *Preventive Medicine,* 1975, *4,* 417–425.

Greene, B. T. Sequential use of drugs and alcohol: A reexamination of the stepping-stone hypothesis. *American Journal of Drug and Alcohol Abuse*, 1980, *7*, 83–99.

Gritz, E. R., & Siegel, R. K. Tobacco and smoking in animal and human behavior. In R. S. Davidson (Ed.), *Modification of pathological behavior*. New York: Gardner Press, 1979.

Gutmann, M. C., Pollock, M. L., Schmidt, D. H., & Dudek, S. Symptom monitoring and attribution by cardiac patients. *Clinical Research*, 1981, *29*, 320A.

Haggerty, R. J. Changing lifestyles to improve health. *Preventive Medicine*, 1977, *6*, 276–281.

Hall, J. A., Roter, D. L., & Rand, C. S. Communication of affect between patient and physician. *Journal of Health and Social Behavior*, 1981, *22*, 18–30.

Hall, J. H., & Zwemer, J. D. *Prospective medicine*. Indianapolis: Methodist Hospital of Indiana, 1979.

Hamilton, S. B., & Bornstein, P. H. Broad-spectrum behavioral approach to smoking cessation: Effects of social support and paraprofessional training on the maintenance of treatment effects. *Journal of Consulting and Clinical Psychology*, 1979, *47*, 598–600.

Harris, D. M., & Guten, S. Health-protective behavior: An exploratory study. *Journal of Health and Social Behavior*, 1979, *20*, 17–29.

Hastings, A. C., Fadiman, J., & Gordon, J. S. (Eds.). *Health for the whole person*. Boulder, Colo.: Westview Press, 1980.

Hayes-Bautista, D. E. Modifying the treatment: Patient compliance, patient control and medical care. *Social Science and Medicine*, 1976, *10*, 233–238.

Haynes, R. B. Determinants of compliance: The disease and the mechanics of treatment. In R. B. Haynes, D. W. Taylor, & D. L. Sackett (Eds.), *Compliance in health care*. Baltimore, Md.: Johns Hopkins University Press, 1979.

Haynes, R. B., Taylor, D. W., & Sackett, D. L. (Eds.). *Compliance in health care*. Baltimore, Md.: Johns Hopkins University Press, 1979.

Heller, K., & Monahan, J. *Psychology and community change*. Homewood, Ill.: Dorsey Press, 1977.

Hershey, J. C., Luft, H. S., & Gianaris, J. M. Making sense out of utilization data. *Medical Care*, 1975, *13*, 838–854.

Herzlich, C. *Health and illness: A social psychological analysis*. New York: Academic Press, 1973.

Hirschman, R. S., & Leventhal, H. The behavioral science of cancer prevention. In S. B. Kahn, R. R. Love, C. Sherman, Jr., & R. Chakravorty (Eds.), *Concepts in cancer medicine*. New York: Grune & Stratton, in press.

Hoffman, C., Mischel, W., & Mazze, K. The role of purpose in the organization of information about behavior: Trait-based versus goal-based categories in person cognition. *Journal of Personality and Social Psychology*, 1981, *40*, 211–225.

Hovland, C. I. Reconciling conflicting results derived from experimental and survey studies of attitude change. *American Psychologist*, 1959, *14*, 8–17.

Hunt, S. M., McKenna, S. P., McEwen, J., Backett, E. M., Williams, J., & Papp, E. A quantitative approach to perceived health status: A validation study. *Journal of Epidemiology and Community Health*, 1980, *34*, 281–286.

Hunt, W. A., Barnett, I. W., & Branch, L. G. Relapse rates in addiction programs. *Journal of Clinical Psychology*, 1971, *27*, 455–456.

Hunt, W. A., & Bespalec, D. A. An evaluation of current methods of modifying smoking behavior. *Journal of Clinical Psychology*, 1974, *30*, 431–438.

Hunt, W. A., & Matarazzo, J. D. Three years later: Recent developments in the experimental modification of smoking behavior. *Journal of Abnormal Psychology*, 1973, *81*, 107–114.

Insel, P. M., & Moos, R. H. Psychological environments: Expanding the scope of human ecology. *American Psychologist*, 1974, *29*, 179–188.

Jaccard, J. A. A theoretical analysis of selected factors important to health education strategies. *Health Education Monographs*, 1975, *3*, 152–167.

Janis, I. L., & Feshbach, S. Effects of fear-arousing communications. *Journal of Abnormal and Social Psychology,* 1953, *48,* 78–92.

Jessor, R., & Jessor, S. L. *Problem behavior and psychosocial development: A longitudinal study of youth.* New York: Academic Press, 1977.

Johnston, L. D., Bachman, J. G., & O'Malley, P. M. Drug use among American high school students 1975–1977. Washington, D.C.: DHEW Publication #(ADM)78-619, 1977.

Kandel, D. B., Kessler, R. C., & Margulies, R. Z. Antecedents of adolescent initiation into stages of drug use: A developmental analysis. In D. B. Kandel (Ed.), *Longitudinal research on drug use: Empirical findings and methodological issues.* Washington, D.C.: Hemisphere, 1978.

Kanfer, F. H. Self-management methods. In F. H. Kanfer & A. P. Goldstein (Eds.), *Helping people change.* New York: Pergamon Press, 1975.

Kaplan, R. M., Bush, J. W., & Berry, C. C. Health status: Types of validity and the index of well being. *Health Services Research,* 1976, *11,* 478–507.

Kasl, S. V. A social-psychological perspective on successful community control of high blood pressure: A review. *Journal of Behavioral Medicine,* 1978, *1,* 347–381.

Kasl, S. V. Cardiovascular risk reduction in a community setting: Some comments. *Journal of Consulting and Clinical Psychology,* 1980, *48,* 143–149.

Kasl, S. V., & Cobb, S. Health behavior, illness behavior, and sick-role behavior. *Archives of Environmental Health,* 1966, *12,* 246–266, 531–541.

Katz, E., & Lazarsfeld, P. F. *Personal influence: The part played by people in the flow of mass communication.* Glencoe, Ill.: The Free Press, 1955.

Kegeles, S. Some motives for seeking preventive dental care. *Journal of the American Dental Association,* 1963, *67,* 90–98.

Kelley, H. H. Attribution theory in social psychology. In D. Levine (Ed.), *Nebraska Symposium on Motivation, 1967* (Vol. 15). Lincoln: University of Nebraska Press, 1967.

Kelley, H. H. Moral evaluation. *American Psychologist,* 1971, *26,* 293–300.

Kirschenbaum, D. S., & Ordman, A. M. Preventive interventions for children: Cognitive-behavioral perspectives. In A. W. Meyers & W. E. Craighead (Eds.), *Cognitive behavior therapy for children.* New York: Plenum, 1981.

Knowles, J. H. The responsibility of the individual. In J. H. Knowles (Ed.), *Doing better and feeling worse.* New York: Norton, 1977.

Kopel, S., & Arkowitz, H. The role of attribution and self-perception in behavior change. *Genetic Psychology Monographs,* 1975, *92,* 175–212.

Kornzweig, N. *Behavior change as a function of fear arousal and personality.* Unpublished doctoral dissertation, Yale University, 1967.

Korsch, B. M., & Negrete, V. F. Doctor–patient communication. *Scientific American,* 1972, *227,* 66–74.

LaLonde, M. *A new perspective on the health of Canadians.* Ottawa: Information Canade, 1975.

Lando, H. A., & McCullough, J. A. Clinical application of a broad-spectrum behavioral approach to chronic smokers. *Journal of Consulting and Clinical Psychology,* 1978, *46,* 583–585.

Langer, E., Blank, A., & Chanowitz, B. The mindlessness of ostensibly thoughtful action: The role of "placebic" information in interpersonal attraction. *Journal of Personality and Social Psychology,* 1978, *36,* 635–642.

Langlie, J. K. Interrelationships among preventive health behaviors: A test of competing hypotheses. *Public Health Reports,* 1979, *94,* 216–225.

Leon, G. R. Cognitive-behavior therapy for eating disturbances. In P. C. Kendall & S. D. Hollon (Eds.), *Cognitive-behavioral interventions.* New York: Academic Press, 1979.

Lerner, M. J., & Matthews, G. Reactions to suffering of others under conditions of indirect responsibility. *Journal of Personality and Social Psychology,* 1967, *5,* 319–325.

Leventhal, H. Findings and theory in the study of fear communications. In L. Berkowitz (Ed.), *Advances in experimental social psychology* (Vol. 5). New York: Academic Press, 1970.

Leventhal, H. Changing attitudes and habits to reduce risk factors in chronic disease. *American Journal of Cardiology,* 1973, *31,* 571–580.

Leventhal, H. The integration of emotion and cognition: A view from the perceptual-motor theory of emotion. In M. S. Clark & S. T. Fiske (Eds.), *Affect and cognition: The 17th annual Carnegie symposium on cognition.* Hilldale, N.J.: Lawrence Erlbaum, in press.

Leventhal, H. Applied social psychological research: The salvation of substantive social psychological theory. In R. F. Kidd & M. J. Saks (Eds.), *Advances in applied social psychology.* Hilldale, N.J.: Lawrence Erlbaum Associates, 1980.

Leventhal, H., & Cleary, P. D. Behavioral modification of risk factors: Technology or science? In M. L. Pollock, *et al.* (Eds.), *Heart disease and rehabilitation: State of the art.* Boston: Houghton Mifflin, 1979.

Leventhal, H., & Cleary, P. D. The smoking problem: A review of the research and theory in behavioral risk reduction. *Psychological Bulletin,* 1980, *88,* 370–405.

Leventhal, H., & Everhart, D. Emotion, pain and physical illness. In C. E. Izard (Ed.), *Emotion and psychopathology.* New York: Pergamon Press, 1979.

Leventhal, H., Jones, S., & Trembly, G. Sex differences in attitude and behavior change under conditions of fear and specific instructions. *Journal of Experimental Social Psychology,* 1966, *2,* 387–399.

Leventhal, H., Meyer, D., & Gutmann, M. The role of theory in the study of compliance to high blood pressure regimens. In R. B. Haynes, M. E. Mattson, & T. O. Engebretson (Eds.), *Patient compliance to prescribed antihypertensive medication regimens: A report to the National Heart, Lung, and Blood Institute.* U.S. Dept. of Health and Human Services, NIH Publication # 81–2102, October, 1980.

Leventhal, H., Meyer, D., & Nerenz, D. The common sense representation of illness danger. In S. Rachman (Ed.), *Medical psychology* (Vol. 2). New York: Pergamon Press, 1980.

Leventhal, H., & Nerenz, D. A model for stress research and some implications for the control of stress disorders. In D. Meichenbaum & M. Jaremko (Eds.), *Stress prevention and management: A cognitive behavioral approach.* New York: Plenum Press, in press.

Leventhal, H., Nerenz, D., & Straus, A. Self-regulation and the mechanisms for symptom appraisal. In D. Mechanic (Ed.), *Psychosocial epidemiology.* New York: Neale Watson Academic Publications, 1980.

Leventhal, H., & Niles, P. A field experiment on fear arousal with data on the validity of questionnaire measures. *Journal of Personality,* 1964, *32,* 459–479.

Leventhal, H., Safer, M. A., Cleary, P. D., & Gutmann, M. Cardiovascular risk modification by community-based programs for life-style change: Comments on the Stanford study. *Journal of Consulting and Clinical Psychology,* 1980, *48,* 150–158.

Leventhal, H., Singer, R., & Jones, S. Effects of fear and specificity of recommendations upon attitudes and behavior. *Journal of Personality and Social Psychology,* 1965, *2,* 20–29.

Leventhal, H., Watts, J. C., & Pagano, F. Effects of fear and instructions on how to cope with danger. *Journal of Personality and Social Psychology,* 1967, *6,* 313–321.

Leventhal, H., Zimmerman, R., & Gutmann, M. Compliance: A topic for behavioral medicine research. In D. Gentry (Ed.), *Handbook of behavioral medicine.* New York: Guilford Press, in press.

Ley, P. Towards better doctor-patient communications. Contributions from social and experimental psychology. In A. E. Bennet (Ed.) *Communications in medicine* London: Oxford University Press, 1976.

Ley, P. Psychological studies of doctor–patient communication. In S. Rachman (Ed.), *Contributions to medical psychology* (Vol. 1). New York: Pergamon Press, 1977.

Ley, P., & Spelman, M. S. *Communicating with the patient.* London: Staples Press, 1967.

Lilienfeld, A. M., & Lilienfeld, D. E. *Foundations of epidemiology.* New York: Oxford University Press, 1980.

Love, R. R., & Stone, H. L. Instructional objectives for a teaching program in cancer for primary care physicians. *The Journal of Family Practice*, 1978, *6*, 1253–1257.

MacLean, P. D. The triune brain, emotion, and scientific bias. In F. O. Schmitt (Ed.), *The neurosciences. Second study program*. New York: Rockefeller University Press, 1970.

McAlister, A. L., Perry, C., & Maccoby, N. Adolescent smoking: Onset and prevention. *Pediatrics*, 1979, *63*, 650–658.

McCamy, J. D., & Presley, J. *Human life styling*. New York: Harper & Row, 1975.

McClelland, D. C. Managing motivation to expand human freedom. *American Psychologist*, 1978, *33*, 201–210.

McClelland, D. C., Atkinson, R. A., Clark, R. A., & Lowell, E. L. *The achievement motive*. New York: Appleton, 1953.

McClure, L., Cannon, D., Allen, S., Belton, E., Connor, P., D'Ascoli, C., Stone, P., Sullivan, B., & McClure, G. Community psychology concepts and research base: Promise and product. *American Psychologist*, 1980, *35*, 1000–1011.

McGuire, W. J. The nature of attitudes and attitude change. In G. Lindzey & E. Aronson (Eds.), *Handbook of social psychology* (Vol. 3) (2nd ed.). Reading, Mass.: Addison-Wesley, 1969.

McKennell, A. D., & Thomas, R. K. Adults and adolescents' smoking habits and attitudes (Government Social Survey). London: Her Majestys' Stationery Office, 1969.

McKeown, T. *The role of medicine: Dream, mirage, or nemesis*. London: Nuffield Provincial Hospital Trust, 1976.

McKinlay, J. B. Who is really ignorant—physician or patient? *Journal of Health and Social Behavior*, 1975, *16*, 3–11.

McKinlay, J. B., & McKinlay, S. M. Medical measures and the decline of mortality. In P. Conrad & R. Kern (Eds.), *The sociology of health and illness: Critical perspectives*. New York: St. Martin's Press, 1981.

Mahoney, M. J., & Mahoney, K. *Permanent weight control: A total solution to the dieter's dilemma*. New York: Norton, 1976.

Marlatt, G. A., & Gordon, J. R. Determinants of relapse: Implications for the maintenance of behavior change. In P. O. Davidson & S. M. Davidson (Eds.), *Behavioral medicine: Changing health lifestyles*. New York: Brunner/Mazel, 1980.

Marston, M. Compliance with medical regimens: A review of the literature. *Nursing Research*, 1970, *19*, 312–323.

Masserman, J. H. Evolution vs. revolution in psychotherapy: A biodynamic integration. *Behavioral Science*, 1957, *3*, 89–100.

Mechanic, D., & Volkart, E. H. Stress, illness behavior, and the sick role. *American Sociological Review*, 1961, *26*, 51–58.

Meichenbaum, D. *Cognitive behavior modification*. Morristown, N.J.: General Learning Press, 1974.

Meichenbaum, D. Self-instructional methods. In F. H. Kanfer & A. P. Goldstein (Eds.), *Helping people change*. New York: Pergamon Press, 1975.

Melzack, R. *The puzzle of pain*. New York: Basic Books, 1973.

Meyer, A. J., Nash, J. D., McAlister, A. L., Maccoby, N., & Farquhar, J. W. Skills training in a cardiovascular health education campaign. *Journal of Consulting and Clinical Psychology*, 1980, *48*, 129–142.

Meyer, D. L. *The effects of patients' representations of high blood pressure on behavior in treatment*. Unpublished doctoral dissertation, University of Wisconsin-Madison, 1981.

Meyer, D. L., Leventhal, H., & Gutmann, M. Symptoms in hypertension: How patients evaluate and treat them. *New England Journal of Medicine*, in press.

Minuchin, S., Rosman, B., & Baker, L. *Psychosomatic families*. Cambridge, Mass.: Harvard University Press, 1978.

Monk, M., Tayback, M., & Gordon, J. Evaluation of an anti-smoking program among high school students. *American Journal of Public Health,* 1965, *55,* 994–1004.

Mortimer, E. A. Immunization against infectious disease. *Science,* 1978, *200,* 902–907.

Mullen, B., & Suls, J. "Know thyself": Stressful life changes and the ameliorative effect of private self-consciousness. *Journal of Experimental Social Psychology,* 1982. *18,* 43-55.

Nathan, P. E., & Goldman, M. S. Problem drinking and alcoholism. In O. F. Pomerleau & J. P. Brady (Eds.), *Behavioral medicine: Theory and practice.* Baltimore, Md.: Williams & Wilkins, 1979.

National High Blood Pressure Education Program. *Hypertension Information and Education Advisory Committee. Executive summary of the task force reports to the hypertension information and advisory committee* (Department of Health Education and Welfare Publication # NIH 74-592). Washington, D.C.: U.S. Government Printing Office, 1973.

Nerenz, D. R. *Control of emotional distress in cancer chemotherapy.* Unpublished doctoral dissertation, University of Wisconsin-Madison, 1980.

Newman, I., Martin, G., & Petersen, C. *Attitudinal and normative factors associated with adolescent cigarette smoking.* Paper presented at the annual meeting of the American Public Health Association, Los Angeles, 1978.

Pechacek, T. F., & Danaher, B. G. How and why people quit smoking: A cognitive behavioral analysis. In P. C. Kendall & S. D. Hollon (Eds.), *Cognitive behavioral interventions.* New York: Academic Press, 1979.

Pelletier, K. R. *Holistic medicine: From stress to optimum health.* New York: Delacorte Press, 1979.

Perri, M. G., Richards, C. S., & Schultheis, K. R. Behavioral self-control and smoking reduction: A study of self-initiated attempts to reduce smoking. *Behavior Therapy,* 1977, *8,* 360–365.

Piper, G. W., Jones, J. A., & Mathews, V. L. The Saskatoon smoking study: Results of the second year. *Canadian Journal of Public Health,* 1974, *65,* 127–129.

Pratt, L. A., Seligman, W., & Reader, G. Physicians' view on the level of medical information among patients. *American Journal of Public Health,* 1957, *47,* 1277–1283.

Proshansky, H. M., Ittelson, W. H., & Rivlin, L. G. *Environmental psychology: Man and his physical setting.* New York: Holt, Rinehart & Winston, 1970.

Ringler, K. *Process of coping with cancer chemotherapy.* Unpublished doctoral dissertation, University of Wisconsin-Madison, 1981.

Robinson, D. *The process of becoming ill.* London: Routledge & Kegan Paul, 1971.

Rogers, E. S. Public health asks of sociology . . . *Science,* 1968, *159,* 506–508.

Rogers, R. W., & Mewborn, C. R. Fear appeals and attitude change: Effects of a threat's noxiousness, probability of occurrence, and the efficacy of coping responses. *Journal of Personality and Social Psychology,* 1976, *34,* 54–61.

Rogot, E., & Murray, J. Smoking and causes of death among U.S. veterans: 16 years of observation. *Public Health Reports,* 1980, *95,* 213–222.

Rosen, G. Historical evolution of primary prevention. *Bulletin of the New York Academy of Medicine,* 1975, *51,* 9–26.

Rosen, T. J., Terry, N. S., & Leventhal, H. The role of esteem and coping in response to a threat communication. *Journal of Research in Personality,* 1982, *16,* 90–107.

Rosenzweig, S. Learning to be your own M.D. *The New Times Magazine,* 1978, *2,* 42–46.

Russell, M. A. H., Wilson, C., Taylor, C., & Baker, C. D. Effect of general practitioners' advice against amoking. *British Medical Journal,* 1979, *2,* 231–235.

Sackett, D. L. Screening for early detection of disease: To what purpose? *Bulletin of the New York Academy of Medicine,* 1975, *51,* 39–52.

Safer, M. A., Tharps, Q. J., Jackson, T. C., & Leventhal, H. Determinants of three stages of delay in seeking care at a medical care clinic. *Medical Care,* 1979, *17,* 11–29.

Salber, E., Goldman, E., Buka, M., & Welsh, B. Smoking habits of high school students in Newton, Massachusetts. *New England Journal of Medicine*, 1961, *265*, 969–974.

Salloway, J. C., & Dillon, P. B. A comparison of family networks and friend networks in health care utilization. *Journal of Comparative Family Studies*, 1973, *4*, 131–142.

Saward, E., & Sorensen, A. The current emphasis on preventive medicine. *Science*, 1978, *200*, 889–894.

Schoenberger, J., Stamler, J., Shekelle, R., & Shekelle, S. Current status of hypertension control in an industrial population. *Journal of the American Medical Association*, 1972, *222*, 559–562.

Schwartz, G. E. The brain as a health care system. In G. C. Stone, F. Cohen, & N. E. Adler (Eds.), *Health psychology*. San Francisco: Jossey-Bass, 1979.

Schwartz, G. E., & Beatty, J. (Eds.). *Biofeedback: Theory and research*. New York: Academic Press, 1977.

Schwartz, J. L., & Dubitzky, M. Requisites for success in smoking withdrawal. In E. F. Borgatta & R. R. Evans (Eds.), *Smoking health and behavior*. Chicago: Aldine, 1968.

Segall, A., Barker, W., Cobb, S., Jackson, G., & Carey, J. A general model for preventive intervention in clinical practice. *Journal of Medical Education*, 1981, *56*, 324–333.

Sehnert, K. S., & Eisenberg, H. *How to be your own doctor (sometimes)*. New York: Grosset & Dunlap, 1975.

Shapiro, D., Tursky, B., Schwartz, G. E., & Snidman, S. R. Smoking on cue: A behavioral approach to smoking reduction. *Journal of Health and Social Behavior*, 1971, *12*, 108–113.

Shapiro, S. Screening for early detection of cancer and heart disease. *Bulletin of the New York Academy of Medicine*, 1975, *51*, 80–95.

Shuval, J. T. *Social functions of medical practice: Doctor–patient relationships in Israel*. San Francisco: Jossey-Bass, 1970.

Silverstein, B., Feld, S., & Kozlowski, L. T. The availability of low-nicotine cigarettes as a cause of cigarette smoking among tennage females. *Journal of Health and Social Behavior*, 1980, *21*, 383–388.

Solomon, R. L., & Corbit, J. D. An opponent-process theory of motivation: I. Temporal dynamics of affect. *Psychological Review*, 1974, *81*, 119–145.

Spelman, M. S., & Ley, P. Knowledge of lung cancer and smoking habits. *British Journal of Social and Clinical Psychology*, 1966, *5*, 207–210.

Sternthal, B., & Craig, C. S. Fear appeals: Revisited and revised. *Journal of Consumer Research*, 1974, *1*, 22–34.

Steuert, G. W. The people: Motivation, education, and action. *Bulletin of the New York Academy of Medicine*, 1975, *51*, 174–185.

Stimson, G. V. Obeying doctor's orders: A view from the other side. *Social Science and Medicine*, 1974, *8*, 97–104.

Stunkard, A. J. Behavioral treatment for obesity: Failure to maintain weight loss. In R. B. Stuart (Ed.), *Behavioral self-control*. New York: Brunner/Mazel, 1977.

Stunkard, A. J. Behavioral medicine and beyond: The example of obesity. In O. F. Pomerleau & J. P. Brady (Eds.), *Behavioral medicine: Theory and practice*. Baltimore, Md.: Williams & Wilkins, 1979.

Suchman, E. A. Stages of illness and medical care. *Journal of Health and Social Behavior*, 1965, *6*, 114–128.

Svarstad, B. L. Physician–patient communication and patient conformity with medical advice. In D. Mechanic (Ed.), *The growth of bureaucratic medicine: An inquiry into the dynamics of patient behavior and the organization of medical care*. New York: Wiley Interscience, 1976.

Taylor, J. A. A personality scale of manifest anxiety. *Journal of Abnormal and Social Psychology*, 1953, *48*, 285–290.

Taylor, S. E., Crocker, J., Fiske, S. T., Sprinzen, M., & Winkler, J. D. The generalizability of salience effects. *Journal of Personality and Social Psychology*, 1979, *37*, 357–368.

Thomas, L. On the science and technology of medicine. In J. H. Knowles (Ed.), *Doing better and feeling worse: Health in the United States*. New York: Norton, 1977.

Thomas, W. I., & Znaniecki, F. *The Polish peasant in Europe and America*. Boston: Badger Publishing Company, 1918.

Thompson, E. L. Smoking reduction programs 1960–1976. *American Journal of Public Health*, 1978, *68*, 250–255.

Tomarken, A. J., & Kirschenbaum, D. S. Self regulatory failure: Accentuate the positive? *Journal of Personality and Social Psychology*, in press.

Ward, G. *Keynote address*. National Conference on High Blood Pressure Control, Washington, D.C., 1977.

Ware, J., & Snyder, M. Dimensions of patient attitudes regarding doctors and medical care services. *Medical Care*, 1975, *13*, 669–682.

Warner, K. E. The effects of the anti-smoking campaign on cigarette consumption. *American Journal of Public Health*, 1977, *67*, 645–650.

Weiner, B. *Theories of motivation*. Chicago, Il.: Markham, 1972.

Weinstein, N. D. Cognitive processes and information seeking concerning an environmental health threat. *Journal of Human Stress*, 1978, *4*, 32–42.

Weiss, W. Effects of the mass media of communication. In G. Lindzey & E. Aronson (Eds.), *New handbook of social psychology* (Vol. 5). Reading, Mass.: Addison-Wesley, 1969.

White, C. W., & Albanese, M. A. Changes in cardiovascular health knowledge occurring from childhood to adulthood: A cross-sectional study. *Circulation*, 1981, *63*, 1110–1115.

White, K. L. Life and death and medicine. *Scientific American*, 1973, *229*, 23–33.

Williams, A. F., & Wechsler, H. Interrelationships of preventive actions in health and other areas. *Health Service Reports*, 1972, *87*, 969–976.

Williamson, J. D., & Danaher, K. *Self-care in health*. New York: Neale Watson Academic Publications, 1978.

Wingard, J., Huba, G., & Bentler, P. The relationship of personality structure to patterns of adolescent substance use. *Multivariate Behavioral Research*, 1979, *14*, 131–143.

Winkelstein, W. Contemporary perspectives on prevention. *Bulletin of the New York Academy of Medicine*, 1975, *51*, 27–38.

Wong, P. T. P., & Weiner, B. When people ask "why" questions, and the heuristics of attributional search. *Journal of Personality and Social Psychology*, 1981, *40*, 650–663.

Zola, I. Problems of communication, diagnosis, and patient care. *Journal of Medical Education*, 1963, *38*, 829–838.

Zola, I. Culture and symptoms: An analysis of patients presenting complaints. *American Sociological Review*, 1966, *31*, 615–630.

8 Burnout in Health Professions: A Social Psychological Analysis

Christina Maslach
Susan E. Jackson
University of California, Berkeley

The practice of medicine has long been regarded as one of the noblest of occupations. To cure illness, repair injury, promote health, and even forestall death are skills that are highly esteemed in our society. However, although the personal rewards and satisfactions of a health career are many, it is not without its problems. The available evidence is by no means definitive, but health professionals appear to have a disproportionate share of stress-related difficulties, including coronary heart disease, drug abuse, and suicide (see Cartwright, 1979, for a review of this literature). Similarly, some health professions, such as nursing, have high rates of attrition (Kramer, 1974).

Taken together, these indices are evidence of sources of stress[1] within a health career, and efforts are now being made to discover just what those sources are (cf. Cartwright, 1979). Recent research on occupational stress has focused attention on job factors (i.e., characteristics of the work itself or of the setting in which the work takes place) that might be related to individual dysfunction (Beehr & Newman, 1978; Cooper & Marshall, 1976). Such job factors include poor working conditions, work overload, role conflict, ambiguity, and minimal

[1]The term *stress* has been defined in widely varying ways by different theorists and researchers. Some view stress as the *stimulus* for dysfunctional reactions (e.g., threats or negative aspects of the environment), others consider it to be the *response* itself (e.g., physical and/or psychological disturbances), and still others conceive of stress in terms of the interaction between stimulus and response. For the purposes of this chapter, we follow the lead of Selye (1956) and others of the stress-as-response position and define stress as a personal or internal experience that is a consequence of any external event (stressor) that places special physical and/or psychological demands upon the individual (see Ivancevich & Matteson, 1980).

decision-making power. Within a health occupation, these factors might translate into the strain of working with too many patients (as a result of hospital understaffing), the need to make critical decisions even in the midst of ambiguous information, the potentially serious consequences of these decisions and the attendant pressure to not make any mistakes, and so forth. According to this point of view, the actual work of health care is inherently stressful, and thus personal dysfunction may be as much a product of the job as it is of individual characteristics (e.g., personality, training).

By definition, most health careers involve a great deal of contact with people—patients, patients' families or friends, and other medical personnel. Often this interpersonal contact is emotionally charged, with feelings of tension, anxiety, embarrassment, fear, or even hostility underlying the verbal exchange. This source of chronic emotional stress can lead to the development of *burnout*—a syndrome of emotional exhaustion, depersonalization, and reduced personal accomplishment. Emotional exhaustion refers to a depletion of one's emotional resources and the feeling that one has nothing left to give to others at a psychological level. The depersonalization phase of burnout is the development of negative and callous attitudes about the people one works with. This depersonalized perception of others can lead one to judge them as somehow deserving of their troubles (Lerner, 1980; Ryan, 1971). A third aspect of burnout is the perception that one's accomplishments on the job fall short of personal expectations, and thus it involves a negative self-evaluation.

Burnout is not unique to health professions but is a potential hazard for any "people-work" occupation, including human services, education, and personnel work. It can have very serious implications for providers, for their recipients, and for the larger institutions in which they interact. Burnout may lead to a decline in the quality of care or service that is provided. It appears to play a part in job dissatisfaction, absenteeism, and job turnover. It is also correlated with various self-reported indices of personal dysfunction, such as physical exhaustion and illness, increased use of alcohol and drugs, marital and family conflict, and psychological problems.

In our research on burnout (Jackson & Maslach, 1982b; Maslach, 1976, 1978a, 1978b, 1979, 1982; Maslach & Jackson, 1978, 1979, 1981a, 1981b; Maslach & Pines, 1977, 1979; Pines & Maslach, 1978, 1980), the underlying thesis has been that social psychology can provide a general orientation, theoretical models, and a methodological approach that will aid in understanding the dynamics of this syndrome. It is an approach that identifies the crux of the problem not as psychological stress per se, but as a particular type of stress arising from the *social* relationship between providers and recipients. It directs attention to certain classes of variables, such as perceptual biases, attributional inferences, and group processes, which provide many insights into possible solutions for burnout. Moreover, the traditional focus of social psychology on the context of individual behavior provides an important framework for understanding the situational causes of the burnout syndrome.

In this chapter, we present a social psychological analysis of burnout, which has evolved over several years of research on this phenomenon and is based on findings from a wide variety of people-workers. However, we illustrate our points with data from several recent studies that we have conducted with physicians and nurses (Jackson & Maslach, 1982a). These studies were all questionnaire surveys, in which participants were contacted through the medical facility where they worked or through medical conferences.

Each of these surveys included the Maslach Burnout Inventory (MBI) as a measure of experienced burnout (Maslach & Jackson, 1981a, 1981b). The MBI yields independent scores of the three aspects of burnout—emotional exhaustion, depersonalization, and reduced personal accomplishment (see Table 8.1 for sample items). It also assesses both the frequency and the intensity of these feelings. A comparison of the MBI scores of our nurse and physician subjects with those of a normative sample reveals some interesting differences between these health practitioners and other people-oriented professionals (see Table 8.2). The nurses reported the same levels of emotional exhaustion as the normative group, but they scored lower on depersonalization and personal accomplishment. However, the physicians scored higher than the normative group on emotional exhaustion and personal accomplishment, though showing a similar level of depersonalization. In other words, the aspects of burnout that were most prominent for nurses were emotional exhaustion and reduced personal accomplishment, whereas for physicians they were emotional exhaustion and depersonalization. Although levels of emotional exhaustion were similar for nurses and physicians, there was a

TABLE 8.1
Sample Items from the Maslach Burnout Inventory (MBI)

Emotional Exhaustion subscale
I feel emotionally drained from my work.
Working with people all day is really a strain for me.
Depersonalization subscale
I've become more callous toward people since I took this job.
I worry that this job is hardening me emotionally.
Personal Accomplishment subscale (reverse scoring)
In my work, I deal with emotional problems very calmly.
I feel I'm positively influencing other people's lives through my work.

TABLE 8.2
Percentage of Health Practitioners Scoring in the Low, Moderate, and High Ranges of the MBI Subscales[a]

	Emotional Exhaustion					
	Low		*Moderate*		*High*	
	Freq. (32)[b]	*Inten.* (33)	*Freq.* (33)	*Inten.* (33)	*Freq.* (35)	*Inten.* (34)
Nurses[c]	34	32	31	35	35	33
Physicians[d]	26	30	39	42	35	28
	Depersonalization					
	Low		*Moderate*		*High*	
	Freq. (36)	*Inten.* (31)	*Freq.* (31)	*Inten.* (34)	*Freq.* (33)	*Inten.* (35)
Nurses	48	42	32	35	20	23
Physicians	33	33	34	34	33	33
	Personal Accomplishment					
	Low		*Moderate*		*High*	
	Freq. (32)	*Inten.* (33)	*Freq.* (34)	*Inten.* (31)	*Freq.* (34)	*Inten.* (36)
Nurses	39	39	29	32	32	29
Physicians	21	24	40	50	39	26

[a]Higher levels of burnout are reflected in higher scores on Emotional Exhaustion and Depersonalization, and lower scores on Personal Accomplishment.

[b]Numbers in parentheses are comparative percentages from a normative sample of 1025 helping professionals (Maslach & Jackson, 1981b).

[c]$n = 169$.

[d]$n = 43$.

striking difference in depersonalization. The much lower scores for nurses may be linked to their professional focus on patients or to their use of certain coping strategies. It may also reflect a sex difference in orientation or empathy toward people. Females in the normative samples (Maslach & Jackson, 1981a, 1981b) were consistently lower than males on depersonalization, and almost all of the nurses were female (whereas most of the physicians were male). As for the major difference between nurses and physicians in their sense of personal accomplishment, this may be linked to other differences between these two professions in terms of pay, promotion, prestige, and performance feedback. These points are discussed later.

In addition to the MBI, our studies included questionnaire assessments of other relevant variables (i.e., demographic information, job characteristics, job satisfaction, coping techniques). However, only selected findings from these studies are presented in this chapter as a way of illustrating our arguments. These findings are always presented in terms of the three different aspects of burnout, rather than as some single overall score. Inasmuch as so little is known about the interrelationships among these three aspects, they should be considered separately instead of combined in some arbitrary way. The global term of "burnout" is reserved for discussion of the syndrome as a whole.

THE JOB SETTING AS A SOURCE OF BURNOUT

When the quality of the care provided by health practitioners declines, all too often people are blamed rather than the work environment. It is either staff or patients who are held to be at fault for spoiling the idealistic relationship between concerned giver and appreciative recipient. Among health practitioners, it is not uncommon to perceive certain people as "bad patients" (Lorber, 1975), such as those who constantly complain and make demands, fail to follow instructions, violate hospital rules, or waste the practitioner's time. By pointing a damning finger at patients, health practitioners may develop hostility and resentment toward them. Moral justifications for a more dehumanized relationship with patients are then easier to come by once it is evident that *they* are the "problem" (Bandura, Underwood, & Fromson, 1975).

On the other hand, by turning the heat on themselves, health practitioners may begin to make more self-deprecatory remarks, to question their suitability for this line of work, and in general to lose such essential qualities as self-confidence, a sense of humor, and a balanced perspective. The alleged personal flaws of practitioners do not go unnoticed by critics who are willing to argue whether the matter involves a lack of ability, a motivational deficit, or a character defect. "He's such an arrogant dictator." "She's just stupid." "They're basically lazy." Such are the diagnostic assessments made by some staff members about each other.

Whether the brunt of the blame is carried by staff or by patients, blaming allows the contribution made by the properties of the situation to be either minimized or ignored. Such dispositional explanations limit, and even misguide, attempts toward solutions to burnout. Although personality variables are certainly an important factor in burnout (see Gann, 1979; Heckman, 1980), our research has led us to the conclusion that the problem is best understood (and modified) in terms of the social and situational sources of job-related stress (see Maslach, 1976; Maslach & Jackson, 1981b; Maslach & Pines, 1977; Pines & Maslach, 1978). The prevalence of the phenomenon and the range of seemingly disparate professionals who are affected by it suggest that the search for causes is better directed away from the unending cycle of identifying the "bad people" and toward uncovering the operational and structural characteristics of the "bad situations" where many good people function. We have reached the point at which the number of rotten apples in the barrel warrants examination of the barrel itself.

Dealing with People

A key aspect of the work situation, in terms of the development of burnout, is the amount and degree of contact with the recipients of one's services. In health settings, this refers to direct care of patients (as opposed to other professional duties, such as teaching, administrative work, staff meetings, etc.). Although patient care is the raison d'etre of health professions and can be very challenging and rewarding, it is also emotionally demanding (Maslach, 1979). The more time spent in direct care, the greater the risk of the emotional exhaustion of burnout. An example of this point can be found in a survey of staff physicians at a health maintenance organization (Jackson & Maslach, 1982a). These physicians gave us estimates of the percentage of their working time that they spent in various professional activities. The greater the percentage of time spent in direct contact with patients, the higher the physicians' scores on the MBI subscale of emotional exhaustion.[2] The scores were lower for those who spent some of their working hours in teaching or administration. Similarly, in a study of cystic fibrosis caregivers (Lewiston, Conley, & Blessing-Moore, 1981), the amount of time they spent with sick, hospitalized patients was the single difference between those scoring high and those scoring low on an overall index of burnout (the MBI subscales combined). Caregivers who scored above the mean spent 28% of their time with patients, whereas those scoring below the mean spent 17% of their time with them.

Direct patient care can be emotionally demanding in a number of ways. Some of this is attributable to the patients' own feelings and behaviors. Patients may be worried, anxious, or even frightened about what is happening to them. They may be embarrassed by the questions they have to answer or the procedures they have to undergo. They may become upset at the news that the health practitioner gives them, or they may deny that it is true. They may misinterpret what is told to them or fail to follow instructions. They may get angry or even abusive. They may

[2]The correlations for all the findings discussed in this chapter are presented in Table 8.3.

have trouble in articulating their thoughts and fears. They may make excessive complaints or become impatient and unreasonable regarding care. Some patients may be rude or obnoxious in their personal style.

The nature of the patient's health problem is also a factor in the emotional strain of direct patient care. Some illnesses or injuries may be especially difficult to look at or work with (e.g., severe burns, facial cancer), whereas in other cases patients may have poor prognoses for recovery. Direct care of such patients often involves nurses in what Hay and Oken (1972) refer to as "intimacy with the frightening, repulsive, and forbidden [p. 110]." Working with dying patients can pose several other emotional problems for health practitioners. First of all, because death is usually viewed as an adversary to be fought and overcome, a dying patient becomes a visible sign of the practitioner's failure and powerlessness. This is especially true when the practitioner is operating with a "rescue fantasy" of saving patients, as opposed to helping them (Bugen, 1979). Dying patients can also arouse disturbing thoughts about one's own death or the death of significant others, such as a relative or close friend. If the practitioner begins to identify with the patient or is reminded of a loved one (e.g., "this guy is just like my father"), then the emotional strain of working with that patient is even more pronounced (Koocher, 1979).

Communication problems with patients are another source of emotional stress. As mentioned before, the patients themselves may have trouble in expressing their thoughts and feelings to medical staff. However, the reverse can also be true. Medical staff may experience difficulties in communicating directly with patients, especially about emotionally laden topics (for themselves, as well as for the patients). "Bad news" constitutes one category of such topics, and very few people ever feel comfortable being the bearer of such tidings (Tesser & Rosen, 1975). For example, the practitioner may have to tell the patient that a treatment is going to be painful or risky, or that the treatment was unsuccessful, or that there will be permanent disabilities or future problems, or that there is nothing more that the practitioner can do. The bad news that is the worst to deliver, however, concerns death and dying. Conveying this information to terminal patients and their families is the task viewed as most threatening by medical students (Saul & Kass, 1969), and it is often avoided and left undone by medical staff (Kastenbaum, 1967; Lasagna, 1970; Oken, 1961; Pearlman, Stotsky, & Dominick, 1969).

The emotional strain of working with any one patient can be multiplied by the need to deal with the patient's family as well. Family members may be upset or frightened by what is happening to the patient, they may want immediate answers to questions about the patient's care, they may make demands or complaints on the patient's behalf, and so forth. Even though the needs of the family are well recognized, providing supportive care for these people can be an additional emotional burden for the practitioner (Cassem & Hackett, 1972; Hay & Oken, 1972).

TABLE 8.3
Correlational Data for the MBI Subscales

	Frequency	*Intensity*
Job Setting		
Physicians (n = 43)		
higher Emotional Exhaustion:		
more time spent in direct contact with patients	.31[a]	.30[a]
less time spent in teaching	−.26[a]	−.33[a]
less time spent in administration	−.21[a]	−.36[a]
Nurses (n = 74)		
higher Emotional Exhaustion:		
less influence on policies and decisions	−.30[b]	−.34[c]
more bureaucratic hassles	.25[a]	ns
fewer opportunities to be creative	−.34[c]	−.26[b]
Nurses (n = 95)		
higher Emotional Exhaustion:		
less feedback about work	−.24[a]	−.38[c]
less knowledge about results	−.31[b]	−.21[a]
higher Depersonalization:		
less knowledge of results	−.32[b]	−.28[b]
less feedback about work	−.44[c]	−.38[c]
lower Personal Accomplishment:		
less feedback about work	.38[c]	.29[b]
Negative Biases		
Nurses (n = 74)		
higher Depersonalization:		
less positive feedback from patients	−.30[b]	ns
felt less successful with patients	−.34[c]	−.32[b]
higher Emotional Exhaustion:		
felt less successful with patients	−.29[b]	−.27[b]
Coping with Burnout		
Physicians (n = 43)		
higher Emotional Exhaustion:		
spend time away from people	.42[b]	.37[a]
do work that does not involve people	.31[a]	.25[d]
avoid thinking about job after leaving hospital	.39[b]	.45[b]
avoid contacting hospital during off-hours	.50[c]	.47[c]
higher Depersonalization:		
avoid thinking about job after leaving hospital	.29[a]	.30[a]
avoid contacting hospital during off-hours	.28[a]	ns
Nurses (n = 95)		
higher Emotional Exhaustion:		
spend time away from people	.29[b]	.35[c]
engage in solitary activities	.32[c]	.21[a]
higher Depersonalization:		
do tasks that avoid contact with people	.25[b]	.25[b]
engage in solitary activities	.23[a]	.22[a]

(*continued*)

TABLE 8.3—*Continued*

	Frequency	*Intensity*
Physicians ($n = 43$)		
lower Emotional Exhaustion:		
seek advice of other staff	−.39[b]	−.34[a]
talk with co-workers about difficulties	−.30[a]	ns
higher Personal Accomplishment:		
discuss relationship with patients	.40[b]	.44[b]
read others' accounts of problem	.36[b]	.23[d]
talk to spouse and/or friend	.28[a]	.32[a]
Nurses ($n = 95$)		
higher Personal Accomplishment:		
think of patients' viewpoint	.27[b]	.23[a]
consider patients' problems objectively	.28[b]	.22[a]
use humor with patients	.20[a]	.25[b]
Nurses ($n = 74$)		
lower Emotional Exhaustion:		
perceive support and recognition from co-workers	−.36[c]	−.25[a]
perceive support and recognition from supervisors	−.38[c]	−.30[b]
higher Personal Accomplishment:		
discuss job with friends	.37[c]	.35[c]
perceive support from friends	.34[c]	.34[c]

Note: All p-values are two-tailed.
[a] $p < .05$.
[b] $p < .01$.
[c] $p < .001$.
[d] $p < .10$.

Success and Failure

The health practitioners' expectations for what they will accomplish in their work are important determinants of the emotional strains they are likely to experience. Especially among new staff members, the anticipation of saving patients from the pain and sadness that accompany illness is a strong motivating force (Cartwright, 1979; Kramer, 1974). As the more experienced professional knows, however, such expectations are unrealistic—failure to reach such idealistic goals is inevitable.

That feelings of failure are related to stress reactions is a prominent theme in the stress literature (Howard & Scott, 1965; McGrath, 1970, 1976; Mechanic, 1962, 1974). Recent studies of the learned helplessness phenomenon have been especially useful for advancing our understanding of the failure-stress relationship. In experimental studies of learned helplessness, subjects first go through a training phase during which they experience repeated failure on some task (which usually involves learning to avoid an aversive stimulus, such as shock or noise). The subject eventually learns that he or she is "helpless," that escape from the aversive stimulus is impossible, and that failure is unavoidable. Subsequently, when these subjects are placed in another, similar situation, their performance is poorer than subjects not previously exposed to the helplessness training (Seligman, 1975).

Of particular interest here are learned helplessness studies in which affective reactions are assessed in addition to changes in performance. In the original formulation of learned helplessness theory as well as in recent reformulations (Abramson, Seligman, & Teasdale, 1978; Miller & Norman, 1979), repeated failure has been hypothesized to induce emotional disturbances such as anxiety, stress, and depression. There are now several studies that relate failure to anxiety and tension, both as reported by the subject (Gatchel, Paulus, & Maples, 1975; Griffith, 1977; Krantz, Glass, & Snyder, 1974; Roth & Kubal, 1975) and as indicated by lowered electrodermal activity (Gatchel & Proctor, 1976; Krantz et al., 1974). These studies suggest that the feelings of disillusionment experienced by health professionals early in their careers may result from a similar experience of repeated encounters with failure. In the early years of one's career in the health field, unrealistic expectations about what can be accomplished in one's work make the new practitioner especially vulnerable to learned helplessness and emotional strain. But even after experience teaches the idealistic practitioner to readjust his or her criteria for measuring success and failure and to take into account the limits of medical technology and bureaucratic procedures, additional sources of emotional stress remain inherent in the job itself—most notably, lack of control and ambiguity.

Control and Lack of Control

The importance of being able to control, or at least predict, outcomes is well-recognized by psychologists (Averill, 1973; Gal & Lazarus, 1975; Miller & Norman, 1979). Having opportunities to be self-determining, combined with the freedom and the ability to influence events in one's surroundings, can be intrinsically motivating and highly rewarding (Deci, 1980; Vroom, 1964). When opportunities for control are absent and people feel trapped in an environment that is neither controllable nor predictable, both psychological and physical health are likely to suffer (Janis & Rodin, 1979).

In health care settings, many aspects of the professional's environment are beyond his or her control. Perhaps most salient are the ever-present reminders that modern medicine is not yet sufficiently advanced to control the diseases of all patients, although such control is its mission. More frustrating, however, is that even when the methods for successfully treating a patient are known, the practitioner's control over the success of the treatment may be sabotaged by an uncooperative patient who refuses to follow prescribed treatments.

However, the restrictions placed on health practitioners by the state of their art and the uncooperativeness of their patients may be less disruptive than the lack of control they exercise over their immediate environment. Nurses often feel unable to exercise control, either over the behavior of the physicians with whom they are closely interdependent or over the decisions of the administrators who determine the hours and conditions of their work. In a study of hospital nurses (Jackson & Maslach, 1982a), we found that feelings of emotional exhaustion were linked to feelings of lack of control. Emotional exhaustion was higher for nurses who were less able to influence policies and decisions and for those who had more bureaucratic hassles. Emotional exhaustion was also higher for nurses who had fewer opportunities to be creative in carrying out their work. Like the decisions of administrators, the decisions of physicians often determine the daily activities of the nurse. Thus, we heard frequent complaints about doctors who failed to show up for regular appointments, scheduled surgery without informing the nurses, "skipped out" when a patient died (thus leaving the nurse to counsel and comfort the patient's family), or disappeared without leaving word of where they could be reached in an emergency.

But if nurses lack control over their immediate work environment, they do seem to have one advantage over many physicians: They have more freedom to cope with the stress of their jobs by taking time off to recuperate. In our research (Jackson & Maslach, 1982a), nurses were much more likely than doctors to report taking time off as a way of coping with job-related stress (61% of the nurses, compared to 12% of the doctors). Nurses may also feel freer to choose the patients with whom they will spend more time. When asked whether they ever rescheduled their work in order to spend more time with those patients with whom they were being more successful, 83% of the nurses said yes as compared to 48% of the doctors. By being able to engage in such rescheduling, nurses may be able both to increase their feelings of autonomy and control and to shield themselves from higher levels of emotional strain in direct patient care.

Ambiguity

Somewhat related to the relative lack of control experienced by nurses are feelings of ambiguity and uncertainty about their roles. Ambiguity has been cited as a major cause of both poor performance and psychological stress by researchers with diverse interests (e.g., Kahn, Wolfe, Quinn, Snoek, & Rosenthal, 1964; McGrath, 1976; Schuler, 1980). Ambiguous job settings—settings in which there is a perceived lack of relevant information—induce feelings of tension and anxiety. Two types of information identified as particularly important in determining stress reactions are: (1) information about the tasks a person is expected to perform; (2) information about how others evaluate the person (feedback). When these two types of information are unavailable, workers experience role ambiguity, which in turn is related to job dissatisfaction, higher blood pressure, physical symptoms of stress, turnover, and poorer job performance (Beehr, Walsh, & Taber, 1976; Brief & Aldag, 1976; Caplan & Jones, 1975; Kahn et al., 1964; Lyons, 1971; Rizzo, House, & Lirtzman, 1970).

That the role of the health practitioner is to maintain and restore the health of patients seems clear, but the uncertainty that exists about how best to carry out this role has been the topic of several articles (Bates, 1970; Johnson & Martin, 1958; Schulman, 1958). The traditional distinction between the medical and nursing professions asserts that the roles of physician and nurse are clearly defined and separated, with physicians functioning to cure patients and nurses functioning to give care. However, observations of nurses at work suggest that such a clear distinction between roles is more theoretical than real. Nurses are often found giving medical advice to physicians, albeit in subtle ways (Stein, 1967), and carrying out procedures that are supposed to be the exclusive domain of the physician.

In and of themselves, the overlapping roles played by physician and nurse need not be a source of role ambiguity. It is the covert nature of this role-sharing that creates ambiguity. Stein (1967) describes this role-sharing as a game in which the objective is for the nurse to: "be bold, have initiative, and be responsible for making significant recommendations, while at the same time she must appear passive. This must be done in such a manner so as to make her recommendations appear to be initiated by the physician [p. 699]." Because of its covert nature, the doctor-nurse game can be learned only through trial and error. Although clear sanctions will signal when the game has been played badly, no explicit recognition can ever be given for a game played well. When playing the doctor-nurse game, then, the nurse is likely to feel uncertainty and ambiguity about the quality of her or his performance.

The importance of being given feedback about one's performance was clearly evident among nurses in our study (Jackson & Maslach, 1982a). Using the Job Diagnostic Survey (Hackman & Oldham, 1975), we assessed the amount of feedback these nurses received about their work as well as the extent to which they had knowledge about the results of their efforts. Emotional exhaustion was higher among nurses who received little feedback and among nurses who felt they had little knowledge about the results of their endeavors. Furthermore, nurses scored higher on depersonalization when they had little knowledge of results and little feedback. Feedback about how one is doing on the job is especially important for the maintenance of a positive self-evaluation. When feedback was minimal for these nurses, they had low scores on feelings of personal accomplishment. Unlike many jobs where pay and promotion are routinely used to acknowledge good performance, recognition from others is one of the few potential sources of feedback for nurses. We have already noted some reasons why feedback from physicians is not always forthcoming; as we see in a later section, there are other forces inhibiting positive feedback from patients.

Thus, there are several aspects of a health professional's job that are related to the burnout syndrome, including a mismatch between ideals and reality, lack of control within the job setting, ambiguities about what defines appropriate job behavior, a lack of feedback about the value of one's efforts, and continuous direct contact with people. However, the context of the job is often overlooked by practitioners who are embedded in it and who are trying to make sense out of their experiences.

PERCEIVING SITUATIONAL STRESS IN DISPOSITIONAL TERMS

As stated earlier, there is a common tendency among health practitioners to make dispositional interpretations with respect to burnout in spite of evidence for the importance of situational determinants. Such dispositional attributions can be made in reference to oneself, as well as to others.

The "Mea Culpa" Reaction

Although the actor-observer hypothesis (Jones & Nisbett, 1971) would predict that health professionals would tend to see their own behavior as a product of situational forces and constraints, it is not unusual for them to interpret their responses as reflections of some basic personality traits (Maslach, 1979). The perception that "I am not cut out for this job"; "Something is wrong with me"; or "I have become a cold, unfeeling person" is not uncommon and appeared to be one factor that propelled several professionals into some form of individual therapy or led them to quit their job. Even when they recognized the special situational stresses of their work, people were still prone to lay blame on some flaw within themselves ("I should have been able to handle it"). Consequently, they experienced a sense of failure and a loss of self-esteem, and a state of depression would often set in.

Why should there be a bias toward a dispositional self-attribution? Just like other people, health professionals have a tendency to overestimate the importance of personal or dispositional variables relative to environmental influences, a tendency known as the fundamental attribution error (Ross, 1977). Moreover, people are often unable to identify accurately the situational variables that influence their behavior (Nisbett & Wilson, 1977). In addition, there are several factors in the health professions that steer the process of causal inference in an ad hominem direction, including the chronicity and gradual escalation of sources of emotional stress, pluralistic ignorance shared by co-workers, and misguided administrative reactions.

First of all, the burnout syndrome appears to be a response to chronic (as opposed to acute) sources of stress. The emotional pressure of working closely with people is a constant, relatively stable part of the daily routine. What varies is the tolerance of the practitioner for this continual stress, a tolerance that gradually wears away under the neverending onslaught of emotional tensions. As a result, when problems begin to occur in the practitioner's relationship with patients or staff, there is no discrete situational discontinuity to which the person can key this response. To put it in terms of Kelley's attribution theory (1967, 1971), the practitioner is unable to see a situational cause that covaries with the observed effect. Therefore, he or she is often left with a choice of dispositional attributions: The problems are caused either by the patient or by oneself.

A dispositional attribution to self is more likely if the person believes that his or her reaction is a unique one not shared by others. Such a belief is likely to occur in many health professions as a result of pluralistic ignorance. Our observations uncovered a tendency to deny or to avoid revealing any personal thoughts or feelings that would be considered "unprofessional" and to behave instead as if one were in control of the job and doing well (Maslach, 1979). When everyone puts on this facade of "I'm doing just fine" and fails to share their true reactions with each other, then any one of them is liable to make the erroneous assumption that he or she is the only one experiencing such problems. This attributional error is further enhanced by the fact that the individual who believes he or she is alone in having these feelings will be especially careful not to reveal this "deviant" response to others and will work harder to maintain the facade of a professional demeanor.

A dispositional attribution to self may also occur as a function of administrative response. When difficulties arise in the delivery of health care, administrators and supervisors are prone to see the problem in terms of people who are not doing their job well, rather than in terms of shortcomings in the institution itself (for which they might be implicated). They assume that many of the hassles are due to errors, faulty judgments, or laziness on the part of the staff and that a major aspect of their job as administrator is to get the employees to improve their job performance or else to get better employees. Thus, when health practitioners complain to administrators about the emotional stress of their work, the common (dispositional) response is, "What's the matter, can't *you* take it?" By assigning causal responsibility to the health professional for his or her reactions, the administrator reinforces and maintains that person's tendency to make dispositional attributions to self.

Putting the Blame on the Patients

The bias of health professionals toward dispositional, rather than situational, attributions for personal experiences can extend to their judgments about recipients as well. They may view patients as having been the cause of their own problems, rather than as suffering from situational circumstances. "You wouldn't be in this predicament if you had taken care of yourself (stopped smoking, lost weight, not gotten into a fight, etc.)." Although members of the medical staff are often expected to be nonjudgmental and accepting of patients' actions ("ignore the behavior, but don't ignore the patient"), it is sometimes difficult not to blame patients for their circumstances (Storlie, 1979). In addition, there are other factors that contribute to the bias toward dispositional attributions.

Casting causal blame among patients becomes more frequent and probable when the operational paradigm is a medical model and when record keeping excludes contextual information but highlights personal problems.

One source of bias toward dispositional attributions about patients lies in the fact that health practitioners usually see patients on an individual basis about their problems. This contact with separate individuals (as opposed to simultaneous exposure to groups of people with the same problem) can lead the practitioners to do a personal analysis that is more likely to identify the causes of the problem internally. They opt for the medical model of diagnosis and treatment rather than the public health model. In other words, when dealing with a single person the health professional tends to focus on what it is about that person that is causing the problem. This is true even when the professional sees a series of individuals who have the same difficulties. However, it is probable that if all of these individuals were to appear en masse to see the practitioner then he or she would be more inclined to look for the situational causes of this apparent epidemic.

The very structure of the records and charts kept on each patient can also contribute to this dispositional bias. The forms to be filed typically ask for a trait characterization of the patient: his or her problem, critical incidents, staff assessments, and other person-centered evaluations. There may be no place in the report form for listing eliciting circumstances for the behaviors noted. Situational circumstances, if not ignored totally or minimized, are often given the status of excuses and rarely that of explanations. As the institutional structure becomes more formalized and the staff–patient ratio grows larger, such records take on a historical validity and become the standard of biographical "truth" against which the patient is subsequently measured. Moreover, they can exert a powerful controlling influence over the allegedly independent judgments made by staff in their face-to-face encounters with patients. That is, they may function as stereotypes or first impressions in shaping later judgments (Schneider, Hastorf, & Ellsworth, 1979). A parallel process has been shown to occur in the job interview situation, where evaluations tend to be made on the basis of a written résumé, and interview information that does not confirm this expectation is discounted (Webster, 1964). Thus, patient records may create not only individual differences but a spurious consistency between the past person of record and the present person at hand.

NEGATIVE BIASES IN PERCEPTIONS OF PATIENTS

A hallmark of the burnout syndrome, across a wide range of helping professions, is a shift from a positive and humanized orientation in the perception of recipients to a negative and depersonalized one (see Wills, 1978). The patients or clients are viewed in more cynical and derogatory terms, and the practitioner begins to develop a lower opinion of their capabilities and their worth as human beings. This process of "moral evaluation" (Roth, 1972) is further enhanced by attempts to underscore and exaggerate the differences between "us" and "them."

In most cases, the structure of the helping relationship is such that it promotes and maintains a negative perception of patients. In particular, four aspects of this relationship seem to be especially critical: (1) the focus on problems; (2) the lack of positive feedback; (3) the type of patient contact; (4) the probability of change or responsiveness by patients.

Primary among these is the fact that, by definition, most patients are people with problems. Whether they are sick, injured, unable to care for themselves, or experiencing some other type of difficulty, this negative part of themselves and their life is what the practitioner sees. What is good and healthy about themselves is often given less attention by the practitioner because it is rarely of immediate relevance to the problem under consideration. Moreover, many health care relationships are set up so that when the patients' problems disappear, so do the patients. That is, once patients are healthy and functioning well, they have no further need for the health professional, and thus the relationship is terminated. From the practitioner's point of view, this consequence further reduces his or her opportunity to see patients in good times as well as bad. Indeed, the practitioner may be unaware of whether terminated patients have given up in despair or are no longer in need of health services because of successful resolution of their problems. Because of this continuous and limited focus on negative aspects of the patients, it is not surprising that health professionals might begin to develop a rather cynical view of human nature.

An exclusive focus on patients' problems is more likely as the number of patients increases. The more people the practitioner has to be concerned about, the less time he or she can give to any one of them. Consequently, what little time exists is spent only on the most serious and urgent problems of the patients; spending time on the positive aspects of patients' lives is a luxury that simply cannot be afforded. This means that health practitioners will inevitably have an incomplete knowledge and understanding of any single patient—in a sense, they cannot see the trees for the forest. This focus on problems exacerbates the tendency of practitioners to see patients as symptoms instead of as individuals (e.g., "the coronary in room 412") and to treat them in more depersonalized ways.

A second factor that adversely biases perception of patients is the negative feedback that health practitioners may get from patients. They hear complaints and criticisms about the job they are doing, and in some instances they are the targets of hostile remarks or even threatening actions. Although some of this feedback may be a justifiable response to errors they have made, it is also the case that the health practitioners are on the receiving end of some very strong emotions of fear, anger, and frustration. In addition to this negative feedback, patients do not always give positive feedback, however minimal, for things that the practitioner does well (Koocher, 1979). One reason for this may be that the practitioner's work is taken for granted by the patients ("that's what you're being paid to do"), and so there is no need to provide feedback except when things fall short of these expectations. Also, when people are ill, their attention is focused on the illness and the disruption it is causing in their life. Consequently, their concern for others (even to the extent of ordinary politeness) may be much less than usual because of this egocentric focus.

The upshot of this bias in patient feedback is that the practitioners' contact with patients can become unpleasant and unrewarding, and they begin to feel more negatively about the patients themselves. In our study of a hospital nursing staff (Jackson & Maslach, 1982a), nurses who reported less amounts of positive feedback from patients did indeed score higher on depersonalization. For those whose major motivation to enter a health profession was to make people's lives happier and healthier, the lack of positive feedback or "strokes" from patients for one's accomplishments along this line is a particularly bitter pill to swallow.

Depersonalized perceptions of patients are also a function of the type of contact practitioners have with them. In some medical settings, such as the intensive care unit, the state of the patients is such that they appear almost nonhuman (Hay & Oken, 1972). Moreover, their comatose condition makes it impossible for staff to communicate with them in the way they would with people who were alert and functioning. Depersonalized perceptions are heightened when patients have prolonged stays in such a unit and/or their prognoses are poor. In contrast, when the contact with patients involves normal conversations and is thus more pleasant at an interpersonal level (e.g., the practitioner can joke with the patient, converse about common interests, discuss current issues), then there are more positive (as well as more humane) elements in the practitioner's perception of the patient.

Finally, perceptions of patients are related to responsiveness and change on their part. Health practitioners may develop more negative views of patients who do not respond to them, either as a professional or as a fellow human being. If the patients do not acknowledge their presence, fail to follow their advice or guidance, and do not provide positive feedback, then they are dehumanizing the health practitioners, and it becomes easier for the practitioners, in turn, to dehumanize them and develop depersonalized attitudes toward them. Furthermore, if the efforts of the health practitioner fail to make any appreciable difference in the patients' lives, then he or she can ward off feelings of failure and ineffectiveness by blaming the patients for their problems, perceiving them as inherently defective, unmotivated to change, bad, or weak. As an example, hospital nurses who felt less successful in their work with patients scored higher on the MBI subscale of depersonalization as well as on the subscale of emotional exhaustion (Jackson & Maslach, 1982a). Viewing the patient as the problem reflects not only the bias toward negative perceptions but the bias toward dispositional attributions discussed earlier. An important consequence of this depersonalized perception of patients is that the quality of patient care may decline. Practitioners may avoid some patients as much as possible, take longer to respond to their call lights, "forget" to do certain tasks (e.g., get lab specimens, provide medication on time), and react with sarcasm or hostility to patient requests or complaints.

COPING WITH BURNOUT

One goal of our research is to discover how people deal effectively with burnout. There are a variety of coping strategies, some of which are individual techniques while others are done at a social or institutional level (see Maslach, 1976, 1978a, 1978b, 1979, 1982). Most of these have been gleaned from self-report measures (interviews and questionnaires) rather than through direct observations of behavior. It is possible to discern correlational patterns between certain coping responses and various aspects of burnout, but we cannot yet specify the underlying causal relationships. Although different levels of experienced burnout could lead people to engage in different activities, it is also possible that different coping styles could precipitate, exacerbate, or alleviate various aspects of burnout. Or, some third factor may be responsible for the correlations (e.g., certain personality traits may mediate both feelings of burnout and coping style). Furthermore, it should be noted that there has been no systematic longitudinal research evaluating the actual effectiveness of different solutions for burnout (or for any other type of job-related stress; see Newman & Beehr, 1979). Thus, any conclusions about how best to deal with burnout must be made with some caution.

Because involvement with people is central to the experience of burnout, it is not surprising that the role of other individuals is central to several strategies for coping with it. In some instances, the key element of the coping activity is the complete absence of other people so that the practitioner is handling the stress on his or her own. In other cases, the presence of specific people is essential for helping the practitioner deal with burnout in a social context.

Getting Away from Others

Since much of the emotional exhaustion of burnout arises from close contact with people, one approach toward reducing that source of stress is to get away from them (Koocher, 1979). By being alone, the health professional can begin to unwind from the tension and pain of the work by relaxing physically and stopping all thoughts of the day's problems. In other words, when the practitioner is suffering from an overload of social input, those inputs can be reduced through techniques of planned, temporary social isolation. This can be accomplished through such techniques as physical withdrawals (e.g., reduction of contact hours, work breaks or absences, vacations); psychological withdrawals (e.g., not thinking about the job, focusing on distracting thoughts or activities); and shifting to work tasks that do not involve direct contact with people (e.g., paperwork). In some of these cases, the health professional has no actual contact with people on the job, whereas in others the professional is in physical contact with people (e.g., they may be in the same room) but can be psychologically alone in his or her thoughts and feelings.

An illustration of this tendency to pull away from others is found in one study of the coping styles of physicians (Jackson & Maslach, 1982a). We asked physicians how frequently they used various activities as a way of coping with tension, and how effective they thought each activity was as a coping technique. Physicians scoring high on emotional exhaustion were more likely to rate various withdrawal strategies as effective ways of coping with stress and tension. These strategies included: finding a way to spend more time away from people, finding work that needs to be done that does not involve working directly with people, trying not to think about the job after leaving the hospital, and making a point not to contact the hospital during off-hours. The latter two strategies were also the ones rated as effective by physicians scoring high on depersonalization. Similarly, a survey of nurses (Jackson & Maslach, 1982a) revealed that those scoring high on depersonalization gave higher effectiveness ratings to tasks that avoid contact with people.

In addition to withdrawal from people on the job, it appears that withdrawal from people in one's private life can also occur. There are times when the individual needs to get away from all human contact, regardless of who the people are (Maslach, 1982). In these instances it appears that *any* form of social input is enough to contribute to a condition of emotional overload. The practitioner does not want to hear anything more from anyone, at least for a while. This desire for total peace, quiet, and isolation can come at the expense of relationships with family and friends, who may not understand why they are sometimes being left out of the practitioner's life. A better alternative is a "decompression routine" between leaving work and arriving home, a time in which practitioners can engage in some solitary activity in order to unwind, relax, and take their mind off the events of the day (Maslach, 1979, 1982). Some of these reported decompression activities involve physical exercise, and others include reading, naps, music, meditation, soaking in a hot bath, and so on. The perceived effectiveness of such activities for reducing stress is rated more highly by practitioners who score high on emotional exhaustion and on depersonalization. By being alone for a while, practitioners are then more ready to be with people again, and especially those people who are important to them.

Turning Toward Others

As opposed to coping techniques that rely on an absence of people, alternative strategies depend on their presence. Other people (e.g., one's peers) can be a very valuable resource for the practitioner experiencing burnout (Koocher, 1979;

Maslach, 1976, 1979, 1982). They can provide a direct reduction of stress by getting the person to withdraw from a difficult or upsetting situation and by giving comfort and emotional support. They also aid indirectly in stress reduction by helping the person to gain some perspective on the situation and to intellectualize about it. By sharing their own feelings and alternative responses to similar problems, they can serve as a social comparison referent, providing the person with information as to what are normal reactions to these types of situations. A sense of shared responsibility can also develop from the person's contact with peers, so that he or she feels less isolated and "on the spot" for any particular course of action. Finally, peers can provide the sort of positive feedback that is often missing from the practitioner's work with patients.

All of these valuable coping functions provided by peers are often best realized within the context of an organized social-professional support system. Not only are various supportive interpersonal behaviors explicitly modeled and reinforced, but such a support system serves to shift people's attributional bias away from exclusively dispositional judgments and toward a more situational orientation. In addition to formally organized groups, such social support can be provided through more informal group gatherings, such as coffee and lunch breaks or the socializing that may take place after the workday is over.

Whereas emotional exhaustion and depersonalization were associated with strategies of turning away from people, strategies of turning toward people were associated with personal accomplishment and low emotional exhaustion. In our study of physicians (Jackson & Maslach, 1982a), those scoring low on emotional exhaustion gave high effectiveness ratings to seeking the advice of other staff regarding specific problems and talking with their co-workers about any difficulties they were having. Physicians scoring high on personal accomplishment reported that effective coping strategies included discussing with patients the limitations of their professional relationship with them, reading accounts of how others have handled specific problems, and talking to their spouse and/or close friend about what has happened at work. Among a sample of nurses (Jackson & Maslach, 1982a), those scoring high on personal accomplishment gave higher effectiveness ratings to various patient-centered techniques such as thinking about how patients view things, considering patients' problems as objectively as possible, and using humor in one's contacts with patients.

In another study with hospital nurses (Jackson & Maslach, 1982a), we assessed the extent to which nurses felt they received support and recognition from their co-workers. The more perceived support, the lower the nurse's score of emotional exhaustion. Similarly, lower rates of emotional exhaustion were associated with greater support and recognition from supervisors. In contast to this support from work peers, support from people outside of the job (friends, family) had little relationship to the experience of emotional exhaustion. However, nurses feeling a strong sense of personal accomplishment were more likely to discuss their job with friends and to feel supported by them.

CONCLUSION

The goal of this chapter has been to extend the domain of social psychology to a new and important problem area—the burnout syndrome—which has received little previous attention from the social sciences. Both social psychology and the helping professions can benefit from such an extension; the former by the development of new hypotheses and a "real world" test of various theoretical models, and the latter by the unique analysis and proposals for specific solutions that are provided by a social psychological perspective.

Social psychology has much to contribute to the analysis of burnout, and it also has much to gain. The often-quoted goal of translating research findings into application and "giving psychology away" has been approached, in this case, not by deriving practical implications from a series of experimental studies but by focusing on an important social problem and working toward an explanation of it in terms of existing theories. One measure of the utility of various theoretical frameworks is the extent to which they can be successfully applied to this all-too-real-world phenomenon.

However, this new use of existing models goes beyond ad hoc explanations to offering predictive power as well. On the basis of this analysis, it is possible to propose hypotheses about differences in the extent and pattern of burnout as a function of specifiable variables. Our future research will test a variety of these hypotheses in both natural field studies and controlled laboratory experiments. For example, in situations where there is no sharing of emotional reactions and thus a greater potential for pluralistic ignorance, there should be higher rates of negative dispositional attributions to self. As another example, negative self-attributions should be higher in situations where it is difficult to make dispositional attributions to clients or patients (i.e., where they simply cannot be viewed as being "at fault," as in the case of pediatric cancer patients). A further prediction would be that people with access to a social-professional support system would display more situational attributions relative to dispositional ones, have a less negative perception of patients, and report less emotional exhaustion and depersonalization than would people who were isolated from such peer support.

In serving as the basis for these and other hypotheses about the social nature of emotional stress, the burnout syndrome can direct the field of social psychology to a new client in desperate need of new solutions to an ageless problem: Who will help the helper? We think that social psychology can and should accept that responsibility.

ACKNOWLEDGMENTS

The research on which this chapter is based was supported by Biomedical Sciences Support Grant 3–S05–RR–07006–08S1. We wish to thank Jennifer Chatman, Brenda Donahoe, and Regina Torrance for their help with the data collection. Parts of this chapter were first presented by Christina Maslach in an address entitled "Burnout: A social psychological analysis" at the annual convention of the American Psychological Association, San Francisco, August 1977.

REFERENCES

Abramson, L. Y., Seligman, M. E. P., & Teasdale, J. D. Learned helplessness in humans: Critique and reformulation. *Journal of Abnormal Psychology*, 1978, *87*, 49–74.

Averill, J. R. Personal control over aversive stimuli and its relationship to stress. *Journal of Personality and Social Psychology*, 1973, *80*, 286–303.

Bandura, A., Underwood, B., & Fromson, M. E. Disinhibition of aggression through diffusion of responsibility and dehumanization of victims. *Journal of Research in Personality*, 1975, *9*, 253–269.

Bates, B. Doctor and nurse: Changing roles and relations. *The New England Journal of Medicine*, 1970, *283*, 129–134.

Beehr, T. A., & Newman, J. E. Job stress, employee health, and organizational effectiveness: A facet analysis, model, and literature review. *Personnel Psychology*, 1978, *31*, 665–699.

Beehr, T. A., Walsh, J. T., & Taber, T. D. Relationships of stress to individually and organizationally valued states: Higher order needs as a moderator. *Journal of Applied Psychology*, 1976, *61*, 35–40.

Brief, A. P., & Aldag, R. J. Correlates of role indices. *Journal of Applied Psychology*, 1976, *61*, 468–472.

Bugen, L. A. Emotions: Their presence and impact upon the helping role. In C. A. Garfield (Ed.), *Stress and survival: The emotional realities of life-threatening illness*. St. Louis: Mosby, 1979.

Caplan, R. D., & Jones, K. W. Effects of workload, role ambiguity, and Type A personality on anxiety, depression, and heart rate. *Journal of Applied Psychology*, 1975, *60*, 713–719.

Cartwright, L. K. Sources and effects of stress in health careers. In G. C. Stone, F. Cohen, & N. E. Adler (Eds.), *Health psychology*. San Francisco: Jossey-Bass, 1979.

Cassem, N. H., & Hackett, T. P. Sources of tension for the CCU nurse. *American Journal of Nursing*, 1972, *72*, 1426–1430.

Cooper, C. L., & Marshall, J. Occupational sources of stress: A review of the literature relating to coronary heart disease and mental ill health. *Journal of Organizational Psychology*, 1976, *49*, 11–28.

Deci, E. L. *The psychology of self-determination*. Lexington, Mass.: D. C. Heath, 1980.

Gal, R., & Lazarus, R. S. The role of activity in anticipating and confronting stressful situations. *Journal of Human Stress*, 1975, *1*, 4–20.

Gann, M. L. *The role of personality factors and job characteristics in burnout: A study of social service workers*. Unpublished doctoral dissertation, University of California, Berkeley, 1979.

Gatchel, R. J., Paulus, P. B., & Maples, C. W. Learned helplessness and self-reported affect. *Journal of Abnormal Psychology*, 1975, *84*, 732–734.

Gatchel, R. J., & Proctor, J. D. Physiological correlates of learned helplessness in man. *Journal of Abnormal Psychology*, 1976, *85*, 27–34.

Griffith, M. Effects of noncontingent success and failure on mood and performance. *Journal of Personality*, 1977, *45*, 442–457.

Hackman, J. R., & Oldham, G. R. Development of the Job Diagnostic Survey. *Journal of Applied Psychology*, 1975, *60*, 159–170.

Hay, D., & Oken, D. The psychological stresses of intensive care unit nursing. *Psychosomatic Medicine*, 1972, *34*, 109–118.

Heckman, S. J. *Effects of work setting, theoretical orientation, and personality on psychotherapist burnout.* Unpublished doctoral dissertation, California School of Professional Psychology, Berkeley, 1980.

Howard, A., & Scott, R. A. A proposed framework for the analysis of stress in the human organism. *Behavioral Science,* 1965, *10,* 141–160.

Ivancevich, J. M., & Matteson, M. T. *Stress and work.* Glenview, Ill.: Scott, Foresman, 1980.

Jackson, S. E., & Maslach, C. *Burnout and the medical work environment.* Unpublished manuscript, 1982. (a)

Jackson, S. E., & Maslach, C. After-effects of job-related stress: Families as victims. *Journal of Occupational Behaviour,* 1982, *3,* 66–77. (b)

Janis, I. L., & Rodin, J. Attribution, control, and decision making: Social psychology and health care. In G. C. Stone, F. Cohen, & N. E. Adler (Eds.), *Health psychology.* San Francisco: Jossey-Bass, 1979.

Johnson, M. M., & Martin, H. W. A sociological analysis of the nurse role. *American Journal of Nursing,* 1958, *58,* 373–377.

Jones, E. E., & Nisbett, R. E. The actor and the observer: Divergent perceptions of the causes of behavior. In E. E. Jones, D. E. Kanouse, H. H. Kelley, R. E. Nisbett, S. Valins, & B. Weiner (Eds.), *Attribution: Perceiving the causes of behavior.* Morristown, N.J.: General Learning Press, 1971.

Kahn, R. L., Wolfe, D. M., Quinn, R. P., Snoek, J. D., & Rosenthal, R. A. *Occupational stress: Studies in role conflict and ambiguity.* New York: Wiley, 1964.

Kastenbaum, R. Multiple perspectives on a geriatric "death valley." *Community Mental Health Journal,* 1967, *3,* 21–29.

Kelley, H. H. Attribution theory in social psychology. In D. Levine (Ed.), *Nebraska Symposium on Motivation* (Vol. 15). Lincoln: University of Nebraska Press, 1967.

Kelley, H. H. Attribution in social interaction. In E. E. Jones, D. E. Kanouse, H. H. Kelley, R. E. Nisbett, S. Valins, & B. Weiner (Eds.), *Attribution: Perceiving the causes of behavior.* Morristown, N.J.: General Learning Press, 1971.

Koocher, G. P. Adjustment and coping strategies among the caretakers of cancer patients. *Social Work in Health Care,* 1979, *5*(2), 145–150.

Kramer, M. *Reality shock: Why nurses leave nursing.* St. Louis: Mosby, 1974.

Krantz, D. S., Glass, D. C., & Snyder, M. L. Helplessness, stress level, and the coronary-prone behavior pattern. *Journal of Experimental Social Psychology,* 1974, *10,* 284–300.

Lasagna, L. Physicians' behavior toward the dying patient. In O. G. Brim, H. E. Freeman, S. Levine, & N. A. Scotch (Eds.), *The dying patient.* New York: Russell Sage, 1970.

Lerner, M. J. *The belief in a just world: A fundamental delusion.* New York: Plenum Press, 1980.

Lewiston, N. J., Conley, J., & Blessing-Moore, J. Measurement of hypothetical burnout in cystic fibrosis caregivers. *Acta Paediatrica Scandinavica,* 1981, *70,* 935–939.

Lorber, J. Good patients and problem patients: Conformity and deviance in a general hospital. *Journal of Health and Social Behavior,* 1975, *16,* 213–225.

Lyons, T. F. Role clarity, need for clarity, satisfaction, tension, and withdrawal. *Organizational Behavior and Human Performance,* 1971, *6,* 99–110.

Maslach, C. Burned-out. *Human Behavior,* 1976, *5*(9), 16–22.

Maslach, C. The client role in staff burn-out. *Journal of Social Issues,* 1978, *34*(4), 111–124. (a)

Maslach, C. Job burn-out: How people cope. *Public Welfare,* 1978, *36,* 56–58. (b)

Maslach, C. The burn-out syndrome and patient care. In C. A. Garfield (Ed.), *Stress and survival: The emotional realities of life-threatening illness.* St. Louis: Mosby, 1979.

Maslach, C. *Burnout: The cost of caring.* Englewood Cliffs, N.J.: Prentice-Hall, 1982.

Maslach, C., & Jackson, S. E. Lawyer burn-out. *Barrister,* 1978, *5*(2), 8; 52–54.

Maslach, C., & Jackson, S. E. Burned-out cops and their families. *Psychology Today,* 1979, *12*(12), 59–62.

Maslach, C., & Jackson, S. E. *The Maslach Burnout Inventory.* Palo Alto, Cal.: Consulting Psychologists Press, 1981. (a)

Maslach, C., & Jackson, S. E. The measurement of experienced burnout. *Journal of Occupational Behaviour,* 1981, *2,* 99–113. (b)

Maslach, C., & Pines, A. The burn-out syndrome in the day care setting. *Child Care Quarterly,* 1977, *6,* 100–113.

Maslach, C., & Pines, A. Burn-out: The loss of human caring. In A. Pines & C. Maslach (Eds.), *Experiencing social psychology.* New York: Knopf, 1979.

McGrath, J. E. (Ed.). *Social and psychological factors in stress.* New York: Holt, Rinehart & Winston, 1970.

McGrath, J. E. Stress and behavior in organizations. In M. D. Dunnette (Ed.), *Handbook of industrial and organizational psychology.* Chicago: Rand McNally, 1976.

Mechanic, D. *Students under stress.* New York: Free Press, 1962.

Mechanic, D. Social structure and personal adaptation: Some neglected dimensions. In G. U. Coelho, D. A. Hamburg, & J. E. Adams (Eds.), *Coping and adaptation.* New York: Basic Books, 1974.

Miller, I. W., & Norman, W. H. Learned helplessness in humans: A review and attribution theory model. *Psychological Bulletin,* 1979, *86,* 93–118.

Newman, J. E., & Beehr, T. A. Personal and organizational strategies for handling job stress: A review of research and opinion. *Personnel Psychology,* 1979, *32,* 1–44.

Nisbett, R. E., & Wilson, T. D. Telling more than we know: Verbal reports on mental processes. *Psychological Review,* 1977, *84,* 231–259.

Oken, D. What to tell cancer patients. *Journal of the American Medical Association,* 1961, *175,* 1120–1128.

Pearlman, J., Stotsky, B., & Dominick, J. Attitudes toward death among nursing home personnel. *Journal of Genetic Psychology,* 1969, *114,* 63–75.

Pines, A., & Maslach, C. Characteristics of staff burn-out in mental health settings. *Hospital & Community Psychiatry,* 1978, *29,* 233–237.

Pines, A., & Maslach, C. Combatting staff burn-out in a day care center: A case study. *Child Care Quarterly,* 1980, *9,* 5–16.

Rizzo, J. R., House, R. J., & Lirtzman, S. I. Role conflict and ambiguity in complex organizations. *Administrative Science Quarterly,* 1970, *15,* 150–163.

Ross, L. The intuitive psychologist and his shortcomings: Distortions in the attribution process. In L. Berkowitz (Ed.), *Advances in experimental social psychology* (Vol. 10). New York: Academic Press, 1977.

Roth, J. A. Some contingencies of the moral evaluation and control of clientele: The case of the hospital emergency service. *American Journal of Sociology,* 1972, *77,* 839–856.

Roth, S., & Kubal, L. Effects of noncontingent reinforcement on tasks of differing importance: Facilitation and learned helplessness. *Journal of Personality and Social Psychology,* 1975, *32,* 680–691.

Ryan, W. *Blaming the victim.* New York: Pantheon, 1971.

Saul, E. V., & Kass, T. S. Study of anticipated anxiety in a medical school setting. *Journal of Medical Education,* 1969, *44,* 526–532.

Schneider, D. J., Hastorf, A. H., & Ellsworth, P. C. *Person perception* (2nd ed.). Reading, Mass.: Addison-Wesley, 1979.

Schuler, R. S. Definition and conceptualization of stress in organizations. *Organizational Behavior and Human Performance,* 1980, *25,* 184–215.

Schulman, S. Basic functional roles in nursing: Mother surrogate and healer. In E. G. Jaco (Ed.), *Patients, physicians and illness: Sourcebook in behavioral science and medicine.* Glencoe, Ill.: The Free Press, 1958.

Seligman, M. E. P. *Helplessness: On depression, development, and death.* San Francisco: Freeman, 1975.

Selye, H. *The stress of life.* New York: McGraw-Hill, 1956.

Stein, L. I. The doctor-nurse game. *Archives of General Psychiatry,* 1967, *16,* 699–703.

Storlie, F. J. Burnout: The elaboration of a concept. *American Journal of Nursing,* 1979, *19*(12), 2108–2111.

Tesser, A., & Rosen, S. The reluctance to transmit bad news. In L. Berkowitz (Ed.), *Advances in experimental social psychology* (Vol. 8). New York: Academic Press, 1975.

Vroom, V. H. *Work and motivation.* New York: Wiley, 1964.

Webster, E. *Decision-making in the employment interview.* Montreal: McGill University Press, 1964.

Wills, T. A. Perceptions of clients by professional helpers. *Psychological Bulletin,* 1978, *85,* 968–1000.

IV ENVIRONMENTAL INFLUENCES

9 Social Support, Interpersonal Relations, and Health: Benefits and Liabilities

Jerry Suls
State University of New York at Albany

In the 1970s a considerable amount was written about the help and assistance people receive from informal support systems such as family, friends, and neighbors. Many scholars (Cassel, 1976; Cobb, 1976; Dean & Lin, 1977; Kaplan, Cassel, & Gore, 1977) have argued that persons who are part of a social network are less negatively affected by stressful life problems and are less likely to fall ill. It is also widely maintained that naturally existing support systems facilitate coping and recovery if the person should succumb to some form of illness.

The broad consensus held about the preventive and ameliorative effects of informal kinds of support has led some scholars to propose that it may be more feasible to attempt to improve and strengthen social supports in the interest of health than to reduce exposure to stressors or pathogens. For example, Cassel (1976) has written:

> With advancing knowledge it is perhaps not too far-reaching to imagine a preventative health service in which professionals are involved largely in the diagnostic aspects—identifying families and groups at high risk by virtue of their lack of fit with their social mileau and determining the particular nature and form of social supports that can and should be strengthened if such people are to be protected from disease outcomes [p. 121].

But although there may be a large consensus about the benefits of social support, there is considerable diversity about how it should be defined or operationalized. Let us consider some representative definitions.

For Caplan, Robinson, French, Caldwell, and Shinn (1976) social support is defined: "as any input directly provided by another person (or group) which moves the receiving person towards goals toward which the receiver desires [p. 39].'' Kaplan et al. (1977) point out that most studies define social support as: ''. . . the 'metness' or gratification of a person's basic social needs (approval, esteem, succorrance, etc.) . . . which can be satisfied through social interaction with others [p. 50].'' *Or* ''as the relative presence or absence of psychosocial support resources from significant others [pp. 50–51].'' The reader no doubt recognizes the expansiveness of the first definition offered by Kaplan et al. and the circularity of the second.

Potentially, a more fruitful approach is to move away from social support as a unitary concept. Silver and Wortman (1980) have gleaned at least five components from recent research:

1. The expression of positive affects.
2. The expression of agreement with or acknowledgment of the appropriateness of a person's beliefs, interpretations, or feelings.
3. Encouraging the open expression of such beliefs and feelings.
4. The provision of material aid.
5. Providing information that the distressed person is part of a network or system of mutual obligation or reciprocal help [p. 312].

Given the diversity of definition and elements that may comprise social support, it is not surprising that a wide variety of measures and instruments have been used to assess this critical concept. But even though there is a plethora of instruments, scales, and indices, in a recent review Dean and Lin (1977) point out: ''A thorough search in the social and psychological inventories of scales has failed to uncover any measures of social support with either known and/or acceptable properties of reliability and validity [pp. 408–409].''

Despite the problems of definition and the need for reliable and valid measures of social support, large claims have been made for the healthful effects of being part of a social network. However, in the early 1960s Mechanic (1962) pointed out that family and friends can also increase stress. Mechanic gives the example of a graduate student facing crucial examinations with a spouse who denies any possibility of failure: ''I'm not worried; I'm sure you'll pass.'' In this case, the student has to worry not only about failing the exam, but about losing respect in the eyes of the spouse. More recently, Wortman and her colleagues (Coates & Wortman, 1980; Silver & Wortman, 1980; Wortman & Dunkel-Schetter, 1979) and Heller (1979) have begun to point to ways that social support may have counterproductive results. This work is clearly in the minority however. In part, advocates of social support have applied the concept tautologically. Support has been defined in such a way as to include only helpful behaviors. We think that this emphasis misses the mark for two reasons: (1) it ignores well-intended behaviors that may have harmful effects; (2) there has been a tendency to overlook behaviors and effects accompanying supportive actions—necessary concomitants of being a part of a social network—which may have serious consequences for the individual's health.

When one takes into consideration the unintended effects of supportive actions and the broader consequences of being part of a social network, it becomes clear that the presence and behavior of others can have some detrimental effects on health and coping. Therefore, it seems necessary to examine carefully whether in fact being a part of an informal support network and all that it entails is actually beneficial to health. The aim of this chapter is to describe how the presence of a social network may have negative as well as positive effects. At the outset, I emphasize that the contention is not that social support is necessarily detrimental but that the positive case for social support may have been argued too strongly.

The paper is organized in the following way: I begin by reviewing briefly some studies reporting positive effects of social support; then, I consider some ambiguous and even negative findings. Following this section, I attempt to describe in some detail ways in which social support can be a positive or negative influence on the three phases of health behavior: prevention, coping, and recovery. In a final section, I suggest how these observations may be incorporated into public health policy and what benefits they may have.

REPRESENTATIVE RESEARCH

Positive Effects

In this section, I describe some representative studies of the stress-buffering effects of social support. My primary purpose here is to convey to the reader the flavor of the work that has been done. Let us begin with some indirect evidence implicating the absence of social supports in disease genesis. Holmes (cited in Kaplan et al., 1977) in an epidemiological study showed that the highest rates of tuberculosis in Seattle occurred in those people who, because of their ethnic group, were distinct, unaccepted minorities in the neighborhoods in which they lived. High incidence of tuberculosis also was found among those persons, irrespective of ethnic group, who were living alone in one room, who had made multiple occupational and residential moves, and who were single or divorced. Thus, disease was more common in people who had no friends, family, or intimate social group to which they could relate. Similar findings have been reported with respect to other respiratory diseases and schizophrenia. Perhaps the strongest claims have been made by Lynch (1977), who employs mortality figures and argues that the socially isolated die prematurely because of loneliness. His evidence, however, is indirect because loneliness was not measured in his investigation. For example, he compared mortality figures indicating that married people experience a lower mortality rate (for all diseases) than unmarried people.

Studies of this sort possess a variety of problems, which have not gone unidentified. As they are based on correlational data, we cannot be assured that the positive relationship between social support and health is not due to some third, unexamined factor or set of factors. Another problem is that people who are poorly adjusted or in ill health may underestimate the amount of support available to them (Heller, 1979). Finally, Silver and Wortman (1980) have pointed out that coping and social support may be causally related but that one's coping or prognosis may determine the amount of support available.

Prospective studies have the potential to resolve these problems, but few have been done. One prospective study by Nuckolls, Cassel, and Kaplan (1972) is frequently cited as evidence for the beneficial effects of social support. These investigators were interested in identifying the relationship between social stresses, psychosocial assets, and the prognosis of pregnancy. The subjects were pregnant married women of similar age and class. Early in pregnancy (prior to the 24th week), psychosocial assets were assessed by an instrument developed to measure the subject's feelings or perceptions of herself (with reference to this pregnancy) and her relationship with her husband, her extended family, and immediate community in terms of the support she was receiving or could anticipate receiving. At 32 weeks, subjects completed the Schedule of Recent Experience (Holmes & Rahe, 1967), a questionnaire designed to measure life changes or readjustments. Scores were calculated for the life change during pregnancy and for the 2 years preceding it. Following delivery, the medical record was used to score each pregnancy as *normal* or *complicated.* The results were interesting in that neither life change nor psychosocial assets were related to complications. However, women with high life change scores both before and during pregnancy, but favorable psychosocial assets, had only one third the complication rate of women who also experienced much change but had unfavorable psychosocial assets. These findings have been interpreted as strongly implicating social support as an important moderating influence over whether social stressors have a negative impact on health. However, there are some grounds to reserve judgment. Specifically, the measure of psychosocial assets tapped a number of factors. Although most refer to family or community ties, one refers to personal assets such as self-esteem, hostility, ego strength, and so on. Inasmuch as the total score for psychosocial assets was based on all the categories (factor scores were not reported or used in the data analyses), we cannot be sure that it was the social ties *or* self-dimensions or both in conjunction that were responsible for the beneficial effects. An added complication is that we cannot be assured that self-perceptions did not influence the degree of perceived support or vice versa. These ambiguities of the data make it difficult to draw any strong conclusions.

The preceding studies dealt with how social support may ameliorate the effect of stressful life events and prevent illness. What evidence is available about the effects of social support for the individual who has succumbed to some form of chronic or acute illness? This question has received a great deal of attention, particularly with reference to patient compliance with their prescribed medical regimen. In a review of the literature on patient compliance, Haynes and Sackett (1974) considered 25 studies dealing with predictors that can be taken as indicators of social support (e.g., influence of family and friends, family stability, and social isolation). Sixteen of these studies reported findings consistent with the thesis that social support encourages compliance; one study showed a negative relationship. Eight others showed no significant relationship; however, Haynes and Sackett questioned the quality of four of these eight studies on the basis of the measures employed.

A more recent review by Baekeland and Lundwall (1975) found nineteen of nineteen studies showing that social isolation or lack of affiliation was a major cause of dropping out of treatment. Given the large number of positive findings reported in the literature, it is not surprising that health researchers have been encouraged by the benefits of social supports. But again, it is important to note that most of the studies are correlational in nature and thus suffer from the problems already described. Nevertheless, it must be admitted that the sheer number of positive findings does lend strength to any optimism.

Ambiguous or Negative Effects

As noted, although the bulk of the available evidence suggests a beneficial effect for social support, there are exceptions that should be considered. For example, Lieberman and Mullan (1978) collected data from a representative sample of Chicago area adults concerning one of three transitions (e.g., birth of a child) or four crises (e.g., death of a spouse) occurring during the interval between 1972 and follow-up 1976–1977 interviews. Subjects were classified into three groups according to their help seeking behavior: those who went to professionals, those who went only to their social networks (their mates, friends, relatives, etc.), and those who sought no help. A variety of measures of adaptation were included: symptoms of anxiety and depression; perceived stress in the marital, occupational, economic, and parental roles. With the use of statistical controls, the groups were equated on demographic characteristics, perceived stress, personal resources, and access to help as well as elapsed time since the event. Surprisingly, no evidence was found that seeking help from either professionals or one's social network had positive adaptive consequences. Those who obtained help showed no significant reduction in symptoms of distress compared to those who did not seek help. The authors make a strong case that these surprising findings are not likely due to result from an inadequate sample, outcome measures, or statistical control. They do concede that they may not have adequately assessed data about kind, quality, and duration of the help provided. We return to this point later.

Whereas Lieberman and Mullan's research found ambiguous effects of social support, Pearlin and Schooler (1978) reported negative effects. In their study, interviews were conducted with a sample of 2300 people who were asked about a variety of life strains connected with their occupation, income, parenting, and marriage. The ways in which the individuals reported coping to deal with strains were also assessed. Finally, symptoms of depression and anxiety were assessed. Most of the results are not appropriate to the present context, but one pattern (Pearlin & Schooler, 1978) is especially noteworthy:

> A somewhat surprising result is that self-reliance is more effective in reducing stress than the seeking of help and advice from others in the two areas in which it is possible to observe its effects, marriage and parenthood. . . . At any rate it is evident we do not yet know the conditions under which help from others can be effective [p. 10].

These negative and ambiguous results stand in contrast to the results of studies reviewed earlier. Of course, it could be argued that we are comparing apples with oranges. The other studies tended to examine specific illness, outcomes, or treatment maintenance. The studies by Lieberman and Mullan and Pearlin and Schooler surveyed nonhospitalized populations and assessed psychological symptoms—depression and anxiety. Also, these negative and ambiguous results come from studies that were correlational in design, thus rendering them as vulnerable to criticism concerning causal inference as were the others.

Hence, in this context it is instructive to turn to experimental studies of the effects of social support. Unfortunately, little is available. An exception is work initiated by Caplan and his colleagues at the University of Michigan (Caplan et al., 1976). These researchers were particularly interested in studying ways in which hypertensives' adherence to their treatment regimen can be increased. In their first study, after identifying a population of hypertensives, an experimental study was designed with three groups: (1) a control group of patients who received no treatment other than the normal care provided by their physicians; (2) a group of patients who attended a series of four weekly lectures on the nature of high blood pressure and its treatment; (3) a group of patients who were assigned to a social support treatment. This condition provided the same factual information as was provided to the lecture group patients, but in addition each patient brought a buddy to the meetings. In the course of the meetings, social-emotional support was provided through various discussion techniques and playing roles dealing with compliance. Pretest measures and posttest (6–8 weeks later) self-reports of adherence, physicians' records, and blood pressure were the primary dependent variables. Caplan et al. reported that patients in the social support program and the lecture program were superior to the control group. The former groups showed gains in information about health care between pre- and posttests, higher motivation to adhere, and greater levels of adherence as measured by self-report data. However, there were no differences in the amount of blood pressure levels among the three groups for the interval between pre- and posttest, although the sample as a whole showed a significant drop in systolic and diastolic blood pressure levels. Perhaps of greatest relevance is that the lecture and social support groups showed the same pattern of results. Caplan et al. (1976) argue that: "This may be because the lecture group had been run in a little too supportive manner to introduce clear differences between it and the social support group [p. 9]." Nevertheless, it is certainly not encouraging that a program instituted to increase social support had no greater beneficial effects than a lecture program. But clearly the greatest disappointment is that neither treatment had an impact on the most critical variable—the patient's blood pressure.

A second study has also been reported by Caplan and his associates (Caplan, Harrison, Wellons, & French, 1980) again concerning social support and adherence on the part of hypertensives. The study had three conditions: Some patients were provided with social support from a nurse attending the case. Nurses were trained to explain the medical regimen and how to follow it, provide encouragement by praising the patient for adherence, allow the patient to express worry and anxiety, and to be warm and friendly. Subjects in a partner condition received this support but, in addition, were asked to bring a partner for their second visit (typically 3 months later). The partner was given information by the nurse about the patient's regimen, a booklet containing background information about high blood pressure, and guidelines about the type of support that was to be provided by the partner. These guidelines included such things as the benefits to the family that could accrue from the patient's health, the need to provide encouragement, reassurance, and praise regarding the taking of medicines, and the other aspects of the treatment. A control group of patients received the care and instruction they typically received prior to the start of the study. A variety of measures were taken at four points in time from pretest to 1 year later. These measures included blood pressure, meeting of clinical appointments, self-reports of adherence, self-reports of anxiety and depression, and self-reports of motivation to adhere to the regimen. Subjects were also asked to report on how much social support they received. Nurse's and partner's perceptions of patient adherence were also assessed as well as the extent to which they supplied social support. The reader is referred to Caplan et al. (1980) for the details.

The results of this study are particularly surprising given the care and apparent thoroughness of the investigators. There were no significant changes in diastolic or systolic blood pressure due to the interventions (all groups improved). Also, there was no evidence that social support either by the nurse or a partner increased objective adherence; subjects in the experimental groups were no more likely to keep appointments than were controls. Similarly, there were no effects on self-reported adherence. Of course, one might argue that perhaps the manipulations failed to increase support. This seems unlikely however. The data from patient reports of perceived support suggested that patients did see the nurse or partner as supportive as the manipulations intended. We are left with an apparent puzzle: Perceived support increased, but no tangible treatment gains were demonstrated.

It is readily acknowledged that perhaps better outcome measures would have detected effects. Also the sample may have had high initial levels of support, motivation, and adherence, making it hard to detect experimental differences. As it turned out, patients did enter the program with high levels of support, motivation, and adherence. However, Caplan et al. (1980) point out that because "all groups showed an improvement in blood pressure . . . it was not the case that we had a sample with no room for improvement at pre-test [p. 203]."

The experimental studies that have been reviewed do not offer strong support for the contention that social support has a beneficial effect on health outcomes. Of course, more carefully designed experimental studies are needed. Recognizing the scarcity of experimental results and the imprecision that is almost unavoidable in human studies, many reviewers refer to experimental investigations with animals, which allow for greater control of extraneous variables and report a protective effect on the presence of other members of the same species. For example, Conger, Sawrey, and Turrell (1958) have shown that an unanticipated series of electric shocks given to animals previously conditioned to avoid them produced high rates of peptic ulcers on animals shocked in isolation. In contrast, animals shocked in the presence of littermates showed a lower rate of ulcers. Although such data are interesting, the literature on the protective effects of animal cospecifics is actually quite mixed in its conclusions. Apropos is a statement by Ader (1980), a leading researcher in this area:

> Relative to those that are housed individually, group housed animals are more susceptible to a variety of pathologic processes, but are more resistant than individually housed animals to a variety of others. In the case of still other pathologic processes, there are no apparent differences between group and individually housed animals [p. 311].

Given these problems, it seems appropriate to reexamine the social support concept carefully. Perhaps social support is not as helpful as initially thought. We might note that this is not the first time that presumed help does not always help. As Lieberman and Mullan (1978) note, despite hundreds of studies, the issue of whether psychotherapy helps is not resolved. Granting that the bulk of the evidence suggests that various kinds of psychotherapy are moderately effective, it is also true that a proportion of those entering psychotherapy become worse (Hartley, Roback & Abramouitz, 1976; Lieberman, 1976; Smith & Glass, 1977).

In light of the fact that professional help may fail to have a beneficial effect, should we expect informal forms of support to be more successful? I suspect that some scholars would say "yes"—that the support of significant others in the person's everyday life may be of more potential benefit. Nevertheless, existing data do not make as strong a case as might have been expected. It is appropriate at this time to consider how an informal social network can have detrimental as well as beneficial effects on health outcomes.

THE POSITIVE AND NEGATIVE EFFECTS OF SOCIAL SUPPORT

In this section, I attempt to describe both the potentially facilitative and potentially detrimental aspects of social support. A point to be made at the outset is that, presumably, although members of a social network intend their behavior to be helpful, sometimes their effect may not be what they intended. A second critical point is that we are going to consider behaviors that are broader than support per se. As noted earlier, it is important to consider the effects of the presence of others' behaviors that may accompany "supportive" actions.

It is useful in examining social support to consider its effects at three major phases: (1) prevention—the phase in which the individual can take steps to avoid becoming ill; (2) coping—the phase in which the individual has fallen ill; (3) recovery—the phase in which the individual is getting better and might soon expect to return to normal life.

Prevention

During the prevention phase, a large class of actions can be taken to avoid ill health. Such behaviors include getting regular medical examinations, obtaining appropriate inoculations during the flu season, eating the proper foods, keeping to a regular schedule of exercise, refraining from cigarette smoking, and so forth. Also, we should include coping behaviors that may ameliorate the effects of significant life events and situations (Dohrenwend & Dohrenwend, 1974; Holmes & Rahe, 1967)—the relentless boss who is provoking an ulcer, a death in the family, and so on. One substantial problem with identifying prevention behaviors is that there are so many. The sheer number of pathogens, environmental health risks (noise, pollution, carcinogens), and potential accidents intensifies the emotion associated with the question: "What do I do to maintain good health?"

There are several ways in which other people can be helpful or not helpful during the prevention phase. Some of these are indicated in Table 9.1. Let us begin with the positive or beneficial aspects of being part of an informal social support network. In the prevention phase, other people can serve as significant informational resources. Suppose, for instance, that an influenza epidemic is forecast or that the individual expects to experience some substantial readjustments in his or her life. Other people may be very helpful in reducing uncertainty

TABLE 9.1
Possible Positive and Negative Effects of Social Support

	Positive Effects	Negative Effects
Prevention	reduce uncertainty and worry	create uncertainty and worry
	set good example	set bad example
	share problems	create new problems
	calm model	calm model
	distract	distract
		germs
Coping	label beneficial	label negative
	provide sympathy	subject to irritation and resentment
	give helpful information	give misleading information
Recovery	maintain regimen	discourage regimen
	contrast with health (incentive)	contrast with health (depressant)
	create desire to stop being a nuisance	create power/dependence need

and worry by providing information about inoculations, expected symptoms, and so forth. Festinger's theory of social comparison (1954; Latane, 1966; Suls & Miller, 1977) suggests that other's opinions are sought in times of uncertainty. A considerable amount of research supports this proposition (see Sanders, Chapter 5, this volume). For example, Schachter (1959) reported that when subjects were highly fearful of electric shocks they expected to receive in an experiment, they were more likely to choose to wait with other people, presumably in order to reduce their uncertainty.

Other people may also set good examples or serve as models. By observing their health-related prevention behaviors, we may be encouraged to take a similar course of action (Bandura, 1977). For instance, research shows that individuals are more likely to take medicine as directed by their physicians if family members have been good models of medicine use (Osterweis, Bush, & Zuckerman, 1979).

In addition to reducing uncertainty and serving as models of health-related behaviors, the presence of others may also have a direct anxiety-reduction effect. This is probably important because there is evidence that extreme stress reactions may impair the immunological system and thus reduce bodily resistance (e.g., Amkraut & Solomon, 1975). In this regard, Wrightsman (1960) found that waiting for painful injections with fellow subjects reduced self-reported anxiety. Other studies examining physiological responses to stress such as heart rate and GSR have also suggested that the presence of others reduces stress reactions. It should be noted however that in a review of the literature, Epley (1974) concluded that socially mediated stress reduction is particularly likely when a modeling companion shows a calm response to the stressor (Cottrell & Epley, 1977).

The presence of others can also serve as a distraction and alleviate fear or worry (Moore, Byers, & Baron, 1981). Distraction may be especially valuable in times of great stress or readjustment. When the individual is surrounded by aversive circumstances that he or she cannot do anything about, other people may provide a respite from these problems.

Finally, persons who are part of a social network may share many problems. The feeling of a common fate, of all being in the "same boat," may transform a health threat into a challenge. Also a "buddy system" may encourage such behaviors as inoculations, smoking cessation, and so on. Organizations like Weight Watchers can be seen as providing a social network of individuals who share a common problem that encourages mutually beneficial actions. Clearly, the preceding discussions of modeling and fear reduction are relevant here, but we should not ignore the emotional catharsis that may be engendered by knowing and talking to other people who have the same problem (see Wortman & Dunkel-Schetter, 1979).

The preceding discussion emphasizes the benefits of being part of a social network, but a closer examination shows how many negative effects can be generated by others in the prevention phase. Rather than reducing worry, other people can create worry and anxiety. Our companions are not always fully knowledgeable or responsible. Talking about an impending epidemic or salient health risks can create or increase the existing level of uncertainty. For the layperson the causes of illness are somewhat mysterious, and as the medical profession becomes more sophisticated its language and forecasts are likely to increase confusion. Unless one is knowledgeable, a discussion of a particular illness may breed more questions than answers. Clearly, in these complex matters, sometimes silence may be appropriate. However, as Sanders (Chapter 5, this volume) indicates, laypeople have strong opinions and recommendations about health even when their knowledge is scanty at best. If members of a family or poker chums all have questions about a new inoculation or a recent fad diet, feelings of uncertainty and worry may be exacerbated through behavioral contagion.

Just as other people can be good examples, they can also be bad examples or models. We have probably all seen the father who smokes a pack of cigarettes a day and tells his teen-age children never to smoke. Epley (1974) notes that others either as observers or as fellow sufferers may overreact to stressful situations and thus serve as models of fearful and counterproductive behavior. It is difficult to assess, but people with close interpersonal relationships may be exposed to as many bad models as good models.

Earlier in our discussion, we mentioned the stress-reducing effect of the presence of other people, but it is important to realize that in some instances fear or anxiety might be necessary to instill appropriate instrumental actions. Work dating from the 1950s (e.g., Janis & Feshbach, 1953) has examined the effects of fear-arousing communications on health-related behaviors (e.g., cessation of smoking, inoculations, proper dental care, etc.). There is still some question about what level of fear is most efficacious (Leventhal, 1970), but it seems clear that at least a moderate level is required to motivate the individual to adopt preventive actions. In this respect then, the presence of others could have the effect of reducing fear and thereby discouraging the instigation of health-related behaviors. Also, the presence of others can produce embarrassment and thus increase stress reactions (Bucke & Parke, 1972; Epley, 1974). Health risks associated with sexual difficulties or with excretory bodily functions are likely candidates, which may engender embarrassment.

The distraction provided by the presence of others can also be counterproductive. Although our relatives, friends, and associates may mean well by trying to get our minds off our problems, such distraction may prevent the kind of actions that in the long-run would be efficacious for good health and illness prevention (Mullen & Suls, in press).

When discussing beneficial aspects of a social network, it was suggested that being part of a network would allow the sharing of problems. But we should recognize that the more people we have as associates and the more intimate the social network, the more one is likely to find the number of problems increasing. In a real sense, the more people one knows and interacts with, the greater the probability that problems will surface and the more likely that other people's problems touch or create new ones for the individual.

Although the list of positive and negative features of social support at this phase can be extended, I expect that the reader already has a substantial idea of the problem with considering social support as *necessarily* facilitative of health preventive actions. Each positive element is balanced by a negative element that could just as easily arise. This is not to say that this must always be the case. The difficulty in whether a given behavior has an ultimate facilitative or detrimental effect is largely situational. For example, some illnesses may be inevitable because of constitutional predispositions. For these instances, a calm model or the distraction provided by others may reduce worry and thus the probability of additional physical or emotional problems. On the other hand, where instrumental actions may be useful and the individual initially has a fear so debilitating that he or she cannot take action, then exposure to a calm model may sometimes reduce fear to a level that is both manageable and arousing to action. Because there are so many unknowns (e.g., what level of fear is appropriate to arouse action without debilitating specific individuals, to what degree will inoculations, drugs, exercise, or diet serve as preventive measures), it is difficult to know a priori what the consequences of well-intended and, for that matter, unintended social behaviors will be.

There is an element associated with the presence of others that should uniformly have a negative effect. Specifically, being a part of a social network should bring the individual into closer contact with germs, viruses, and so forth. In contrast, social isolates should receive less exposure to communicable diseases. If anything, the isolates have this advantage over those with close social associations. Of course, things are complicated by the fact that isolation can itself be a stressful life occurrence.

Coping

The vast majority of research on social support has examined its effects during the coping phase. As the selective review indicated, although most studies report a positive relationship, problems of causal inference as well as some negative and ambiguous results suggest that social support may not always be as helpful during this phase as frequently maintained. In this section, we consider how being part of a social network can have positive and negative effects when one has fallen ill.

First, it should be noted that the points discussed in the previous section apply to the coping phase as well. When one is ill, others can reduce worry, but they can also increase worry. They can act calm, tell you everything will be all right, and encourage you to stop worrying when some worry might be energizing and useful.

There are some behaviors of close associates that are unique to this stage. On the positive side, relatives and friends can supply sympathy and affection when one has fallen victim to illness or injury. This aspect of social support has been given emphasis by Cobb (1976). It appears obvious that displays of affection and concern reflecting that the ill person is valuable and important to others should buoy his or her spirits and provide a reason to fight the illness. But just how displays of affection and sympathy translate into improved physiological functioning remains unclear. Along with sympathy, it is normative for close associates to take over the responsibilities of the ill person, to provide help with expenses, to take care of children, and so on. The positive effects of these forms of social support cannot be underemphasized, although, as we discuss later, there are some problems associated with being the recipient of assistance, especially from one's peers.

Another positive aspect of social support is that others may provide helpful information about how to adjust to one's illness and what symptoms or difficulties to expect. Close associates may also be better able to comprehend the information and recommendations of physicians and nursing staff than the distressed patient. If friends or relatives have had similar bouts with illness, they may be able to share useful facts and advice.

During the coping phase, members of one's social network may provide beneficial labels to the patient. Telling ill persons that they are strong and capable and that they are the kind of people who pull through may provide confidence just when it is most needed.

On the negative side, relatives and friends may signal irritation and resentment rather than sympathy. This is especially likely if the illness is long-term. As the patient becomes more dependent on his or her physician and associates, friends and family may find their time and effort being monopolized. Their frustration and increased responsibilities may lead to a veiled or perhaps open irritation (Coyne, 1976), which should exacerbate the patient's sense of dependence and destroy the quality of interaction with family and friends. In this regard, O'Brien (1980) has reported a prospective study of dialysis patients, which found that although the amount of interactional behavior between the patient and family and friends increased, the quality of such interactions decreased with time.

A closely related problem is that the patient may receive a negative label rather than a beneficial one. Becoming ill, as Goffman (1963) has discussed, is a form of stigma. Further, there is ample research to suggest that people form negative attributions about people who are hurt or suffering. Specifically, Lerner (1970) has proposed that people need to believe that the world is a fair place where individuals get what they deserve and deserve what they get. Research findings demonstrate that when we confront others who are hurt or suffering, we may convince ourselves that the person somehow earned his or her pain either by careless behavior or because of undesirable personal characteristics. To think otherwise would be to admit that decent people like ourselves could suffer a similar fate. Given these considerations, it is highly possible that friends and associates may have extremely negative views of the patient. Of course, these feelings may coexist with feelings of sympathy, love, and affection. In short, the patient's friends and relatives may possess very mixed feelings about him or her. We might expect that their nonverbal messages may reveal discomfort and irritability.

Another negative element at the coping stage is that members of the social support network may give the patient misleading information about his or her illness, prognosis, or regimen. As Sanders indicates in Chapter 5, the layperson frequently offers all sorts of medical advice despite a lack of expertise. Given the complexity of illness and modern medical practice, it would not be surprising that friends or relatives offer biased and inappropriate information, which could lead to detrimental actions or thoughts on the part of the patient.

Recovery

Just as in the other phases, social support may have positive and negative effects on health during recovery. Many of the pluses and minuses described for the preceding phases apply to this phase as well. However, in this section, we describe aspects associated with being a part of a social network that may show themselves plainly during the patient's recovery.

On the positive side, friends and associates may encourage the maintenance of the patient's medical regimen—diet, exercise, the dos and don'ts outlined by the physician or other medical staff. Some reviews have emphasized this aspect of social support. To quote Cobb (1976): "As data on such matters go, this association of cooperative patient behavior with various components of the social support complex is one of the best established facts about the social aspects of medical practice [p. 306]." It must be noted, though, that the bulk of the evidence is correlational in nature and is subject to problems of causal inference.

Another way in which people may have a facilitative function is by providing a contrast between good health and poor health. By perceiving the difference between other's (good) health with one's own (poor) health, the patient may feel more incentive to recover. This added incentive to get well may instill greater motivation to comply to the medical regimen and relinquish the sick role (Parsons, 1951).

Members of one's social network may also create a desire to stop being dependent. This can take a variety of forms ranging from the encouragement to a return to normal life to signaling irritation that one's dependence is becoming a nuisance. Note that the latter aspect may have deleterious effects during the coping phase. However, when the patient is on the road to recovery, it may be helpful for the patient to be told (verbally or nonverbally) that it is expected that he or she begin to take appropriate actions to return to normal life.

On the negative side, there are a variety of ways in which others may discourage compliance to the medical regimen. After all, many aspects of a patient's recovery regimen may complicate or interfere with one's friends or family's own life circumstances (e.g., special diets, exercise regimens, frequent visits to the clinic). To the extent these prescriptions make life more difficult for one's close associates, the more likely they are to communicate their displeasure or put stumbling blocks in the way of compliance. It seems likely also that once it appears the patient is over the serious phase of illness, the patient as well as others may perceive less reason to listen to and heed the physician's advice.

Just as the contrast between other's (good) health and the patient's (ill) health can serve as an incentive for the patient, it can also be a depressant. We know from adaptation level theory (Helson, 1964) that the perceived intensity and valence of a stimulus depends in part on the intensities and valence of other stimuli that are present; so a 60-watt light bulb appears brighter in the presence of a 25-watt light than it does in the presence of a 100-watt bulb. In the same fashion, the patient may perceive his or her own health as very poor when contrasted with that of healthy family and friends. Even if the patient's health has progressed significantly, the negative contrast may be a depressant, impair motivation, and further encourage maintenance of the sick role.

Finally, especially after a long and serious illness, other people may instill and perpetuate the dependence role of the patient. Instead of creating the desire to stop being a dependent, others may just as likely behave in such a way as to produce the opposite behavior. To the extent that others are overly worried about the patient's health or have actually grown used to making decisions and acting on behalf of the patient, it may be difficult to relinquish this responsibility. In part, this may result from the fear that the illness could recur. In the case of many chronic illnesses (e.g., heart disease, cancer, etc.), this possibility is not unlikely. Also, significant others may be weary of allowing the patient to make decisions again especially if they feel that the patient behaved in certain ways that helped to increase vulnerability to illness in the first place.

At this point, it is to be noted that there is little empirical evidence that allows us to determine the extent to which these detrimental behaviors occur. However, there are distinct possibilities that they should increase in probability as the size and intimacy of the patient's social network grows. We would add that whether the incentive effects of contrast predominate over the depressant effects is probably situational depending in part on how large a difference there is between other's actual and the patient's actual health, how realistic a possibility it is that the patient can fully return to normal health, and so forth. There are a myriad of factors that need to be taken into account. The lesson here seems to be that much more fine-tuned empirical analyses of social support need to be performed before it can be concluded with any confidence that social support is facilitative of health.

ADDITIONAL PROBLEMS OF SOCIAL SUPPORT

Before I consider the implications of this analysis for health care policy and future research, it is necessary to consider two additional elements of social support, which have been overlooked by most of those scholars who emphasize the positive effects.

The Attributional Problem

The first element that pervades all attempts by others to console or help the patient concerns the fact that the provision of such assistance is normatively appropriate. That is, all of us know that we should be sympathetic and helpful to those who fall victim to illness. To ignore the sick is to be unfeeling and callous. However, this norm is in fact a double-edged sword. Inasmuch as giving help is the normative behavior—is in fact expected—patients cannot know whether they are the recipients of assistance because they are loved and cared for or whether their family and friends are only behaving in a way dictated by social convention. According to attribution theory (Jones & Davis, 1965; Kelley, 1967), one cannot unambiguously discern the sincerity of a help giver when there are other plausible reasons for his or her behavior, in this case social pressures to assist the sick. In a sense, this attributional problem undermines just what social support is, in part, supposed to achieve. For instance, Cobb (1976) emphasizes that social support provides information leading subjects to believe they are cared for and loved, esteemed, and part of a network. But how can one's associates provide this information without evoking the possibility that their concern only represents an execution of their duty? Only when the amount of help exceeds what would be normatively expected can the recipient be assured that family and friends are not simply behaving out of a sense of duty, but indeed value him or her as a unique and loved human being.

Of course, we hasten to add that if close associates make only infrequent visits to the hospital or signal some irritation, then the patient can make an unambiguous attribution: "They don't care about me, they have more important things to attend to, etc." Thus, when assistance is not offered or is offered with some irritation or reluctance, it may have a strong negative effect.

It is difficult to know at this point how preoccupied the patient may be with whether help givers are sincere and truly concerned about his or her condition. We can easily imagine, however, how patients may covertly and overtly question the motives of associates. They might even make excessive demands to test their friends and families. These could backfire and produce real anger and irritation just when the patient is seeking love and consideration.

The Aversive Effects of Receiving Help

A large portion of what comprises social support consists of rendering help or assistance to the ill person. It is commonly assumed that the recipients of this assistance will be appreciative of the donor. A growing body of research literature (e.g., Fisher, DePaulo, & Nadler, 1981) indicates that under many conditions the recipient of aid may respond with: "feelings of tension and obligation, decrements in self esteem and social status, and derogations of the helper, [and] the help [p. 368]." On first glance this may seem paradoxical, but there are a wide variety of social psychological theories that suggest just such negative reactions. For instance, reactance theory (Brehm, 1966) posits that people prefer to maximize a motivational state (reactance), which is characterized by negative feelings and which is directed toward the reestablishment of the lost freedoms. In applying this theory to the aid recipient, Fisher et al. (1981) suggest: ". . . to the extent that help limits the recipient's present or future actions (e.g., because they will have to act kindly toward the benefactor), it will arouse reactance. Recipients can reduce reactance by acting as though their behavior has not been restricted by help (e.g., by avoiding any actions based on perceived obligation toward the donor, and/or by derogating the source of the threat [p. 369]."

A threat to self-esteem theory developed by Fisher and Nadler (1974) is perhaps most relevant to the present discussion. These researchers argue that it is the self-related consequences of aid that are critical in understanding a recipient's reactions to assistance. To be more specific, Fisher and Nadler observe that aid contains a mixture of self-supportive qualities (e.g., evidence of caring and concern) as well as self-threatening qualities (e.g., evidence of failure, inferiority, and dependence). Which qualities predominate depends on particular aspects of the helping situation.

In examining the literature on reactions to assistance, a number of empirical findings have relevance for social support in the health context. For instance, when the donor is someone with whom the recipient compares his or her own abilities, the recipient of aid may highlight failure and dependence relative to the donor. Fisher and Nadler (1974) have in fact shown that self-esteem is decreased more after receiving assistance from a similar rather than dissimilar other. Given that friends and peers are plausibly the ones used for comparison, the suggestion is that assistance from members of one's social network may engender a certain amount of threat and lowered self-esteem. It has been suggested that these negative effects of aid from a social-comparison other might be mitigated when the other is someone with whom the recipient has a long-term relationship (DePaulo, 1978). However, this is because the other is obligated to help. This means that, although help from a close similar other may not be threatening, it at best has an ambiguous meaning.

Other research has shown that people who have high self-esteem are more disturbed by receipt of aid than low self-esteem persons. Presumably this is because receiving and accepting aid suggests that one has failed and cannot cope by oneself, which should be more inconsistent for the high than the low self-esteem individual. This finding has mixed implications for patients because it depends on their level of self-esteem. The problem is that during the coping and recovery phases the patient is likely to be fluctuating in self-regard. Although family, friends, and doctors encourage patients to lift their spirits, their physical condition may engender a wide variety of negative self-conceptions. To the extent patients are feeling good about themselves, the receipt of aid may be threatening; on the other hand, to the extent patients are feeling negative self-regard, they may not perceive the aid as a threat. These circumstances provide a no-win situation, problematic in either case.

Another factor that influences whether aid is experienced as threatening or supportive is the recipient's level of sensitivity to nonverbal cues. DePaulo and Fisher (1980) have shown that individuals who are attuned to covert nonverbal cues (e.g., signs of annoyance that a donor might "leak" while overtly expressing a willingness to help) are likely to experience aid as aversive. In this regard, Coates and Wortman (1980) have suggested that depressed persons may be especially sensitive to such cues in an attempt to discern what their family and friends are really thinking and feeling about their illness and recovery. It is plausible that people who are physically ill may also be overly sensitive to nonverbal cues. Thus, taken together, it appears likely that the patient may be tuned in and threatened by the receipt of aid from friends and relatives just at those times when it is most needed.

A final consideration is that research shows that recipients of aid respond most favorably (i.e., accept the assistance and suffer no deficits in self-esteem) when they feel they can reciprocate the help (Gergen, 1974). In the case of the gravely ill patient, the probability that one will be able to return the favor in the future may be extremely low. So, in still another way, patients may accept assistance with ill effects—lowered self-esteem, derogation of the donor or perhaps even rejection of the assistance because he or she feels that the obligation cannot be fulfilled.

IMPLICATIONS

In the preceding sections, we have described some of the potentially positive and negative effects of social support on health outcomes during the prevention, coping, and recovery phases. We have not made any attempt to be comprehensive in this analysis. Doubtless there are other positive *and* negative elements that may be associated with being part of a social support network. Our major purpose will be achieved if we conveyed to the reader that the effects of social support, no matter how well-intended, may not always be facilitative of prevention, coping, and recovery.

Of course, it must be acknowledged that the present analysis appears to contradict the findings of a very substantial number of studies that report social support to be helpful. The sheer number of positive findings in the literature suggests that the facilitative effects of support are not entirely blocked out by the detrimental effects. We expect that informal social support systems may act much as psychotherapy does (e.g., Smith & Glass, 1977); that is, in general most people are helped, but a significant proportion may not change or get worse.

As noted earlier, what seem to be required are fine-tuned empirical investigations of just exactly how family and friends behave when an associate becomes sick. Too often, assessment of social support has simply involved measurements of the availability of other persons rather than the quality of their interactions and assistance to those that are ill. It is interesting in this regard to mention a study reported by Sandler and Barrara (1980), who used multiple measures to examine the stress-buffering role of social support. These included: (1) measures derived from social network analysis (network size); (2) reports of satisfaction with received support; (3) reports of actual supportive transactions. Sandler and Barrara reported that neither the total quantity of helping behavior received nor the number of helpers in the social network operate as buffers. However, support that was rated as satisfying did provide effective assistance in coping with stress. As this study was retrospective in nature, we must be careful in drawing strong conclusions, but the suggestion again is that not all help is indeed helpful. It would be instructive in future research to examine just what helping behaviors are perceived by patients as satisfying and facilitative of health and what helping behaviors have the opposite effect.

At a speculative level, we can identify some situations where the social support system is more likely to have an adverse effect. First, the more debilitating the disease, the more likely that family and friends will want to help but feel powerless to have any success. Under these circumstances, it may be most difficult for them to hide their pessimism. Nevertheless, they will probably try to act like things will be all right. These behaviors will make communication with family and friends difficult and may prompt the patient to avoid talking about his or her feelings and physical condition. As Wortman and Dunkel-Schetter (1979) point out, there is considerable evidence with cancer patients to show that interpersonal communication problems with family and friends only exacerbate their depression and sometimes interfere with their compliance to important aspects of their medical regimen.

It might also be expected that the more mysterious and/or rare the disease, the greater the likelihood that family and friends will offer inappropriate or incorrect advice or information. In addition, their own uncertainty may increase the worry and fears of the patient. To the extent the illness can be tied to the patient's behavior (e.g., emphysema to cigarette smoking), the family may signal irritation and resentment because the patient was responsible for his or her illness.

Where might the positive features of social support be most likely to predominate? The positive features of support may predominate in situations where help is not one-sided, that is, where the ill person can be of aid to the other person as well, and so will not feel lowered self-esteem from merely being the recipient of assistance. Circumstances such as these may be most likely to occur between the patient and other patients who have shared many of the same experiences. Here both partners act as cohelpers and thus minimize the problem of merely being a recipient of aid. Also, someone in a similar situation is not likely to distract the individual from the kinds of compliance behaviors necessary for coping and recovery. Other people who are suffering from the same illness can share problems (as in Alcoholics Anonymous) without feeling that things are one-sided. Research by Binger, Ablin, Feuerstein, Kushner, Zoger, and Mikkelson (1969) and Bozeman, Orbach, and Sutherland (1955) have documented that discussions with similar others have beneficial effects. In the Bozeman study, parents of leukemic children were regarded by most mothers participating in the study as the most important source of emotional support. Finally, we might add that interaction with similar others would reduce the probability of negative labels. Copatients are not likely to derogate each other because they both have fallen victim to the same illness. For these reasons as well as others, it is not surprising that so-called self-help groups such as Reach for Recovery for mastectomy patients, Weight Watchers, and the Mended Heart Society for heart surgery patients have grown in popularity (Levy, 1976). It remains for future study, however, to evaluate their effectiveness.

The broader implication of the present arguments for health care policy is probably obvious by now. For physicians to assume that patients who have large informal social networks will fare better than those who do not is probably not always a safe bet. By the same token, requesting that family and friends enter fully into the patient's situation and offer assistance and concern may not always be to the patient's benefit. Whether it would be fruitful for the physician and staff to point out to family and friends just how they can be helpful and (unwittingly) not helpful remains an important question that needs to be addressed by future study. Perhaps, armed with the knowledge that well-intended actions can have adverse effects, family and friends might be able to avoid some of the behaviors that lead to unfortunate outcomes.

ACKNOWLEDGMENTS

The author is indebted to Glenn S. Sanders for his many suggestions and careful reading of earlier drafts of this chapter.

REFERENCES

Ader, R. Psychosomatic and psychoimmunologic research. *Psychosomatic Medicine*, 1980, *42*, 307–321.

Amkraut, A., & Solomon, G. F. From symbolic stimulus to the pathophysiologic responses: Immune mechanisms. *International Journal of Psychiatry in Medicine*, 1975, *5*, 541–563.

Baekeland, F., & Lundwall L. Dropping out of treatment: A critical review. *Psychological Bulletin*, 1975, *82*, 738–783.

Bandura, A. *Social learning theory*. Englewood Cliffs, N.J.: Prentice-Hall, 1977.

Binger, C. M., Ablin, A. R., Feuerstein, R. C., Kushner, J. H., Zoger, S., & Mikkelson, C. Childhood leukemia: Emotional impact on patient and family. *The New England Journal of Medicine*, 1969, *280*(8), 414–418.

Bozeman, M. F., Orbach, C. E., & Sutherland, A. M. Psychological impact of cancer and its treatment. III. The adaptation of mothers to threatened loss of their children through leukemia. Part I. *Cancer*, 1955, *8*, 1–19.

Brehm, J. *A theory of psychological reactance*. New York: Academic Press, 1966.

Bucke, R., & Parke, R. D. Behavioral and physiological response to the presence of a friendly or neutral person in two types of stressful situations. *Journal of Personality and Social Psychology*, 1972, *24*, 143–153.

Caplan, R. D., Harrison, R. V., Wellons, R. V., & French, J. R. P. *Social support and patient adherence*. Ann Arbor, Mich.: Institute for Social Research, 1980.

Caplan, R. D., Robinson, E. A. R., French, J. R. P., Caldwell, J. R., & Shinn, M. *Adhering to medical regimens: Pilot experiments in patient education and social support*. Ann Arbor, Mich.: Institute for Social Research, 1976.

Cassel, J. The contribution of the social environment to host resistance. *American Journal of Epidemiology*, 1976, *104*, 107–123.

Coates, D., & Wortman, C. Depression maintenance and interpersonal control. In A. Baum & J. E. Singer (Eds.), *Advances in environmental psychology* (Vol. 2). Hillsdale, N.J.: Lawrence Erlbaum Associates, 1980.

Cobb, S. Social support as a moderator of life stress. *Psychosomatic Medicine*, 1976, *38*, 300–314.

Conger, J. J., Sawrey, W., & Turrell, E. S. The role of social experience in the production of gastric ulcers in hooded rats placed in a conflict situation. *Journal of Abnormal Psychology*, 1958, *57*, 214–220.

Cottrell, N., & Epley, S. Affiliation, social comparison, and socially mediated stress reduction. In J. Suls & R. L. Miller (Eds.), *Social comparison processes: Theoretical and empirical perspectives*. Washington, D.C.: Hemisphere, 1977.

Coyne, J. C. Depression and the response of others. *Journal of Abnormal Psychology*, 1976, *85*, 186–193.

Dean, A., & Lin, N. The stress-buffering role of social support. *Journal of Nervous and Mental Disease*, 1977, *165*, 403–415.

DePaulo, B. M. Help-seeking from the recipient's point of view. JSAS *Catalog of Selected Documents in Psychology*, 1978, *8*, 62.

DePaulo, B. M., & Fisher, J. D. The costs of asking for help. *Basic and Applied Social Psychology*, 1980, *1*, 23-35.

Dohrenwend, B. S., & Dohrenwend, B. P. (Eds.). *Stressful life events: Their nature and effects*. New York: Wiley, 1974.

Epley, S. W. Reduction of the behavioral effects of aversive stimulation by the presence of companions. *Psychological Bulletin*, 1974, *81*, 271–283.

Festinger, L. A theory of social comparison processes. *Human Relations*, 1954, *7*, 117–140.

Fisher, J. D., DePaulo, B. M., & Nadler, A. Extending altruism beyond the altruistic act: The mixed effects of aid on the help recipient. In J. P. Rushton & R. M. Sorrentino (Eds.), *Altruism and helping behavior*. Hillsdale, N.J.: Lawrence Erlbaum Associates, 1981.

Fisher, J. D., & Nadler, A. The effect of similarity between donor and recipient on reactions to aid. *Journal of Applied Social Psychology*, 1974, *4*, 230–243.

Gergen, K. J. Toward a psychology of receiving help. *Journal of Applied Social Psychology*, 1974, *44*, 187–194.

Goffman, E. *Stigma: Notes on the management of spoiled identify*. Englewood Cliffs, N.J.: Prentice-Hall, 1963.

Hartley, D., Roback, H. B., & Abramovitz, S. I. Deterioration effects in encounter groups. *American Psychologist*, 1976, *31*, 247–255.

Haynes, R. B., & Sackett, D. L. *A workshop/symposium: Compliance with therapeutic regimens*. Hamilton, Ontario: McMaster University Medical Center, 1974.

Heller, K. The effects of social support: Prevention and treatment implications. In A. P. Goldstein & F. H. Kanfer (Eds.), *Maximizing treatment gains: Transfer enhancement in psychotherapy*. New York: Academic Press, 1979.

Helson, H. *Adaptation level theory*. New York: Harper & Row, 1964.

Holmes, T. H., & Rahe, R. H. The social readjustment rating scale. *Journal of Psychosomatic Research*, 1967, *11*, 213–217.

Janis, I. L., & Feshbach, S. Effects of fear-arousing communications. *Journal of Abnormal and Social Psychology*, 1953, *48*, 78–92.

Jones, E. E., & Davis, K. E. From acts to dispositions: The attribution process in person perception. In L. Berkowitz (Ed.), *Advances in experimental social psychology* (Vol. 2). New York: Academic Press, 1965.

Kaplan, B. H., Cassel, J. C., & Gore, S. Social support and health. *Medical Care*, 1977, *15*, 47–58.

Kelley, H. H. Attribution theory in social psychology. In D. Levine (Ed.), *Nebraska Symposium on Motivation* (Vol. 15). Lincoln: University of Nebraska Press, 1967.

Latane, B. (Ed.) Studies in social comparison. *Journal of Experimental Social Psychology*, 1966, Supplement 1.

Lerner, M. J. The desire for justice and reactions to victims. In J. Macaulay & L. Berkowitz (Eds.), *Altruism and helping behavior*. New York: Academic Press, 1970.

Leventhal, H. Findings and theory in the study of fear communication. In L. Berkowitz (Ed.), *Advances in experimental social psychology* (Vol. 5). New York: Academic Press, 1970.

Levy, S. Self-help groups: Types and psychological processes. *Journal of Applied Behavioral Science, 1976, 12,* 310–322.

Lieberman, M. A. Change induction in small groups. *Annual Review of Psychology,* 1976, *27,* 217–250.

Lieberman, M. A., & Mullan, J. T. Does help help? The adaptive consequences of obtaining help from professionals and social networks. *American Journal of Community Psychology,* 1978, *6,* 499–517.

Lynch, J. J. *The broken heart: The medical consequences of loneliness.* New York: Basic Books, 1977.

Mechanic, D. *Students under stress.* New York: Free Press, 1962.

Moore, D., Byers, D., & Baron, R. S. Socially mediated fear reduction in rodents: Distraction, communication, or mere presence. *Journal of Experimental Social Psychology,* 1981, *17,* 485–505.

Mullen, B., & Suls, J. The effectiveness of attention and rejection as coping strategies: A meta-analysis of temporal differences. *Journal of Psychosomatic Research,* in press.

Nuckolls,K. B., Cassel, J., & Kaplan, B. H. Psychosocial assets, life crisis, and the prognosis of pregnancy. *American Journal of Epidemiology,* 1972, *95,* 431–441.

O'Brien, M. E. Effective social environment and hemodialysis adaptation: A panel analysis. *Journal of Health and Social Behavior,* 1980, *21,* 360–370.

Osterweis, N., Bush, P., & Zuckerman, A. Family context as a predictor of individual medicine use. *Social Science and Medicine,* 1979, *13,* 287–291.

Parsons, T. *The social system.* New York: Free Press, 1951.

Pearlin, L. I., & Schooler, C. The structure of coping. *Journal of Health and Social Behavior,* 1978, *19,* 2–21.

Sandler, I. N., & Barrara, M. *Social support as a stress-buffer: A multi-method investigation.* Paper presented at the annual meeting of the American Psychological Association, Montreal, September, 1980.

Schachter, S. *The psychology of affiliation.* Stanford, Cal.: Stanford University Press, 1959.

Silver, R., & Wortman, C. Coping with undesirable life events. In J. Garber & M. E. P. Seligman (Eds.), *Human helplessness.* New York: Academic Press, 1980.

Smith, M. L., & Glass, G. V. Meta-analysis of psychotherapy outcome studies. *American Psychologist,* 1977, *32,* 752–760.

Suls, J., & Miller, R. L. (Eds.). *Social comparison processes: Theoretical and empirical perspectives.* Washington, D.C.: Hemisphere, 1977.

Wortman, C., & Dunkel-Schetter, C. Interpersonal relationships and cancer: A theoretical analysis. *Journal of Social Issues,* 1979, *35,* 120–155.

Wrightsman, L. S. Effects of waiting with others on changes in level of felt anxiety. *Journal of Abnormal and Social Psychology,* 1960, *61,* 216–222.

10 Environmental Stress and Health: Is There a Relationship?

Andrew Baum
A. Wallace Deckel
Robert J. Gatchel
Uniformed Services University of the Health Sciences

Environmental stress can best be thought of as the process by which environmental conditions such as crowding, noise, temperature, and air pollution threaten or cause harm to people. This process includes the stressor (i.e., the condition that poses potential consequences), the interpretation or appraisal of the stressor, and behavioral, emotional, and physiological response to it (e.g., Lazarus, 1966; Lazarus & Cohen, 1977). Response may be directed to coping, wherein the individual seeks to modify the situation or manage emotional response to it, or it may be more nonspecific physiological arousal (e.g., Lazarus, 1966; Selye, 1956). When environmental conditions evoke appraisals of actual or likely harm, some combination of these responses occurs. If coping is unsuccessful or if threatening conditions persist or recur repeatedly, psychological and physiological damage is possible.

This description of environmental stress belies the complexity of its processes. The number of variables that affect the kind of interpretations made, and hence, determine whether stressful appraisals are made, is very large. Anything that affects an individual's confidence in his or her ability to cope with a stressor successfully, for example, will influence the appraisal process. The many factors defining a particular situation will also affect appraisal and influence the kinds of coping responses that are used. At almost every step, psychosocial variables can exert a tremendous influence on stress. Perceived control (or lack thereof), social support, instrumental assets, previous experience, social dynamics of the setting, and so on can all act to determine whether an environmental stressor will cause a stress response and the form this response will take.

Unfortunately, research on environmental stress has often been more concerned with identifying effects of different stressors without consideration of the processes underlying these effects. In doing so, effects of these conditions are often not found. Thus, studies of crowding that neglected to determine whether physical conditions of density translated into stressful experience, that failed to account for the intervening effects of various psychosocial variables, or that did not consider the role of coping in determining response often reported that crowding had few effects. Inasmuch as research that considered these factors and viewed crowding as a process rather than a physical condition has found effects of crowding, it is probably the case that failure to consider the complexity of crowding often masked its effects. Research now indicates that noise and crowding both have substantial effects on behavior and well-being (e.g., Cohen & Weinstein, 1981; Sundstrom, 1978).

As we see later, much of the research on environmental stress as it influences health is plagued with contradiction. However, we also see that, to some extent, this is due to a failure to assess adequately whether or not a condition is experienced as stress. When it is not, we should not expect many effects, but when it is, these consequences are more likely. Without some assessment or appraisal, including the factors that determine it, these kinds of distinctions cannot be made.

In considering these and other problems, we attempt to determine whether environmental stress does affect our health. There is no question but that environmental conditions are important in the development of illness or the maintenance of good health. High levels of air pollutants such as carbon monoxide, sulfur oxides, or nitrous oxides increase the frequency of respiratory illnesses, decrease pulmonary capacity, and increase distress among cardiovascular patients (Evans & Jacobs, in press). Extremes of temperature or pressure can result in acute physiological disturbances, psychological problems, and behaviors that can pose problems for health (e.g., Bachrach, 1980; Baron, 1977; Bell, 1981). Yet, the ways in which stress affects health are more complex and pervasive than the sum of physiological threats to the organism. By considering research on crowding and noise, by considering their impacts on health, and by viewing these relationships in the context of psychological processes underlying them, we attempt to determine the extent to which environmental stress affects our health.

CROWDING AND HEALTH

Crowding is a well-researched topic. Study of high density animal populations has been supplemented by correlational studies of the relationship between density and pathology, laboratory examinations of response to manipulation of group size or available space, and quasi-experimental field studies of naturalistic response to varying densities. However, research directly concerned with health has not been uniformly applied to different aspects of crowding, and for the most part, research dealing with health-relevant outcome measures has focused on animal populations or has relied largely on correlational methods. Problems inherent in these approaches have made interpretation of their results somewhat tenuous, and many of the same problems that have plagued research on crowding, including slow development of clear frameworks for its study, make it impossible to draw definitive conclusions about the effects of crowding on health.

Central to the reluctant development of coherent perspectives on human crowding phenomena has been the persistence of multiple definitions of crowding. Some researchers consider crowding to be a subjective variable—a label for negative experiences associated with high density. Stokols (1972) distinguished the experience of crowding from density, a physical ratio of people to space antecedent to the experience of crowding. Following from this and the fact that density does not always arouse feelings of crowding, it becomes necessary to assess subjective response in studies of crowding (Epstein & Baum, 1978; Stokols, 1972).

This perspective may be contrasted with a second approach in which density and crowding are equated; subjective response is not included in this more physicalistic view (e.g., Freedman, 1975). Further complicating this definitional conflict, researchers have inconsistently defined crowding in terms of spatial density (i.e., the consequences of restricted space) and in terms of social density (i.e., the consequences of large numbers of people). Inasmuch as response to these two components of density may be different (e.g., Baum & Koman, 1976), the interchangeability of these two definitions is not productive.

As we show when selectively reviewing research on crowding and health, these definitional issues limit interpretation of this research. Most researchers now consider subjective response to density to be important, but most studies of the effects of crowding on health do not assess experience directly. Rather, most index crowding in physical terms. In drawing conclusions from these studies, density may be considered as an imprecise measure of crowding, an indicator of potential crowding. As people vary in their responses to different high density situations, one should not expect all of the people in such situations to experience crowding or show crowding-related effects. However, differences in subjective response have not been assessed and, as a result, these studies yield data based on people who do not feel crowded as well as on people who do. This should cause weakening of observed effects and inconsistent findings. For the most part, it has. Although we do not *know* that these effects would be strengthened if subjective responses were considered, some research suggests that it would.

Crowding as Stress

One of the more important developments in the study of crowding has been consideration of crowding as stress. Stokols (1972) defined crowding as a "syndrome of stress," and studies of naturalistic response to crowding assumed that it constituted stress (e.g., Baum & Valins, 1977; Paulus, McCain, & Cox, 1978). Moreover, research demonstrated that physiological arousal was involved in crowding (e.g., Aiello, Epstein, & Karlin, 1975). Lazarus and Cohen (1978) have discussed the applicability of an appraisal-based view of psychological stress to crowding phenomena, and data have suggested that some of the effects of crowding are similar to those of other stressful conditions (e.g., Cohen, 1980; Sherrod, 1974; Singer, Lundberg, & Frankenhaeuser, 1978).

By considering crowding in the framework of stress research, mechanisms by which health may be affected are revealed. One characteristic of stress is that its effects are physiological as well as psychological. Selye (1976), Mason (1975), Frankenhaeuser (1973), and others have demonstrated that stress is associated with activation of the pituitary and adrenal glands resulting in increased levels of circulating catecholamines (epinephrine and norepinephrine) and corticosteroids (e.g., cortisohaldosterone). Although adaptive in some instances, this arousal, accompanied by increased cardiovascular response, sweating, respiration, and the like, can cause wear and tear on the body (e.g., Selye, 1976). The experience of stress, when repeated, prolonged, or when cognitive and behavioral attempts to cope are not successful, can therefore cause physiological as well as psychological problems. By suppressing immune strength, by weakening organs or the vascular system that feeds them, or by interfering with normal health maintenance, stress may contribute to the etiology of illness (e.g., Bartrop, Luckhurst, Lazarus, Kiloh, & Penny, 1977; Baum, Aiello, & Davis, 1979; Eliot & Buell, 1978; Glass, 1976; Gunderson & Rahe, 1974; Solomon, 1969).

Evidence of a Crowding-Health Link

Armed with at least one good reason to expect crowding to affect health and with some reasons for caution in interpreting research on the subject, we now consider some of the studies that have examined health in crowded settings. Before doing so, however, one further issue must be explored. Although the popular press has suggested it, the effects of crowding are not overwhelmingly negative by themselves. Crowding may affect health and may be an important determinant of well-being, but it is not by itself an overpowering stress. Rather, it may have its most dramatic effects when it is coincident with other problems. Crowding affects people in an environmental and psychosocial context; when poor people are crowded, effects may be more severe than when the affluent are crowded, and when density is but one of many sources of stress, crowding should be more debilitating than when it is encountered alone. The effects of crowding are, as a result, extremely complex and of a lesser magnitude in and of themselves than many expect.

Crowding and Immune Response. Dubos (1970b) has suggested that increased density not only facilitates the transfer of infection by increasing the probability of contact with people who have contagious illness, but also that it modifies response to these pathogens when they are communicated. Crowding is associated with increased corticosteroid secretion, he argued, that can suppress immunological functioning and reduce resistance to infection. He reports evidence for this from a study conducted with mice infected with Trichinella. Mice caged together developed more intestinal worms than mice kept in isolation. Inasmuch as all animals were exposed to the same risk, these results suggest that being caged together reduced resistance to the disease. It is, of course, conceivable that isolation may have strengthened immune response rather than the other way around, but Dubos (1970b) concluded that: "it is probable that the effect of crowding on tissue response accounts for the decrease in resistance to infection, presumably via glucocorticoid production [p. 205]."

These results are consistent with other studies of the effects of crowding on animals' susceptibility to infection or parasitic invasion (e.g., Brayton & Brain, 1974). One study found differences in antibody response between very large and small groups of animals (Edwards & Dean, 1977). Dubos' contentions are limited somewhat, however, by results of another study that he reports in which isolated mice were less resistant than were grouped mice to disturbances in intestinal ecology caused by antimicrobial drugs and other physiological disturbances. Thus, although Dubos gives the greater emphasis to reporting that crowding may affect such diverse physiological systems as adrenal hyperplasia, barbiturate anesthesia, toxicity of central nervous system stimulants, hypertension, resistance to infection, and so on, he also concludes that isolation of laboratory animals can arouse fear and decrease ability to adapt to such problems as cold stressors and food restriction or selection. These findings are not necessarily contradictory, however. They may reflect the fact that there is an ideal range of density and that deviations above (crowding) or below (isolation) this range may lead to illness. This is consistent with depictions of crowding and isolation in human populations (e.g., Altman, 1976).

A number of studies provide rough human parallels for these resistance-to-infection findings. For example, crowding has been linked to childhood and adult respiratory infection (e.g., Fanning, 1967; Sims, Downham, McQuillin, & Gardner, 1976). Research has also noted that increases in residential density are related to increased incidence of hepatitis and meningitis (e.g., Jacobson, Chester, & Fraser, 1977; McGlashan, 1977). However, these and other studies do not allow us to conclude that resistance to infection was affected by crowding. As one might expect, they are complicated by a number of factors that obscure relationships between crowding and illness rates. Cassel (1972) and Stewart and Voors (1968), for example, both considered military populations and found relationships between crowding and infection among recruits. Yet, their findings do not simplistically suggest that crowding alone led to changes in resistance to infection; several other factors, including platoon-specific variables, also varied with illness rates. Conversely, the effect of isolation on resistance was reported to be measurable by Holmes (1956) and Brett and Benjamin (1957). In epidemiological studies, they found that individuals living alone were from three to four times as susceptible as individuals who were living in meaningful social contact with others.

Physiological Dysfunction and Death. In a study that has been widely referenced, Calhoun (1962) reported that high population densities lead to devastating social and physiological pathologies in experimental animals. These pathologies included a 96% pre-weaning infant mortality, decreases in the ability of the females to service delivery or provide adequate mothering, and increasing numbers of overactive, cannibalistic, withdrawn, or sexually deviant males. Calhoun's work was among the first major efforts to examine the effects of crowding, and despite problems, it remains important today.

In an early study, Calhoun (1952) placed a small number of rats into a setting that could "comfortably" accommodate 48 adults. The setting consisted of four pens, each with a capacity of 12 rats, linked together to create two end-pens (access limited to one ramp) and two middle pens with access from two sides. He then allowed the rats to overpopulate the pens, artificially controlling the maximum population so that it never exceeded 80 animals.

Calhoun also manipulated feeding arrangements. Rats were fed with either hard pellets or powdered pellets, and water was distributed either in troughs or from a "water fountain" that allowed only one rat to drink at a time. These feeding conditions were designed to establish conditions of high social density. This would naturally occur as the animals clustered around either the hard pellets or troughs. For a variety of reasons, only the hard pellet condition led to very high densities, creating a "behavioral sink," in which 60–80 rats would assemble around the hard pellets in one of the middle pens during periods of feeding. Further contributing to the development of behavioral sinks was the fact that the two end-pens fell under the control of dominant male rats, which restricted access to these pens and forced more rats into the middle pens.

Calhoun (1962) defined behavioral sinks in terms of their tendency to: "aggravate all forms of pathology that can be found within a group [p. 7]." Environmental conditions (e.g., feeding mechanisms and access to pens) caused many animals to congregate in large numbers, and the presence of other animals became associated with the reinforcing nature of feeding. Thus, animals tended to congregate together in these large groups much of the time. The consequences of exposure to this density were considerable. Dominant males who occupied the more sparsely populated end-pens showed few abnormalities, but rats living in the congested center pens showed decreased ability to discriminate appropriate sexual partners, passivity, and reproductive failures as well as those problems noted earlier.

It is possible that many of these consequences, which Calhoun considered to be pathological, may have represented adaptation to the overpopulated setting. For example, Calhoun interpreted mating aberrations, homosexuality, infant mortality, and the like as evidence of dysfunction. Yet, despite the 96% death rate of rat pups, the number of young that survived was always sufficient to offset the adult mortality rate and actually increase the total population. More recent work (Calhoun, 1970; Marsden, 1972) suggests that this kind of adaptation does not hold for mice. In a large enclosure, a population of mice protected from predators and provided with all the food and water that was required grew rapidly but leveled off at 2200 animals, at which point effects similar to those found with rats were readily observable. As reproductive failures and other problems increased, the population size gradually decreased until all of the animals had died. Even when removed from the crowded setting, reproductive difficulties persisted (e.g., Marsden, 1972). The issue of maintenance/reduction of total population obviously requires additional research attention.

It should be noted that Calhoun's initial studies did not use control groups to allow for consideration of low density populations in these enclosures. As a result, the possibility remains that behavior observed in the behavioral sink is more common than is generally believed. For example, Christian (1963) has noted than many animals congregate in large, sinklike groups even when the areas around them are sparsely populated and available. Thus, it is possible that this behavior is typical rather than abnormal, and it may play a role in natural selection and survival of the species. However, this is speculation, and it is difficult to make any specific predictions. Regardless, Calhoun's work provides evidence of an impact of density on behavior and physiological functioning.

Other research on animal populations exposed to high density suggests that high density is associated with organ damage or change in function (Myers, Hale, Mykytowycz, & Hughes, 1971) and with disruption of social organization (e.g., Southwick, 1955) and learning (Goeckner, Greenough, & Maier, 1974). In addition, research suggests that animal populations pass through fairly regular cycles of growth and shrinkage (cf. Christian, 1963; Christian & Davis, 1964). Populations of animals appear to build to a peak size naturally, decrease precipitously, and then level off before beginning the cycle again. Wilson (1975) describes these cycles as reliant on "density dependent controls," which facilitate the maintenance of optimal population density.

These cyclical variations of population density appear to be independent of such environmental factors as food, water, or disease. Rather, they appear to be mediated by endocrine function that may be related to stress. Christian (1963), for example, describes the growth of a herd of deer living on an island in the Chesapeake Bay. The herd grew to a peak size and then experienced a massive die-off and depopulation. Autopsies on deer that died during the decline revealed that they had enlarged adrenal glands, suggesting stress-related changes in bodily function. Whether stress and associated endocrinological events cause these die-offs or are associated with them in more correlational fashion cannot be determined from these data. However, the linkages between population size cycles and these changes in physiological functioning are suggestive.

These findings, as with those based on other animal studies that we discuss later in this chapter, must be considered with great caution when attempting to apply them to human response to crowding. As Freedman (1975) and others have noted, humans are far more adaptive than most infrahumans, and effects observed in animals may not generalize to humans. Clearly, one would expect people's greater ability to cope to result in reduced vulnerability to crowding and generally less severe consequences. And, as we noted earlier, methodological problems may further weaken any attempt at causal inferences.

Levy and Herzog (1974) conducted a study of the effects of density in the Netherlands and found some effects of high density. Controlling for a number of socioeconomic and cultural factors, they found modest relationships between density and crime, illegitimacy, and divorce rates. However, a number of other studies have found that, when social status factors are controlled, relationships between density and pathology are weak (e.g., Schmitt, 1957; Winsborough, 1965). These differences can partially be reconciled by Levy and Herzog's conclusion that their results could not be generalized across cultures due to the uniform social and economic conditions in the Netherlands. In addition, they could not determine from their results whether density causes pathology or whether persons prone to these pathologies end up living in common areas. Freedman (1975), in reviewing American and Canadian epidemiological statistics similar to those used by Levy and Herzog, concluded that it is more nearly the case that suffering people came to live densely than that density causes suffering.

Levy and Herzog also found that density was related to the overall death rate in a weak but statistically significant fashion. This finding has been replicated in prison populations; McCain, Cox, and Paulus (1980) found that death rates of inmates over 50 years of age were 220% higher in more crowded prisons than the expected death rate for that age group. Furthermore, they found some evidence suggesting that, excluding suicide, violence, and accidents, larger housing units with larger social densities had higher death rates at every age level than did smaller housing units. Paulus et al. (1978) found similar results, noting that for prisoners older than 45, higher death rates due to circulatory disease and neoplasms were observed in years with more highly crowded conditions.

A similar study conducted in Chicago, Galle, Gove, and McPherson (1972) concluded that high population densities may have an effect on mortality, fertility, public assistance, and juvenile delinquency. Further, social consequences of density were implicated in this relationship, as measures of interpersonal press or interpersonal distress were most likely to relate to pathology. When considering census-tract densities as an index of crowding, relationships with pathology independent of social status were weak and unreliable. However, measures reflecting the social consequences of density (e.g., persons per housing unit) yielded stronger and more robust relationships with pathology. Again, conclusions about causality cannot be drawn, but an effect of crowding on pathology is again suggested.

Booth and his associates (e.g., Booth, 1976; Booth & Cowell, 1976; Johnson & Booth, 1976) have reported findings suggesting that some illnesses are associated with crowding. Interviews with residents of a large urban center, supplemented by physical examinations, indicated a modest relationship between crowding and health status.

Blood Pressure. Several studies conducted by Henry and his associates (e.g., Henry, Meehan, & Stephens, 1967; Henry, Stephens, Axelrod, & Mueller, 1971) suggest that density may cause increases in blood pressure and related changes in catecholamine levels. In one study, Henry et al. (1967) manipulated density, group composition, and a number of other variables to study the development of hypertension in mice. Stable social organization, reflected either by caging siblings together or by maintaining constant group membership, was associated with lower blood pressure. Mixing of groups in limited space led to aggressive behavior and a sharp elevation in blood pressure. Further, aggression and increased blood pressure were associated with the pairing of adult male mice under conditions of high spatial density.

In this study, density may have indirectly caused blood pressure change. In many instances, spatial density may lead to aggressive response, which may in turn be related to blood pressure. Another study (Henry & Stephens, 1977) compared crowded mice with mice caged with approximately three times as much space and reported blood pressure differences approaching 20 mmHg. However, their density groups were composed of siblings whereas high density groups were not, limiting any conclusions about density and blood pressure.

Research on humans has also reported a relationship between blood pressure and density (e.g., D'Atri, 1975; D'Atri & Ostfeld, 1973). D'Atri and Ostfeld initially hypothesized that there were three environmental characteristics required in order to produce elevated human blood pressures: (1) a crowded environment; (2) an enforced stay in that environment; (3) a continuous subjection to that environment requiring a high degree of vigilance. Studying these factors in a prison environment, they controlled for health, age, weight, duration of confinement, and total institutional confinement in examining the relationship between crowding and blood pressure. The systolic and diastolic blood pressures of residents of single occupancy cells and dormitory cells were compared. Their data suggested that single occupancy was associated with lower blood pressure than was dormitory housing. Though cautioning against strong causal inferences, D'Atri and Ostfeld (1973) nevertheless concluded that: "A new environmental threat to man's health has been identified [p. 565]." In light of the authors' own caution about the interpretation of their results, such a conclusion may be too strong. Further, the relative impacts of crowding, an enforced stay, and a "continuous subjection to that environment requiring a high degree of vigilance" cannot be separated. Despite a nonsignificant trend indicating a relationship between blood pressure and reported crowding (D'Atri, 1975), the conclusion that "Man in crowded conditions may respond as do several animal species, by exhibiting elevated blood pressures (D'Atri & Ostfeld, 1973) [p. 565]" should probably include some recognition of the possibility of enforcement and vigilance and their interaction with crowding.

Some inconsistencies in the reporting of data in these studies also suggest caution in interpreting the results. More importantly, evidence from other studies is only sometimes consistent; whereas some studies find relationships between density and blood pressure, others do not. For example, Paulus et al. (1978), in a study of 112 prisoners, found that the systolic blood pressures of men in three- and six-person cells were higher than the systolic blood pressures of residents of two-person cells. There were no differences between the three- and six-person cells, and diastolic pressures were not different across any conditions. Strengthening this finding is the fact that all indices of crowding, including social density, spatial density, and self-reports of perceived crowding, were higher in the three- and six-person cells than in the two-person cells.

McCain et al. (1980) examined 1400 inmates in six different federal institutions on a variety of measures, including blood pressure. Although finding scattered positive and negative correlations between social density and blood pressure, they did not find strong evidence of elevated blood pressure in these crowded settings. Consistent patterns relating crowding and blood pressure did not emerge. However, in a state prison, which the authors suggest was more intensely crowded, Paulus et al. (1978) found higher systolic blood pressure among prisoners housed in three- or six-person cells than in two-person cells. Similarly, a study reported by Paulus, Cox, McCain, and Karlovac (1980) indicated a weak but significant relationship between crowding and systolic blood pressure. Research by Baum and Davis (1980) has indicated that partitioning or architecturally segmenting settings characterized by high social density reduced most symptoms of social overload and crowding associated with high social density. Paulus et al. (1980) studied segmented and nonsegmented prison dormitories and found systolic blood pressures averaging 6 mmHg less in cubicles than in open rooms. However, differences between divided and open dormitories at another institution were not found.

Generally speaking, then, the data suggest that crowding may be associated with modest increases in blood pressure. However, they are far from conclusive. Additional research in a number of settings is necessary to evaluate this relationship more fully. Blood pressure is a physiological measure of cardiovascular functioning that can have great significance for health. As a major factor in the etiology of several serious illnesses, chronic high blood pressure associated with crowding would constitute a primary mechanism in affecting health. However, neither the chronicity nor necessary association of blood pressure and crowding has been amply demonstrated.

Health Behavior. Thus far, we have concerned ourselves primarily with physiological mechanisms related to stress that may have consequences for health. Clearly, however, there are problems associated with crowding that impact on health without necessarily involving organic dysfunction. Crowding is associated with a number of behavioral and psychological responses that may contribute to health problems. For example, crowding may cause people to withdraw (e.g., Baum & Valins, 1977), and research has indicated that such inward focusing of attention is associated with increasing experience of somatic symptoms (Pennebaker & Brittingham, in press). Likewise, crowding appears to be linked to the development of learned helplessness (e.g., Baum, Aiello, & Calesnick, 1978; Rodin, 1976; Rodin & Baum, 1978). Briefly stated, learned helplessness is viewed as a phenomenon that develops when an organism learns that responding and reinforcement are independent. This learning is assumed to undermine the motivation for initiating instrumental responses and is suggested to be central to the etiology and treatment of depression. Given the parallels between helplessness and depression (e.g., Seligman, 1975), it is likely that crowding can cause depression as well.

Dean, Pugh, and Gunderson (1975) studied the effects of crowding on U.S. naval vessels. Enlisted men on board 13 ships were given a habitability questionnaire, which assessed crowding in ships' mess areas, sleeping quarters, work areas, sanitary areas, and on the ships in general. Social and spatial factors were considered separately, and correlations with outcome measures were, for the most part, small but statistically significant. For example, illness rates (assessed as a ratio of the number of dispensary visits to length of time on board) were weakly related to both spatial ($r = .12$) and social ($r = .11$) crowding. Only satisfaction with the habitability of the ship showed strong relationships (r's $\geq .55$).

These relationships do not provide much reassurance for those who assume a crowding-health link. Despite the fact that subjective indices of crowding were used, very little of the total variance in illness rates could be explained. And, of course, visits to the dispensary may not necessarily translate into illness rates. Complaint rates or visits to a clinic, physician, or infirmary for volitional, emergency, or scheduled appointments reflect illness behavior rather than illness (e.g., Mechanic, 1978). In prisons, such behavior is rewarded and in some senses desirable in that it is a deviation from the daily routine. The medical record or willingness to seek medical help is as much an index of social behavior as a reflection of experienced symptoms or illness (Baum, Aiello, & Davis, 1979; Mechanic, 1978). In addition, close examination of Dean et al.'s (1975) report indicates 262 men for whom data are not reported; they state that 1200 men were given the questionnaire but that 5% (60) of these subjects were eliminated from the analyses because of their difficulty with the English language or their brief time aboard ship. Since the final sample included only 938 men, it appears that 22% of the men given questionnaires were not considered in the analyses for reasons not mentioned in the article.

Because of these issues, we cannot make strong conclusions about the relationship between crowding and illness complaints based on this research. Other studies have also found some evidence of illness behavior as a function of crowding, but these data are again suggestive rather than conclusive. For example, Baum et al. (1979) reported preliminary findings linking crowding stress to both symptom perception and frequency of visits to physicians, but these relationships were based on relatively few subjects and were complicated by mediation by social support and perceived control. Crowded residents of urban neighborhood settings tended to experience more symptoms of somatic or psychological distress, but visits to physicians were not related to these symptom reports. Rather, residents who did not feel a sense of control over events were less likely to visit the doctor regardless of symptom experience.

McCain, Cox, and Paulus (1976) reported higher rates of illness complaints for prisoners living in dormitory style housing than in one- or two-person cells. Similarly, Paulus et al. (1978) reported a positive relationship between psychiatric commitments and prison density. McCain et al. (1980) report fairly strong evidence for crowding being associated with illness complaint rates, and Paulus et al. (1980) found higher illness complaint rates in open rather than segmented prison dormitories. Again, the meaning of this relationship is not clear and may vary from setting to setting. Data suggest that, for several possible reasons, people who feel crowded or who live in dense settings are more likely to seek medical attention or complain of possible illness than are people who do not feel crowded.

Does Crowding Affect Health?

The answer to this question is, at present, a very tentative "yes." Density and crowding are related to a number of indices of health and illness among animal and human populations. However, these relationships are complex, sometimes inconsistent with one another, and generally not very strong. Some possible reasons for this have already been noted, and others reflect the different ways in which crowding may be experienced.

The literature on animals generally shows stronger relationships between density and measures of health than does the literature on humans. To some extent, this may be due to the limited adaptive abilities of nonhuman subjects or to the more concentrated densities to which animals may be exposed. At another level, one can consider the reasons for dysfunction observed in crowded animal populations. Although reproductive problems, overactive adrenal glands, cannibalism, homosexuality, withdrawal, or massive die-offs may appear pathological at the individual level, they appear to be adaptive at the group or species level. Population crashes, changes in maturational processes, and psychosocial abnormalities, for example, may reflect regulatory mechanisms that serve as a check on population size or density. When density is in an optimal range for a given species, the concentration of animals is ideal for survival of the group. When too low, increased reproductivity may reflect a way of readjusting density upward toward the optimal level (e.g., Calhoun, 1970; Freedman, 1979); death and precipitous drops in reproduction may readjust density downward and facilitiate survival of the remaining animals.

This kind of equilibrium view of animal response to density is consistent with work by Christian (1963), Welch and Welch (1969), and others (see Fig. 10.1). However, it is probably not as suitable to describe human crowding phenomena and their effects on health. One reason for this is that a number of animal species, including humans, are able to modify their environment directly. Hoarding food and building shelters are examples of such behavior. The ability of humans to modify their environment would suggest that many of the species-wide, biological triggers common among animals are of less value in humans and may have been selected out of the gene pool. Obviously, changes in food and water availability do not necessitate population crashes among humans as long as storage of food and water and/or agricultural exchange flourishes. Similarly, during increases in population density, our intellectual skills allow us to structure our environments to reduce the number of interactions or expand "conceptual space" to reduce the press of other people (e.g., Calhoun, 1970). Symbolic thought processes and learning play a predominant role in regulating the extent to which stress reactions result in humans (Lazarus, 1974). Activation of the hypothalmic-pituitary-adrenal axis does not necessarily occur reflexively but rather can result from higher psychological/neurological processes that regulate this axis. Cognitive processes combine with physiological response to determine the intensity and quality of emotional response and directly regulate the extent of subsequent changes accompanying the stress response (Lazarus, 1977b; Mason, 1975). Psychological influences may either raise or lower the levels of pituitary-adrenal-cortical or sympathetic-adrenal-medullary activity; indeed, Mason suggests that central nervous system function is constantly modulated by cerebral processes.

Evidence that cognitive appraisal of threat via cerebrally controlled processes can be involved in the initiation of the body's stress mechanisms is reported by

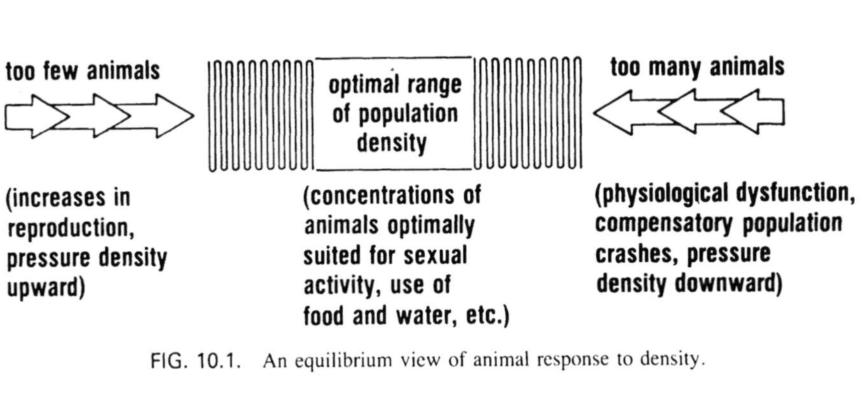

FIG. 10.1. An equilibrium view of animal response to density.

Symington, Currie, Curran, and Davidson (1955). Their research indicated that the adrenal glands of patients dying of cancer who remained conscious during the terminal phase of their illness showed marked adrenal pathologies, whereas those of patients who remained in a coma during the terminal phase of their illness showed normal functioning. Thus, the stress response appeared to be at least partly controlled by cognitive functioning.

It would therefore seem that animal studies are not simply and directly applicable to human experimentation. Rather, one might expect to see greater similarities in physiological changes between animals and those members of human populations whose ability to cope with environmental stressors breaks down and becomes ineffective. As a stressor, crowding should have some effects on health and well-being. But the extent and strength of these effects will be limited by the rather advanced adaptive abilities that most people possess.

In lower species, variability in coping skill is represented by differences in physiological hardiness or different capacities for tolerating physiological extremes. In humans, variability of higher intellectual processes that relate to the adaptation to environmental extremes becomes important. Differences in the skills, capacities, and social supports of different people allow them to deal more or less effectively with the environmental stresses with which they are confronted (e.g., Jenkins, 1979; Mechanic, 1978). If these resources are sufficient, the individual will be able to deal with environmental stress, and physiological changes leading to illness should not be expected. However, when the individual's capacity to adapt is exceeded by the demands of the environment, physiological change or pathological end states are more likely (e.g., Jenkins, 1979; Selye, 1976). Because of differences in coping resources, density is not uniformly related to behavioral or physiological malady.

In many ways, coping responses or "the effects of crowding" represent dynamic attempts to adapt to crowded settings (e.g., Greenberg & Baum, 1979). In considering coping with stress, Lazarus (1977a) suggests that there are two stress regulatory processes: (1) coping; (2) defense or control of emotion. He defines coping as the process that represents the effort taken by the individual to deal directly with and hopefully resolve perceived threat or harm. One method of coping is taking direct action through which the person attempts to directly alter or master the environmental threat and restore a state of homeostasis. To accomplish this, the person tries to demolish, avoid, or fix the problem or prepare to meet the threat directly. Considering crowding, actions such as withdrawal, flight to less crowded settings, aggressive claiming of additional space, or making friends with those in the setting may all represent direct coping.

A second mode of dealing with stress is through the use of intrapsychic defense mechanisms. These palliative coping strategies differ from direct action in that they are focused on control of emotional response rather than the threat causing stress. These defenses are used primarily when direct action is too costly, unsuccessful, or not feasible. Not all environments can be modified or mastered, and when they cannot, response may turn to control of the emotional, visceral, and motor responses that are associated with stress. Ego defenses, cognitive restructuring or labeling of potential threats, selective attention, and the use of tranquilizers, alcohol, and the like represent palliative attempts to reduce the stress of environmental disequilibrium.

Katz, Weiner, Gallagher, and Hellman (1977) studied hydrocortisone production and the use of ego defenses in 30 women who were undergoing breast biopsies. The authors found that six different basic defense reactions were employed by the women to relieve the stress including, displacement, projection, denial with rationalization, stoicism-fatalism, prayer and faith, and a mixture of other defenses. They found that, for this small sample size, patients who used stoicism-fatalism, prayer and faith, and denial with rationalization appeared to experience considerably less psychological and physiological disruption than the other women. Likewise, several studies have examined denial and vigilance defenses in presurgical situations (e.g., Andrew, 1970; Cohen & Lazarus, 1973). These kinds of defenses may play a role in coping with crowding as well.

On a slightly different level, several studies have considered individual response to threat when it is believed that problems can be controlled or predicted. Studies of crowding and other stressors indicate that such control facilitates successful coping (e.g., Fisher & Baum, 1980; Johnson & Leventhal, 1974; Langer & Saegert, 1977). In a review of this literature, Gatchel (1980) concluded that feelings of helplessness and lack of control appear to interfere significantly with the ability to respond adaptively to stressful situations. Lack of control has significant impact upon cognitive, emotional, and motivational responding, which in turn can lead to physiological changes and presumably to illnesses. Noise (Berlyne, 1960; Broadbent 1957; Glass & Singer, 1972; McLean & Tarnopolsky, 1977), crowding (Baron & Rodin, 1978; Baum & Valins, 1979; Rodin, 1976), and other environmental stressors are exacerbated by loss or lack of control and ameliorated when such control is maintained. Of course, this is not a simple relationship, varying with the nature of the situation (e.g., Baum, Fisher, & Solomon, 1981), but even the false perception of control appears to play an important role in coping.

Other coping-related factors may intervene to affect the degree to which the stress of crowding is associated with illness. Studies reported by Cassel (1972) and by Cassel and Tyroler (1961) suggest that preparation for stress is important; poorly-prepared people tend to experience poorer health than well-prepared people when under stress. Similarly, lack of social support—close social ties that provide a person with a reference group, a sense of belonging, and so on—is associated with poor health under stressful conditions (e.g., Cobb, 1976). Thus, studies of the effects of isolation may in part reflect the effects of low levels of social support (e.g., Brett & Benjamin, 1957; Holmes, 1956).

The complexity of the relationships between crowding and health can be illustrated by Baum et al.'s (1979) study of urban neighborhoods. The residents of these areas who reported crowding seemed to experience a syndrome of social overload and loss of regulatory control over local social experience. One apparent cause of these experiences was the inhibition of the development of casual neighborhood groups. Thus, crowding was associated with low levels of perceived control and social support from neighbors. Inasmuch as perceptions of control determined whether people were likely to seek medical assistance (those with low expectations for control did so rarely) and as perception of health was related to social support (low levels were associated with more symptom reporting), crowded individuals were more likely to complain about their health but less likely to do anything about it.

Thus, crowding appears to have some moderate effects on health. The complexities of coping, situational factors, individual differences, and the ranges of acceptable densities aside, one may find significant health impacts of prolonged or repeated crowding episodes. Viewing this relationship out of context, however, invites premature and untenable conclusions regarding the nature and extent of these effects.

NOISE AND HEALTH

Like studies of crowding, studies of the effects of noise on health lead the reviewer to literature that is somewhat contradictory and often tentative in its conclusions. At various times, noise is reported to have a positive, negative, or no effect on physiological functioning and health. Even when effects are found, the extent of these effects is often so small that their measurement is difficult (Kryter, 1970). Perhaps, as Cohen and Weinstein (1981) have implied, this may be due to the fact that noise-induced changes can be considered to be idiopathic and subtle in nature. Illness may result only after long-term exposure to noise or as an aftereffect (Cohen, 1980; Glass & Singer, 1972), which would tend to mitigate against experimental documentation of induced illness. Despite the conclusion reached by a number of authors that there is not enough clear evidence to justify the definite conclusion that noise leads to pathological states and/or tissue damage (Anthony & Ackerman, 1955; Anthony, Ackerman, & Lloyd, 1959b; Bond, 1969; Burns, 1970; Kryter, 1970), there is stronger evidence that noise leads to a host of at least transient autonomic changes. Systems and organs that are known to be affected include the cardiovascular, adrenal, pituitary, thymus, respiratory, digestive, reproductive, vestibular, cochlear, and labyrinth organs. Other changes have been found in glandular secretions, peripheral vasoconstriction, blood pressure, galvanic skin responses, eye movements, and neurotransmitter production (Anthony, 1976; Anthony et al., 1959a; Cohen & Weinstein, 1981; Geber, Anderson, Van Dyne, & Vermillion, 1966; Glass & Singer, 1977; Kryter, 1970; McLean & Tarnopolsky, 1977; Sackler, Weltman,

& Bradshaw, 1959; Sackler, Weltman, & Jurtshuk, 1960; Welch, 1979; Welch & Welch, 1969). Thus, the question to be considered is whether or not the noise-induced physiological changes lead to permanent tissue damage and illness.

Many apparently contradictory experimental results can be explained by the suggestion that physiological response is dose-dependent to noise intensity and bandwidth (McLean & Tarnopolsky, 1977). Paradigms that employ different doses can be expected to yield different results. Noise below 40 db has no real physiological arousal effects, whereas 40–80 db has slight effects (depending on length of time of exposure), and 80–130 db may cause clearly measurable degrees of somatic arousal (Kryter, 1970). Further experimental variance is added by the fact that the noise source and its meaning for the receiver can differentially affect the extent of the physiological arousal (Cohen & Weinstein, 1981; Glass & Singer, 1977; Kryter, 1970; McLean & Tarnopolsky, 1977).

As with crowding, a number of problems have hindered the interpretation of experimental findings; the linkages between noise and health also appear to be complex. Like crowding, noise often shows strong and clear effects in animals but weaker and more suggestive effects among humans. It also appears to be mediated by psychosocial variables such as control or social support and is therefore contextually bound. Further, the effects of noise are affected by coping and by cognitive appraisals of the noise. It is not difficult to understand why the school bell that signifies the start of the school day may be far more aversive to students than the exact same bell ringing 7 hours later to signal the end of the day.

The importance of these parallels between noise effects and crowding effects is clear. The effects of noise are determined in part by the noise, in part by the situational variables defining the setting, and in part by cognitive appraisal and coping. In this section, we do not consider direct effects of noise on sound-sensing organs. Instead, we restrict ourselves to nonauditory effects. Obviously, noise can affect the ear. Less obvious is its effects as a stressor: It can weaken the organism and place it in a state of enhanced susceptibility to illness. However, these effects—the indirect and sometimes dangerous consequences of more chronic exposure to noise—are more difficult to isolate and therefore more likely to show only weak relationships with health. Thus, as with crowding, evidence of observable effects of noise on health are somewhat less than compelling.

The literature on noise also roughly parallels research on crowding in that a range of acceptable levels of noise and extremes above and below these levels is indicated. When acceptable ranges are exceeded or not met, disequilibrium may occur. Steady state and interrupted noise up to levels as high as 120 db frequently have been shown to have no discernible effects on people (as reviewed by Kryter, 1970). At the other extreme, sensory deprivation studies have shown that lack of all stimuli, including sound, leads to a variety of severe mental disturbances (Bachrach, 1980; Zubek, 1973).

Evidence of a Noise-Health Link

Research on noise and its effects on health have not necessarily considered the same problems that were of interest in crowding studies. For example, one would expect noise stress to affect immune response the same way that crowding stress does. Although evidence of this is lacking, some parallel data do exist.

Physiological Dysfunction. As Welch (1979) has noted, the evidence for noise-related cardiovascular changes is very strong. In studies of workers in noisy occupational settings from several different nations, cardiovascular change has been associated with noise. Several studies have reported cardiac dysrhythmias as a major pathological consequence of noise exposure. Jansen (1959) found that workers exposed to 90–115 db of noise suffered more dysrhythmias, extrasystoles, and tachycardia than workers in a 65–90 db zone, although these results were not always statistically significant. Cuesdan, Teganeanu, Yurgu, Raiciu, Carp, and Coatu (1967) found retarded interventricular conductivity and repolarization and conduction anomalies in workers exposed to 85–95 db, whereas workers subjected to 95–106 db showed increased levels of hypertension, cardiac hypertrophy, and ECG abnormalities. Shatalov, Saitanova, and Glotova (1962) also found conduction problems, but they were greater for workers exposed to 85–95 db of sound than for workers in 114–120 db environments. Yazaburskis (1971) and Terentev (1969) found an increase in bradycardias as well as changes in pulse pressure and peripheral blood vessel resistance. Welch reviewed studies by Kangelari, Abramovich-Polyakov, and Rudenko (1966), Sanova (1975), Maugeri and Odescalchi (1974), Capellini and Maroni (1974), Meinhart and Renker (1970), Graff, Bockmuhl, and Tietze (1968), and the Raytheon study (1972), which all reported increases of varying nature in cardiovascular morbidity. Further, varying and discontinuous noise apparently affected cardiovascular functioning more than did relatively unvarying and continuous noise.

Kryter (1970) has researched similar conclusions. He concurred that the majority of studies show increases in cardiovascular pathology in humans with increased exposure to intense broadband industrial noise.

Thus, there appears to be enough evidence to support Welch's (1979) conclusion that prolonged exposure to high intensity sound can be viewed in a much broader sense as a serious threat to general human health.

Blood Pressure. In his review, Welch (1979) noted that in 27 different studies chronically elevated blood pressure was associated with long-term employment in high noise environments. With the exception of a study by Capellini and Maroni (1974), most research suggests a tendency for blood pressure to be elevated during the middle and later years of life in people who have been employed for long periods under intense industrial noise. However, many of these studies did not have adequate statistical controls; for example, some were confounded by the coincident presence of noise and vibration. Further, of the studies that report increases of blood pressure, Welch (1979) notes that six of them report hypotensive effects among noise-exposed workers (Maksimova, Kanevskaya, & Kuzmia, 1974; Meinhart & Renker, 1970; Pokrovskii, 1966; Shatalov, 1965; Shatalov et al., 1962).

Reconciliation for these differential responses is offered by McLean and Tarnopolsky (1977); they suggest that both humans and animals show a vasoconstrictive response to noise. Humans compensate for it with a decrease in stroke volume and thus do not show consistent hypertensive responses. By complication, it is only when the baroreceptors cannot compensate for the vasoconstriction, or when the medullary set-point for blood pressure regulation is shifted upwards, that hypertension would be expected. Such changes would be observed only as a consequence of long-term exposure and would support Welch's claim that the probability of developing hypertension is greatest in the middle and later decades of life.

A number of other reviews have reported conclusions similar to those of Welch (1979) and Kryter (1970). Cohen and Weinstein report that several studies show that children living or attending school near an airport or under a flight path have increased systolic and diastolic blood pressures. Cohen, Evans, Krantz, and Stokols (1980), for example, found elevated blood pressures among children attending noisy schools, compared with matched counterparts who attended schools not under flight paths. In some of the other studies, blood pressure increases were accompanied by increases in electrodermal activity, catecholamine secretions, and peripheral vasoconstriction. Research also indicates that people who already show signs of hypertensive disease are especially prone to the hypertensive reactions to noise (Arguelles et al., 1962, 1970; Finke et al., 1974; Knipschild, 1976; Mosskov, 1976).

Similar results in a rat population were presented by Medoff and Bongiovanni (1945). They found no difference in the incidence of hypertension in younger rats, but there was a significant difference in the older group. In this group, 61% of the rats exposed to noise showed a hypertensive response, compared to only 19% among controls.

Gastro-Intestinal Disturbances. Suggestive but generally inconclusive data exist to support the statement that industrial noise affects gastro-intestinal complaints, ulcers, chronic gastritis, and general digestive problems (Cohen & Weinstein, 1981). Kryter (1970), for example, discusses incidental reports of workers in noisy heavy industries suffering from unusually high percentages of digestive disorders. Similar incidental reports of gastro-intestinal disturbances were reviewed by Welch. However, these reports are scattered, often nonsignificant, and mostly informal in nature.

Peptic ulceration has been reported in guinea pigs exposed to high levels of noise (McLean & Tarnopolsky, 1977), but others have reported no gastro-intestinal ulceration or pathology (Anthony et al., 1959b). We agree with Welch's conclusion that the available data are not sufficient to justify any judgment about the possible induction of gastro-intestinal pathology from long-term exposure to noise.

Sleep Disturbances. As many have stated or implied, one of the greatest hazards of noise is constant or repeated stimulation of the sleeping person (e.g., Grandjean, 1962; Jansen & Schulze, 1964; Kryter, 1970). However, evidence that environmental noise leads to any physiological or mental pathologies in this manner is lacking (Kryter, 1970). Despite this, it appears that in both humans and animals, habituation of any orienting response is suspended during sleep (McLean & Tarnopolsky, 1977). This is in marked contrast to studies showing that habituation to noise occurs rapidly and after short exposure in awake subjects (Glass & Singer, 1972). In awake subjects, the noise, in order not to habituate, must possess at least one of the following properties: novelty, indications of conflict, or learned significance (e.g., McLean & Tarnopolsky). Thus, the sleeping person will consistently show the *N*-response (Kryter, 1970) without decrement. This response includes changes in heart rate, vasoconstriction, increase in skeletal muscle tension, slow deep breathing, and so on. However, a definitive link between nonhabituated *N*-responses and illness has not been established.

Mental Illness. Despite an occasional study that reports a positive correlation between noisy environments and the incidence of mental distress, reviewers of this literature agree that serious attempts to prove or disprove the connection between noise and mental illness are flawed, few, and contradictory (Burns, 1970; Cohen & Weinstein; Kryter, 1970; McLean & Tarnopolsky, 1977). Much of the available information that reports positive correlations between noise and mental illness does not have adequate controls is based on clinical impressions rather than objective evidence and is linked to isolated symptoms (Kryter, 1970). It has been suggested that this lack of effect could be a consequence of the use of measures of illness (e.g., hospital admissions rates) that are not sensitive enough to pick up more subtle changes. Systematic evidence that noise leads to mental disorders is not available at this time.

Does Noise Affect Health?

Although the evidence of a noise-health link is somewhat stronger than for crowding, our conclusions must still remain guarded. Some complex relationship between noise and cardiovascular disease is apparent, both in terms of disease and its precursors. Research still relies primarily on imprecise indices of noise and associated stress, often fails to consider appraisal or coping processes, and generally does not consider mediation of noise stress by psychosocial variables. Despite the fact that noise can be studied in a number of settings, the exact nature of the impact of noise on health is unknown.

SUMMARY AND CONCLUSIONS

Thus far, we have been equivocating whenever conclusions are required. Yes, this appears to be the case, but . . . Unlike many areas of investigation, these *buts* are more than the exceptions that prove the rule. They are legitimate doubts that persist in spite of fairly strong evidence. The ultimate answer to all of these cases—to the question of whether environmental stress influences health—depends on the type of proof that is desired. If an inexorable cause and effect relationship must be demonstrated, the answer is "no." Environmental stress has not been proven to be a cause of changes in health. Because of the relatively long "recruitment" period between exposure to stress and actual tissue damage (i.e., the lengthy interval between stress and observable health effects), such a link may never be proven. However, if one is willing to accept the weight of probable evidence—the repeated demonstration of associations between stress and illness or the parallel changes in stress levels and health status—then prudent people would have to answer "yes."

The problems inherent in studying the effects of stress on health are numerous. Many have already been considered. Because the well-controlled experimental laboratory is of less value in studying such effects than are field settings, absolute control will never be obtained. People cannot be randomly assigned to stressful and nonstressful settings, stress levels are not easily manipulated, and the long-term nature of the stress-illness link makes its study difficult and costly. Improvements and refinements in methodology have and will continue to provide better estimates of the effects of stress on health.

The use of multilevel assessments of stress in field and laboratory settings (e.g., Baum, Gatchel, Fleming, & Lake, 1981; Cohen et al., 1980) promises to provide more reliable estimates of stress levels and should reduce some of the error in relating stress to health. More complete depictions of environmental events and of their continuing influence after their occurrence will also provide more specific and revealing comparisons. Simultaneous assessment of physiological and psychological aspects of response to various stressors should also contribute to understanding the effects of crowding, noise, and other stressful events. Despite problems, the evidence warrants continued investigation of these relationships.

REFERENCES

Aiello, J. R., Epstein, V., & Karlin, R. Effects of crowding on electrodermal activity. *Sociological Symposium*, 1975, *14*, 42–57.

Altman, I. *The environment and social behavior*. Monterey, Cal.: Brooks/Cole, 1976.

Andrew, J. M. Recovery from surgery with and without preparatory instruction, for three coping styles. *Journal of Personality and Social Psychology*, 1970, *15*, 223–226.

Anthony, A. Endocrine and neurohistochemical aspects of noise stress in laboratory animals. In H. D. Johnson (Ed.), *Effects of light, high altitude, noise, electric, magnetic, and electromagnetic fields, ionization, gravity, and air pollution on animals*. Amsterdam: Swels & Zeittinger, 1976.

Anthony, A., & Ackerman, E. Effects of noise on the blood eosinophil levels and adrenals of mice. *Journal of the Acoustical Society of America*, 1955, *27*, 1144–1149.

Anthony, A., Ackerman, E., & Lloyd, D. Effects of chronic noise exposure on sexual performance and reproductive function of guinea pigs. *Journal of the Acoustical Society of America*, 1959, *31*, 1437–1440. (a)

Anthony, A., Ackerman, E., & Lloyd, D. Noise stress in laboratory rodents; behavioral and endocrine responses of mice, rats, and guinea pigs. *Journal of the Acoustical Society of America*, 1959, *31*, 1430–1436. (b)

Arguelles, A. E., Ibeas, D., Ottone, J. P., & Chekherdemian, M. Pituitary-adrenal stimulation by sound of different frequencies. *Journal of Clinical Endocrinology*, 1962, *22*, 846–852.

Arguelles, A. E., Martinez, M. A., Pucciarelli, E., & Disisto, M. V. Endocrine and metabolic effects of noise in normal, hypertensive, and psychotic subjects. In B. Welch (Ed.), *Physiological effects of noise*. New York: Plenum, 1970.

Bachrach, A. J. The human in extreme environments. Naval Medical Research and Development Command, Work Unit No. M0099.PN.00 3.3016. Naval Medical Research Institute, Bethesda, MD, 1980.

Baron, R. A. *Human aggression*. New York: Plenum, 1977.

Baron, R., & Rodin, J. Personal control as a mediator of crowding. In A. Baum, J. E. Singer, & S. Valins (Eds.), *Advances in environmental psychology*. Hillsdale, N.J.: Lawrence Erlbaum Associates, 1978.

Bartrop, R. W., Luckhurst, E., Lazarus, L., Kiloh, L. G., & Penny, R. Depressed lymphocyte function after bereavement. *The Lancet*, April 16, 1977, pp. 834–836.

Baum, A., Aiello, J. R., & Calesnick, L. E. Crowding and personal control: Social density and the development of learned helplessness. *Journal of Personality and Social Psychology*, 1978, *36*, 1000–1011.

Baum, A., Aiello, J. R., & Davis, G. *Urban stress, withdrawal, and health*. Paper presented at the annual meeting of the American Psychological Association, New York, 1979.

Baum, A., & Davis, G. Reducing the stress of high-density living: An architectural intervention. *Journal of Personality and Social Psychology*, 1980, *38*(3), 471–481.

Baum, A., Fisher, J. D., & Solomon, S. K. Type of information, familiarity, and the reduction of crowding stress. *Journal of Personality and Social Psychology*, 1981, *40*, 11–23.

Baum, A., Gatchel, R. J., Fleming, R., & Lake, C. R. Chronic and acute stress associated with the Three Mile Island accident and decontamination: Preliminary findings of a longitudinal study. Technical report submitted to the U.S. Nuclear Regulatory Commission, 1981.

Baum, A., & Koman, S. Differential response to anticipated crowding: Psychological effects of social and spatial density. *Journal of Personality and Social Psychology*, 1976, *34*, 526–536.

Baum, A., & Valins, S. *Architecture and social behavior: Psychological studies of social density*. Hillsdale, N.J.: Lawrence Erlbaum Associates, 1977.

Baum, A., & Valins, S. Architectural mediation of residential density and control: Crowding and the regulation of social contact. In L. Berkowitz (Ed.), *Advances in experimental social psychology*. New York: Academic Press, 1979.

Bell, P. A. Physiological, comfort, performance, and social effects of heat stress. *Journal of Social Issues*, 1981, *37*, 71–94.

Berlyne, D. E. Conflict and information-theory variables as determinants of human perceptual curiosity. *Journal of Experimental Psychology*, 1960, *53*, 399–404.

Bond, J. Effects of noise on the physiology and behavior of farm-raised animals. In B. L. Welch & A. S. Welch (Eds.), *Physiological effects of noise*. New York: Plenum Press, 1969.

Booth, A. *Urban crowding and its consequences*. New York: Praeger Publishers, 1976.

Booth, A., & Cowell, J. Crowding and health. *Journal of Health and Social Behavior*, 1976, *17*, 204–220.

Brayton, A. R., & Brain, P. F. Proceedings: Studies on the effects of differential housing on some measures of disease resistance in male and female laboratory mice. *New England Journal of Medicine*, 1974, *291*, 48–49.

Brett, G. Z., & Benjamin, B. Housing and tuberculosis in a mass radiographic survey. *British Journal of Preventive and Social Medicine*, 1957, *11*(1), 7.

Broadbent, D. E. Effects of noise on behavior. In C. M. Harris (Ed.), *Handbook of noise control*. New York: McGraw-Hill, 1957.

Bronson, F. H., & Eleftherione, B. B. Adrenal response to fighting in mice: Separation of physical and psychological causes. *Science*, 1967, *147*, 627–628.

Buckley, J. P., & Smookler, H. H. Cardiovascular and biochemical effects of chronic intermittent neurogenic stimulation. In B. L. Welch & A. S. Welch (Eds.), *Physiological effects of noise*. New York: Plenum Press, 1969.

Burns, W. *Noise and man*. London: Murray, 1970.

Calhoun, J. B. Population density and social pathology. *Scientific American*, 1962, *206*, 139–148.

Calhoun, J. B. Space and the strategy of life. *Ekistics*, 1970, *29*, 425–437.

Capellini, A., & Maroni, M. Clinical survey on hypertension and coronary disease and their possible relations with the environment in workers of a chemical plant. *Medicina del Lavoro*, 1974, *65*, 297–305.

Cassel, J., & Tyroler, H. A. Epidemiological studies of culture change. I: Health status and recency of industrialization. *Archives of Environmental Health*, 1961, *3*, 25–33.

Christian, J. J. The pathology of overpopulation. *Military Medicine*, 1963, *128*, 571–603.

Christian, J. J., & Davis, D. E. Endocrines, behavior and population. *Science*, 1964, *146*, 1550–1560.

Cobb, S. Social support as a moderator of life stress. *Psychosomatic Medicine*, 1976, *38*, 300–314.

Cohen, F., & Lazarus, R. S. Active coping processes, coping dispositions, and recovery from surgery. *Psychosomatic Medicine*, 1973, *35*, 375–389.

Cohen, J. Aftereffects of stress on human performance and social behavior: A review of research and theory. *Psychological Bulletin*, 1980, *87*, 578–604.

Cohen, S., Evans, G. W., Krantz, D. S., & Stokols, D. Physiological, motivational and cognitive effects of aircraft noise on children: Moving from the laboratory to the field. *American Psychologist*, 1980, *35*, 231–243.

Cohen, S., & Weinstein, N. Nonauditory effects of noise on behavior and health. *Journal of Social Issues*, 1981, *37*, 36–70.

Cox, V. C., Paulus, P. B., McCain, G., & Karlovac, M. The relationship between crowding and health. In A. Baum & J. E. Singer (Eds.), *Advances in environmental psychology* (Vol. 4). Hillsdale, N.J.: Lawrence Erlbaum Associates, in press.

Cuesdan, L., Teganeanu, S., Yurgu, C., Raiciu, M., Carp, C., & Coatu, S. Study of cardiovascular and auditory pathophysiological complications in a group of operatives working in noisy industrial surroundings. *Physiologie*, 1967, *14*, 53–61.

D'Atri, D. Psychophysiological responses to crowding. *Environment and Behavior*, 1975, *7*, 237–252.

D'Atri, D. A., & Ostfeld, A. M. Stress, crowding and blood pressure in man. In Proceedings of the A.P.H.A. 116, November 4–8, 1973.

D'Atri, D. A., & Ostfeld, A. M. Crowding: Its effects on the elevation of blood pressure in a prison setting. *Preventive Medicine*, 1975, *4*, 550–566.

Dean, L. M., Pugh, W. M., & Gunderson, E. K. Spatial and perceptual components of crowding: Effects on health and satisfaction. *Environment and Behavior*, 1975, *7*, 225–236.

Dubos, R. Physiological responses to population density. In H. M. Proshansky, W. H. Ittelson, & L. G. Rivlin (Eds.), *Environmental psychology: Man and his physical setting*. New York: Holt, Rinehart, & Winston, 1970. (a)

Dubos, R. The social environment. In H. M. Proshansky, W. H. Ittelson, & L. G. Rivlin (Eds.), *Environmental psychology: Man and his physical setting*. New York: Holt, Rinehart, & Winston, 1970. (b)

Edwards, E. A., & Dean, L. M. Effects of crowding of mice on humoral antibody formation and protection to lethal antigenic challenge. *Psychosomatic Medicine*, 1977, *39*, 19–24.

Eliot, R., & Buell, J. *Environmental and behavioral influences in the major cardiovascular disorders*. Paper presented at the annual meeting of the Academy of Behavioral Medicine Research, Snowbird, Utah, 1979.

Epstein, Y. M., & Baum, A. Crowding: Methods of study. In A. Baum & Y. M. Epstein (Eds.), *Human response to crowding*. Hillsdale, N.J.: Lawrence Erlbaum Associates, 1978.

Evans, G. W., & Jacobs, S. V. Air pollution and human behavior. *Journal of Social Issues*, 1981, *37*, 95–125.

Fanning, D. M. Families in flats. *British Medical Journal*, 1967, *4*, 382–386.

Finke, H. O., Gusti, R., Martin, R., Rohrmann, B., Schumer, R., & Schumer-Kohrs, A. Effects of aircraft noise on man. Proceedings of the Symposium on Noise in Transportation, Section III, Paper 1. Institute of Sound and Vibration Research, Southampton, England, 1974.

Frankenhaeuser, M. Experimental approaches to the study of catecholamines and emotion. Reports from the Psychological Laboratories, University of Stockholm, 1973 (392).

Freedman, J. *Crowding and behavior*. San Francisco: Freeman, 1975.

Freedman, J. L. Reconciling apparent difference between the responses of humans and other animals to crowding. *Psychological Review*, 1979, *86*, 80–85.

Galle, O. R., Gove, W. R., & McPherson, J. M. Population density and pathology: What are the relations for man? *Science*, 1972, *176*, 23–30.

Glass, D. C. *Behavior patterns, stress, and coronary disease*. Hillsdale, N.J.: Lawrence Erlbaum Associates, 1976.

Glass, D. C., & Singer, J. E. *Urban stress: Experiments on noise and social stressors*. New York: Academic Press, 1972.

Glass, D. C., & Singer, J. E. Environmental stress and the adaptive process. In A. Monat & R. S. Lazarus (Eds.), *Stress and coping*. New York: Columbia University Press, 1977.

Goeckner, D., Greenough, W., & Maier, S. Escape learning deficit after overcrowded rearing in rats: Test of a helplessness hypothesis. *Bulletin of the Psychonomic Society*, 1974, *3*, 54–57.

Graff, Von Ch., Bockmuhl, F., & Tietze, V. Noise exposure and essential arterial hypertension in humans. In S. Witschoff & G. Kriwizkaja (Eds.), *Larmbelastung, Akusticher Reiz und Neurovegetative Storungen*. Leipzig, 1968.

Grandjean, E. The care of the athlete on the day of competition. *Int Z. Vitamin-forsch*, 1962, *32*, 314–333.

Greenberg, C. I., & Baum, A. Compensatory response to anticipated densities. *Journal of Applied Social Psychology*, 1979, *9*(1), 1–12.

Gunderson, E. K. E., & Rahe, R. H. (Eds.). *Life stress and illness*. Springfield, IL: Charles C. Thomas, 1974.

Henry, J. P., Meehan, J. P., & Stephens, P. M. The use of psychosocial stimuli to induce prolonged systolic hypertension in mice. *Psychosomatic Medicine*, 1967, *29*, 408–432.

Henry, J. P., & Stephens, P. M. *Stress, health, and the social environment*. New York: Springer-Verlag, 1977.

Henry, J. P., Stephens, P. M., Axelrod, J., & Mueller, R. A. Effect of psychosocial stimulation on the enzymes involved in the biosynthesis and metabolism of noradrenaline and adrenaline. *Psychosomatic Medicine*, 1971, *33*, 227–237.

Holmes, J. H. Multidiscipline studies of tuberculosis. In P. J. Sparer (Ed.), *Personality, stress, and tuberculosis*. New York: Oxford University Press, 1956.

Jacobson, J. A., Chester, T. J., & Fraser, D. W. An epidemic of disease due to serogroup B Neisseria meningitis in Alabama. *Journal of Infectious Diseases*, 1977, *136*, 104–108.

Jansen, G. On the origin of functional vegetative change due to working under noise. *Archiv. fur Gewerbepathologie und Gewerbehygiene*, 1959, *17*, 238–261.

Jansen, G., & Schulze, J. Beispiele von Schlafstorung durch Gerausche. *Klinwschr.*, 1964, *42*, 132–134.

Jenkins, D. C. Psychosocial modifiers of response to stress. *Journal of Human Stress*, 1979, *5*(4), 3–5.

Johnson, D. R., & Booth, A. Crowding and human reproduction. *Milbank Memorial Quarterly*, 1976, *54*, 321–337.

Johnson, J. E., & Leventhal, H. Effects of accurate expectations and behavioral instructions on reactions during a noxious medical examination. *Journal of Personality and Social Psychology*, 1974, *29*, 710–718.

Kangelari, S. S., Abramovich-Polyakov, D. K., & Rudenko, V. F. The effects of noise and vibration on morbidity rates. *Gigiena Truda i Professional'nye Zabolevaniya*, 1966, *6*, 47–49.

Katz, J. L., Weiner, H., Gallagher, T. F., & Hellman, Z. Stress, distress, and ego defenses: Psychoendocrine responses to impending breast tumor biopsy. In A. Monat & R. S. Lazarus (Eds.), *Stress and coping*. New York: Columbia University Press, 1977.

Knipschild, P. G. Medische gevolgen van Vliegtuilawud. Doctoral dissertation, Amsterdam Coronel Laboratorium, 1976.

Krsiak, M., & Janky, I. The development of aggressive behavior in mice by isolation. In S. Garathini & E. B. Sigg (Eds.), *Aggressive behavior*. Amsterdam: Excerpta Medica Foundation, 1969.

Kryter, K. D. *The effects of noise on man*. New York: Academic Press, 1970.

Langer, E. Y., & Saegert, S. Crowding and cognitive control. *Journal of Personality and Social Psychology*, 1977, *35*, 175–182.

Lawrence, J. E. S. Science and sentiment: Overview of research on crowding and human behavior. *Psychological Bulletin*, 1974, *81*, 712–720.

Lazarus, R. S. *Psychological stress and the coping process*. New York: McGraw-Hill, 1960.

Lazarus, R. S. Cognitive and coping processes in emotions. In A. Monat & R. S. Lazarus (Eds.), *Stress and coping*. New York: Columbia University Press, 1977.(a)

Lazarus, R. S. Psychological stress and coping in adaptation and illness. In Z. J. Lipowski, D. R. Lipsitt, & P. C. Whybrow (Eds.), *Psychosomatic medicine: Current trends and clinical applications*. New York: Oxford University Press, 1977, 14–26. (b)

Lazarus, R. S., & Cohen, J. B. Environmental stress. In S. Attman & J. F. Wohlwill (Eds.), *Human behavior and environment* (Vol. 2). New York: Plenum Press, 1977.

Levy, L., & Herzog, A. N. Effects of population density and crowding on health and social adaptation in the Netherlands. *Journal of Health and Social Behavior*, 1974, *15*, 228–240.

Maksimova, L. I., Kanevskaya, Zh. S., & Kuzmia, G. F. Effect of impulse noise on the body of workers. *Gigiena i Sanitaria*, 1974, *11*, 92–94.

Marsden, H. M. Crowding and animal behavior. In J. F. Wohlwill & D. H. Carson (Eds.), *Environment and the social sciences: Perspectives and applications*. Washington, D.C.: American Psychological Association, 1972.

Mason, J. W. Organization of psychoendocrine mechanisms. *Psychosomatic Medicine*, 1968, *30*(5), 565–791.

Mason, J. W. A historical view of the stress field. *Journal of Human Stress*, 1975, *1*(2), 22–36.

Maugeri, S., & Odescalchi, C. P. The pathology of noise. In E. Guliano (Ed.), *Noise as an occupational hazard: Effects on performance level and health*. Rockville, MD: Informatics, Inc., 1974, p. 43.

McCain, G., Cox, V. C., & Paulus, P. B. The relationship between illness complaints and degree of crowding in a prison environment. *Environment and Behavior*, 1976, *8*(2), 283–290.

McCain, G., Cox, V. C., & Paulus, P. B. The effect of prison crowding on inmate behavior. Final Report, L.E.A.A. grant 78-NIAX-0019, February 29, 1980.

McCann, S. M., Rothhaller, A. B., Yeakel, E. H., & Shenkin, H. A. Adrenalectomy and blood pressure of rats subjected to auditory stimulations. *American Journal of Physiology*, 1948, *155*, 128–131.

McGlashan, N. D. Viral hepatitis in Tasmania. *Social Science and Medicine*, 1977, *11*, 731–744.

McLean, E. K., & Tarnopolsky, A. Noise, discomfort, and mental health. *Psychological Medicine*, 1977, *7*, 19–62.

Mechanic, D. Effects of psychological distress on perceptions of physical health and use of medical and psychiatric facilities. *Journal of Human Stress*, 1978, *4*(4), 26–32.

Medoff, H. S., & Bongiovanni, A. M. Blood pressure in rats subjected to audiogenic stimulation. *American Journal of Physiology*, 1945, *143*, 300–305.

Meinhart, P., & Renker, U. Indicators of morbidity in the heart and circulation as a result of excessive exposure to noise. *Zeitschrift fur die gesamte Hygiene und ihre grenzgebiete*, 1970, *16*, 853–857.

Mosskov, J. I. Experimentelle untersuchungen iiber Lurmwirkungen auf den Menschen. Doctoral dissertation, Amsterdam Coronel Laboratorium, 1976.

Myers, K., Hale, C. S., Mykytowycz, P., & Hughes, R. L. Density, space, sociality and health. In A. H. Esser (Ed.), *Behavior and environment*. New York: Plenum Press, 1971.

Paulus, P. B., McCain, G., & Cox, V. C. Death rates, psychiatric commitments, blood pressure, and perceived crowding as a function of institutional crowding. *Environmental Psychology and Non-Verbal Behavior*, 1978, *3*, 107–116.

Pennebaker, J. W., & Brittingham, G. L. Environmental and sensory cues affecting the perception of physical symptoms. In A. Baum & J. E. Singer (Eds.), *Advances in environmental psychology* (Vol. 4). Hillsdale, N.J.: Lawrence Erlbaum Associates, in press.

Pokrovskii, N. N. On the effect of industrial noise on the blood pressure level in workers in machine building plants. *Gigiena Truda i Professional'nye Zabolevaniya*, 1966, *10*, 44–46.

Raytheon Service Company. Industrial noise and worker medical, absence, and accident records. National Institute of Occupational Safety and Health Contract Report TRL-NIOSH RR-17, 1972.

Rodin, J. Crowding, perceived choice and response to controllable and uncontrollable outcomes. *Journal of Experimental and Social Psychology*, 1976, *12*, 564–578.

Rodin, J., & Baum, A. Crowding and helplessness: Potential consequences of density and loss of control. In A. Baum & Y. M. Epstein (Eds.), *Human response to crowding*. Hillsdale, N.J.: Lawrence Erlbaum Associates, 1978.

Sackler, A. M., Weltman, A. S., Bradshaw, M., & Jurtshuk, P. Endocrine changes due to auditory stress. *Acta Endocrinologica*, 1959, *31*, 405–418.

Sackler, A. M., Weltman, A. S., & Jurtshuk, P. Endocrine aspects of auditory stress. *Aerospace Medicine*, 1960, *31*, 749–759.

Sanova, A. G. The complex effect of low-frequency noise and infra-sound on the bodies of workers. *Vrachebnoe Delo*, 1975, *10*, 133–136.

Schmitt, R. C. Density, delinquency and crime in Honolulu. *Sociology & Social Research*, 1957, *41*, 274–276.

Seligman, M. E. P. *Helplessness: On depression, development, and death*. San Francisco: Freeman, 1975.

Selye, H. *The stress of life*. New York: McGraw-Hill, 1956.

Selye, H. *The stress of life*. New York: McGraw-Hill, 1976.

Shatalov, N. N., Saitanova, A. O., & Glotova, K. V. On the state of the cardiovascular system under conditions of exposure to continuous noise. *Gigiena Truda i Professional'nye Zabolevaniya*, 1962, *6*, 10–14.

Sherrod, D. R. Crowding, perceived control and behavioral aftereffects. *Journal of Applied Social Psychology*, 1974, *4*, 171–186.

Sims, D. G., Downham, M. A., McQuillin, J., & Gardner, P. S. Respiratory syncytial virus infection in northeast England. *British Medical Journal*, 1976, *2*, 1095–1098.

Singer, J., Lundberg, U., & Frankenhaeuser, M. Stress on the train: A study of urban commuting. In A. Baum, J. Singer, & S. Valins (Eds.), *Advances in environmental psychology*. Hillsdale, N.J.: Lawrence Erlbaum Associates, 1978.

Solomon, G. F. Emotions and immunity. *Annals of the New York Academy of Sciences*, 1969, *164*, 461–462.

Southwick, C. H. The population dynamics of confined mice supplied with unlimited food. *Ecology*, 1955, *36*, 212–225.

Stewart, G. L., & Voors, A. W. Determinants of sickness in Marine recruits. *American Journal of Epidemiology*, 1968, *89*(3), 254–263.

Stokols, D. On the distinction between density and crowding: Some implications for future research. *Psychological Review*, 1972, *79*, 275–277.

Sundstrom, E. Crowding as a sequential process: Review of research on the effects of population density on humans. In A. Baum & Y. M. Epstein (Eds.), *Human response to crowding*. Hillsdale, N.J.: Lawrence Erlbaum Associates, 1978.

Symington, T., Currie, A. R., Curran, R. S., & Davidson, J. N. The reaction of the adrenal cortex in conditions of stress. In *Ciba Foundations Colloquia on Endocrinology. Vol. 8. The human adrenal cortex*. Boston, Mass.: Little, Brown, and Company, 1955, 70–91.

Terentev, V. G., Shelvdyakov, Ye. Ye., & Suridova, Ye. Reaction of the human nervous and cardiovascular system to aviation noise. *Vovenno-Meditsinmin Zhurnal*, 1969, *6*, 55–58.

Vinogradova, O. S. The limbic system and registration of information. In R. Hinde & G. Korn (Eds.), *Short term processes in nervous activity and behavior*. Cambridge, England: University Press, 1970.

Welch, B. L. *Extra-auditory health effects of industrial noise*. Aerospace Medical Research Laboratory. Available from N.T.I.S., Springfield, Va. 22161.

Welch, B. L., & Welch, A. S. Aggression and the biogenic amine neurotransmitters. In S. Garattini & E. B. Sigg (Eds.), *Aggressive behavior*. Amsterdam: Excerpta Medica Foundation, 1969.

Wilson, E. O. *Sociobiology*. Cambridge, Mass.: Harvard University Press, 1975.

Winsborough, H. The social consequences of high population density. *Law and Contemporary Problems*, 1965, *30*, 120–126.

Yazaburskis, B. I. Effect of ultrasound and noise on the cardiovascular system of operators of powerful acoustic units. *Hygiene and Sanitation*, 1971, *36*, 455–458.

Zubek, J. P. Behavioral and physiological effects of prolonged sensory and perceptual deprivation: A review. In J. Rasmussen (Ed.), *Man in isolation and confinement*. Chicago: Aldine, 1973.

11 Healthy, Wealthy, and Wise? Health Care Provision for the Elderly from a Psychological Perspective

Robert Kastenbaum
Arizona State University
Tempe, Arizona

"May you have a long life! May you live to be healthy, wealthy, and wise!" These are salutations I remember hearing as a child.

"That geriatric item has to go—we have other priorities!" "No thank you! Working with old people would just be too depressing!" These are salutations I have been hearing for many of my adult years.

Our culture possesses its share of heart-in-the-right-place homilies about the value, dignity, and lovability of the aged. *Honor thy father and mother* may be carved in stone, but in the budgets and bureaucracies of contemporary health care, benefits for the elderly seem to be written instead in vanishing ink. Those concerned with services for the aged have repeatedly seen provisions delayed, reduced, and reallocated "when push comes to shove." This situation should not be simplified into the good guys versus the bad guys. Few are so cruel as to wish suffering and despair on the aged; yet few are so enamored of age that they would themselves prefer to be older, and this includes advanced students in gerontology (Kastenbaum, Derbin, Sabatini & Artt 1972). *Ambivalence* is perhaps the most appropriate term for our attitude toward old people and, for that matter, toward that old man or woman who will shuffle in our own slippers some years hence. It is in our attitudes and expectations as well as in the biology of senescence that we must seek a future in which ideal and reality are less distant.

THREE LETHAL ASSUMPTIONS REGARDING HEALTH CARE OF THE AGED

As a health care administrator, I encounter many assumptions about care of the aged. Often these are voiced not as the questionable assumptions they are, but as established fact. Three of these assumptions have a particularly lethal quality and well reflect our society's mixed feelings toward aging and the aged:

1. Very little can be done to relieve the miseries of old age; it is the most hopeless of cases.
2. The old folk themselves know that they have had their day and now desire only the opportunity to age quietly and gracefully until the angel descends from the clouds.
3. Health care is already so expensive that it would be folly to pour even more money into geriatrics, which would simply absorb all the funds available and with little payoff.

These assumptions all neatly merge into the grand conclusion that there is little that can or should be done to improve health care services for the elderly. An occasional nursing home scandal or personal experience involving an old person dear to the bureaucrat will temporarily suspend the operation of this grand conclusion. But, spasms of conscience and special-interest pressure aside, many decision makers adhere faithfully to the foregoing assumptions and conclusion.

To characterize these assumptions as lethal is not an exercise in hyperbole. When vigorously applied, the assumptions go a long way toward assuring that talented professionals will seldom be attracted to care of the aged; that research, which might develop new concepts and techniques, will have relatively little encouragement; that new concepts and techniques found effective with other populations will not be applied to the aged; and that the self-doubt and borderline despair of many old men and women will be heavily reinforced by the general climate of pessimism. The assumptions tend to operate in the classic self-perpetuating, "vicious cycle" mode. Therapeutic nihilism (Butler, 1975) helps to generate the very conditions that limit the opportunity to test its validity.

A roundup of the reasons for the persistence of these dysphoric orientations would include the following:

1. They serve the interests of fiscal control (i.e., spend less on the elderly so more can be invested in consituencies that will yield a greater return).

2. There is no shortage of observations to support the dysphoric view. Look at how much of the health care budget is already devoted to the elderly! Look at their incredible range of debilities! Look at all the age-associated conditions that do not respond dramatically to treatment! One can easily work up a case for the futility of expensive care if one has the proper motivation and is willing to look away from every example of therapeutic progress that does not fit the desired picture. The primary point here is that the lethal assumptions were not created ex nihilo; they do have substance. With this bit of tough reality acknowledged, we are then in a position to show that this substance is actually rather malleable—the misery is real enough, but not entirely necessary. We must expect, however, that

those who have developed a vested interest in therapeutic nihilism will have to transcend a defensive reflex even to examine the threatening evidence that health and old age can be compatible, given our genuine commitment to make this so.

3. They reinforce the psychological distance between *us* and *them*. It has often been observed that we Americans behave as though we will really never grow old and that we are supported in this self-willed deception by merchants and media. On a philosophical level, we seem to lack a clear, convincing image of what it is to be a *completed person* (Kastenbaum, 1979a). There is really no point in *being* old. Psychiatrists and social scientists also have observed repeatedly (e.g., Feifel, 1959) that the old remind us of death. The image of the aged person burns itself into our awareness as manifestation of almost all that we dread: wrinkles, falterings, sensory deficits, aches and pains, unemployment, uselessness, out-of-dateness, financial woes, and the ever-lengthening shadow of death. The aged represent a mirror that shows ourselves not as we are now and would like to believe we will be forever, but as we actually might become. This reflected vision often repels us. We are eager to put all possible distance and insulation between the relatively youthful immortal we are today and the being who will have felt the touch of decline and mortality. The aversion to recognizing continuity between our own present and future selves contributes to out-grouping those who are the aged of the moment. In this way, we become victims of our own dysphoria, a process that can be discerned in adolescence if not earlier (Kastenbaum, 1959). We just have a terrible time in trying to look freshly and directly into the eyes of age, whether our own or others.

One consequence has been the tendency to invent the old person's orientation toward life and death rather than discover what it really is through intimate contacts on an individual-by-individual basis. We project a readiness if not a rampant desire for death on the part of the old person as a way of alleviating anxiety and guilt we might otherwise experience. Assumptions that it is entirely natural and proper for people to "disengage" from the mainstream of life fit in so well with the politics of low priority that we should beware of too easy an alliance between social gerontological theory and the political marketplace.

THE FINANCIAL IMPERATIVE

The health care establishment as well as the old person must be placed within a socially informed psychological perspective. The octogenerian in Chicago may have the same health problems as a counterpart in Stockholm, but the availability of services is likely to be quite different. Start with a different premise about what citizen and society should expect from each other and how these expectations can be met, and one develops a different system of care for the older person, including but not limited to health. If counseling, home services, and prosthetic devices are readily available to one old person but not another, we cannot explain the subsequent differences in their functioning by referring to the inevitabilities of an intrinsic process of aging.

We focus here on the financial imperative as it influences the health of old people in the United States. This brief discussion is particularly attuned to social and psychological variables associated with financing of health care. Our health care system in general emphasizes short-term treatment. The acute care model dominates. *But* many old people require long-term or continuing care of some kind. Long-term care has come to be associated heavily with institutionalization. *But* most people, the elderly included, would prefer to live in a more homelike, community setting.

Research and clinical priorities usually are targeted on conditions that threaten the well-being and survival of those who are young or in "prime time." *But* the elderly have more health problems than younger echelons in the population. The escalating cost of health services in general is a major national problem. *But* new money is needed to develop better techniques for meeting health needs of the elderly and training an adequate number of competent professionals.

The health care needs of elderly Americans call for resources that our system has become accustomed to invest in other ways. This could develop into a progressively nastier situation. There is already competition for resources among people with various types of problems. Advocacy for the elderly is increasing and is bringing with it an intensification of the competition. Decision makers who have regarded the aged simply as a relatively "ignorable" population now may see them (or their advocates) as downright enemies—another increasingly forceful hand reaching into the till. In the dialectic of competing interests, then, improved advocacy for the elderly is likely to garner a response of annoyance or even hostility, whether or not it actually garners increased resources.

Paradoxically, one major source for improved advocacy is closely tied to the fiscal problems and heightened resistance. There are more elders in the U.S. population than ever before, both in proportional and in absolute terms (Markson & Butra, 1980), a trend that all sayers of sooth believe will become even more pronounced in the future. The increased mass of advocacy draws not only upon a larger number of elders, but also their middle-aged children. Furthermore, each successive wave of men and women reaching the retirement years will bring with them a higher level of education and "Americanization" to make their advocacy efforts more effective. Both the size of the "problem" (if having many people reach old age must be regarded as a problem) and the size of the advocacy have been increasing, and they will probably continue to increase for some time.

Hudson (1978), a keen student of the politics of aging and social welfare, has pursued some of these implications. He concludes that the heyday of new benefits for the elderly may have passed. Widespread public interest in the elderly during the last 2 decades facilitated the enactment of many pieces of favorable legislation. Now, however, in an economy that itself is far from healthy, there is more cost-based pressure and more competition for resources. Attempts to initiate further programs are apt to meet with new and perhaps overwhelming resistance, Hudson predicted, and the trend has been consistent with this assessment. He notes that the built-in expenses will continue to increase even if no new legislation is enacted for the elderly. He sees agencies that serve the elderly coming under exceptionally hard scrutiny because the political climate has changed along with the economy. According to Hudson (1978), these agencies: "have served a number of political agendas as well as . . . the elderly, and these other agendas are changing. As the aging come to be viewed increasingly as a political *problem* and less as a source of political *opportunity,* the role and utility of these agencies will be assessed more in terms of problem resolution than problem recognition [p. 428]."

The attitudinal context for the rise and foreseen decline of benefits for the elderly deserves our attention. Franklin D. Roosevelt (1938) was on safe popular ground when he argued that the problems encountered by old people were not generally a result of their own failings: "Usually it is a mere by-product of modern industrial life. . . . No greater tragedy exists in modern civilization than the aged, worn-out worker who after a life of ceaseless effort and useful productivity must look forward for his declining years to a poor house." The no-fault plight of the elderly could be seen in contrast to the legendary host of lazy, shiftless, and improvident people who line up for welfare benefits because they managed their lives ineffectively. The public gradually warmed to the idea of providing health and other benefits to those who, like themselves, had labored vigorously as part of the all-American work ethic and now were facing illness and destitution for reasons beyond their control. This sentiment persisted and helped put across social security and Medicare legislation. The aged had done all that could have been reasonably expected of them and thus had moral claim on society. In Hudson's terms, there existed a "permissive consensus" in which the needs of elders were acknowledged with little question. With the exception of Medicare, many of the major pieces of legislation were accomplished without much lobbying pressure from the elderly because the permissive consensus was sufficient for this purpose.

Precisely what has happened to this permissive consensus is a matter of conjecture. It still appears to be true that the vulnerable aged are not held culpable for their difficulties. Nevertheless, the "out of sight, out of mind" pseudo-solution of age segregation and institutionalization seems to have taken the place of the previous orientation. Two related factors are easy to identify: (1) the larger numbers of old people; and (2) especially the larger numbers of people reaching advanced old age where losses and disabilities both accumulate and accelerate. Society at large could afford to hold a generous attitude when relatively few people survived to reach the "worn-out worker" phase and were also relatively less likely to survive another 2 decades. It is probable, however, that there are other reasons as well, which are harder to pin down. I think it possible that a miserable old age "sans everything" has become more of a psychological threat to Americans. We have more examples than ever of very aged people among us—people who are too often handicapped further by lack of the necessary resources and supports. It is one thing to feel solidarity with the relatively young aged—those expelled from the work force after many years of hard service—and another to feel at all comfortable with those who appear like a distortion mirror in front of our own eyes. A more comprehensive analysis would also have to consider the overall shift in the texture of social attitudes from depression and New Deal days to the present.

We have already touched on some of the changing circumstances that endanger the favorable legislative climate that had started to meet the challenges posed by the "greying of America." A special emphasis should be given to the formidable pressure being exercised by taxpayers as the cost of social programs literally comes home. The entire social security system has become a major target. Every time the elderly receive their mandated cost-of-living increase benefits, the taxpayer's ambivalence becomes ever more intensified. This is fiscal ambivalence based on rational self-interest (keeping one's own head above water and still trying to do the right thing for elders), but it adds one more level to the existing structure of psychosocial ambivalence. This larger foundation of ambivalence includes the usual grappling for power between old-timers and newcomers and a deeply felt discomfort with life's available options: Grow old or die young.

Sociopolitical changes that place the aged in a deprived condition on any dimension are likely to have deleterious implications for health maintenance. Vulnerabilities increase for the old person who cannot afford to eat well, live in appropriate housing, travel, mingle socially, and generally function as an intact citizen. A person of any age who has these difficulties would be at greater risk from a variety of causes. The situation is intensified for the individual who has such limitations superimposed on biological changes that reduce energy and the margin for error and compensation. To take but one of many possible examples, a short period of malnutrition from which a young person would quickly rebound might in the aged person generate a metabolic imbalance that cascades into serious, perhaps irreversible, decline. Within the health domain specifically, financial problems are immense. Medicare expenditures were a little over $3 billion in the program's first year. By 1976, the expenditures had risen to almost $17 billion. The 1979 budget exceeded $29 billion, and it is projected to fall in the neighborhood of $45 billion by 1983 and up to at least $90 billion by 1990. Obviously, decision makers need not be considered gerontocidal if they prefer not to think about the health problems that remain unmet even with the sizable level of present expenditures. The individual elderly American may be deprived of timely access to the full range of health maintenance services at the same time that the system is struggling to moderate the escalating cost of existing health benefits.

Some individuals have more difficulty than others in finding adequate health care. Hudson (1978) believes that the dissolution of the permissive consensus will have its most pronounced effects on those elderly Americans who are more disadvantaged to begin with—the minority aged, widows, and the old-old (80 and upwards). The familiar dynamics of "the poor get poorer" are likely to become intensified as the most socially connected among the young-old receive the greatest share of resources that are considered too limited to serve everybody's needs.

The situation is further intensified, I believe, by our society's rising expectations regarding the quality of life and freedom from discomfort. Hard times were taken for granted by many of the pioneers and immigrants who laid the foundations for this nation. Deprivation, suffering, and risk could be tolerated to some extent both because these were commonplace and to be expected and because these experiences could be part of the down payment toward a better life. Many of today's old-old are themselves the children of immigrants who accepted self-sacrifice to win a better life for their children if not themselves. With each succeeding generation there has been a lessening of the inclination to accept adversity as life's natural counterpoint. Many of today's aged have had ample experience of hard times, but also some taste of honey. They have, I believe, more ability to tolerate impairment, suffering, and disappointment than do their juniors, in part because they expected fewer guarantees from life to begin with. Expectations continue to rise, however, with every new generation. This general rise in expectations has been stimulated by improvements in health care, labor-saving conveniences, and such amenities as air conditioning. The expectations often seem to increase disproportionately, staying well ahead of the actual accomplishments. This phenomenon has been described in the related area of terminal care, where "healthy dying" has become an ideal verging on a fantasy (Kastenbaum, 1979b).

This rise in expectations might be regarded as a special case of relative deprivation. The deprivation in this instance is not so much the perceived shortfall in benefits when disadvantaged individuals compare themselves with their more fortunate contemporaries. It is, instead, the perceived discrepancy between what one has and what seems to have been promised (to some extent, independent of what others have at the moment). There was once a certain intrinsic value in being able to tolerate pain and adversity without complaint. The social-attitudinal context for private heroics has been weakening, replaced with visions of comfort, freedom from distressing symptoms, and a sense of entitlement. I know a number of old people today who bear their considerable adversities with little complaint, accept with gratitude whatever small comforts society offers, shelter their spirits with religious faith, and personify the stereotype of growing old gracefully. People of this kind, however, are becoming increasingly rare. As

America continues to "grey," more and more old men and women will be expecting everything that has been promised or even implied. Passivity in the face of deprivation is on its way out.

The custodial-institutional solution for old people with significant health problems has been assumed to have the advantage of cost effectiveness, which to some minds is sufficient to counterbalance the many disadvantages. This assumption that "institutional is cheaper" has been challenged by a number of studies reviewed by Koff (1981), but administrators are not renown for their reading habits. It is appropriate, then, to examine the financial imperative as it interacts with the realities of the old person in the institution.

INSTITUTIONALIZATION AS SOLUTION AND PROBLEM

Attempts have been made to minimize the scope of institutionalization and its attendant problems. One still comes across statements to the effect that only 4–5% of elderly Americans reside in an institution. This kind of statement often intends to show that many elders are healthy, vigorous, and independent. The latter proposition can, in fact, be well supported, but not through the low-institutionalization argument. It has been demonstrated (Kastenbaum & Candy 1973) and repeatedly confirmed (e.g., Wershow, 1976) that there has been a "4% fallacy" based upon erroneous generalizations from cross-sectional statistics. Although only 1 elder in 20 or 25 (depending on definitions of institutions) lives in an institution at any given moment, the odds are at least 1 in 4 that a particular person will eventually end up in an institution. Whatever disadvantages are associated with institutionalization of the aged must be understood to affect—sooner or later—a sizable proportion of the population.

Let us consider two of the major types of institution that have become the residence of many older Americans beset by substantial health-related problems: the nursing home and the mental hospital.

The Nursing Home

The bed capacity of American nursing homes more than doubled soon after the introduction of Medicaid and Medicare in 1965. Prior to this time, facilities often provided little if any nursing, but sometimes did have a homelike atmosphere. The new funding program brought with it a set of regulations intended to insure quality standards, although not infrequently experienced by care providers as though a swarm of killer bees were constantly harassing them. Medicare demanded around-the-clock nursing services, an individualized care plan for every client, and medical and dietary supervision. The system was designed for the elderly person who had been successfully treated at an acute hospital and needed the opportunity to convalesce before returning home. Consistent with this idea, Medicare would finance a fixed maximum of days in skilled nursing home care. The old person who is chronically ill and requires continued long-term care is neglected by this system. The long-term care administrative-fiscal system was established in such a way that many elderly who needed such services were either excluded or forced to become wanderers (i.e., relocating from place to place as various benefits expired). Both the original legislation and the various amendments have fallen short of providing a thorough long-term care system (often facing determined opposition by the American Medical Association and other special interest groups). Social workers and other care providers have had to cope with a disheartening labyrinth of regulations in order to determine what benefits were available to which clients and when.

One of the many unfortunate effects has been the exposure of frail elders to the stress of relocation, a process sometimes implicated in increased morbidity and mortality (e.g., Schulz & Brenner, 1977). Another consequence has been the forced closure of nursing homes that were too small to qualify for payments. The facilities that closed their doors to the elderly for this reason included some that were substandard, but others that had maintained a homelike atmosphere more difficult to develop in larger facilities. The tradition of small, family-operated nursing homes with its distinctive mix of pluses and minuses has since given way to larger operations. Increasingly, the profit-oriented nursing home has become a professionally managed operation, often on a franchised or other conglomerate basis.

Alternatives are possible. Funding policies could be revised to give new life to the smaller, more homelike facility. I believe such a move would attract many competent and compassionate people who want no part of large, institutional settings into the nursing home field. Additionally, there is an art to deinstitutionalizing the institution. This is not an easy task to accomplish, but some examples do exist, and there are promising approaches to pursue. When there is to be new or renovated construction, there is the opportunity to design a facility that meets the psychosocial needs of the residents. Architects and decorators can do much to establish an environment that reinforces self-esteem and continuity. Social and environmental psychologists can make effective contributions to the design and redesign of facilities for the aged, as well as recommendations for improved interpersonal processes. Even in the most institutional of physical settings, it is possible to emphasize the individual if one chooses to do so. Residents can be encouraged to take an active part in the life of the facility, making a variety of decisions and exercising all options that are within their reach. The old person who has a real say in such matters as menu, mealtime, scheduling of activities, and—why not?—hiring, firing, and promoting personnel is less likely to withdraw in bitter alienation. The smaller facility has the advantage in such matters, but most of the larger facilities have not done what they might to develop a more humane ambiance.

How adequate is the nursing home solution? It can at least be said that standards exist and that some efforts are made at monitoring quality. Furthermore, individual nursing homes in both the profit and nonprofit sectors have developed humane and effective programs. Models of good quality can be found. Ah, but the problems! Shoddy and even scandalous nursing home management still exists. Somewhat less obvious, perhaps, are problems such as: (1) inadequate distribution across the nation, not in proportion to local needs; (2) regulations and funding formulas that make it very difficult for the most enlightened nursing homes to offer the range of services they recognize as desirable; (3) relative neglect from "fancy" health professionals who have little interest in this clientele; and (4) a fundamental misconception, I would say, about the potential of frail and impaired old people. The people who perhaps have most to gain from sensitive and imaginative care are the very ones consigned to bear custodial staffing patterns in the name of cost effectiveness. This results in a tragic reduction of human possibility—and possibly is even less "cost effective" when the differential outcomes of excellent versus desultory treatment are weighed.

What has already been said suggests that care adequate in quality and scope cannot be counted on in nursing homes and other long-term care facilities, although there are fortunate exceptions to this rule. But it must also be added that many elders would much prefer not to be in any kind of nursing home. Alternatives have been slow in coming, although there is now a more vigorous effort in this direction than ever before. It would be naive to conclude, however, that the search for alternatives comes primarily from a desire to help the frail elderly live with greater independence and contentment. Closer to the truth would be the proposition that the energies behind the search for alternatives are fiscally fueled. Perhaps this should not matter—why should we care what agendas have motivated a valuable course of action? But it does matter, I think, because the already precarious quality of institutional care might well suffer further as priority is given to alternatives. My own knowledge of these dynamics, unfortunately, is more than theoretical. As administrator of a facility for the aged, I have repeatedly encountered low priority within low priority: The aged come after almost everybody else, and the institutionalized (out-of-sight, out-of-mind) aged come after those who are more visible. The dynamics here are attitudinal as well as financial. The public (including most peer advocacy groups) find it less painful to dwell on the prospects of elders who still appear to have a future in contrast to those who are regarded as literally dead-ended in an institution.

The Mental Hospital

The mental hospital has been a curious part of the health care labyrinth for the aged in the United States. Markson (1970) and others have shown that the terminally ill aged have sometimes been routed to the back wards of the mental hospital. The old man or woman might have had no history of mental illness, and the present symptomatology might represent physical distress, enfeeblement, anxiety, and despair. Such a person is not welcome in most nursing homes, nor in acute hospitals. Furthermore, such a person often lacks advocacy and connections. The pathway of ill—even dying—old people into the mental hospital has been facilitated by other health establishment dynamics as well. Deinstitutionalization is part of the picture. "Progressive" states have been emptying out their mental hospitals for some time now. The ethics and effectiveness of these programs is an important matter. Although not our focal concern here, it is a side effect that should be noted: When a mental institution has its census reduced but must still remain in business, there can be a cost effective advantage in stocking up on elderly patients who take up a little space, bring in reimbursements, and require relatively little professional investment. If nobody else wants the physically deteriorating old person, why there's an open bed up on the hill! The mental hospital becomes the depository of "difficult" patients. As Frankfather's study reveals, community-based administrators and clinicians alike have perfected their rationales for declining to serve aged people with substantial disabilities and needs (Frankfather, 1977).

The career of the mental hospital itself is likely to be in decline by the time the old person arrives. Institutions successful in deinstitutionalization often have called upon the services of well-trained, motivated, and innovative staff. This is the phase of the deinstitutionalization process that can be marked by excitement and achievement. Later, when most of the job has been done, the more talented staff members tend to go elsewhere, and the facility is apt to suffer from neglect. It is into this grim environment that a physically ill and emotionally vulnerable old person is likely to enter: a mental hospital past its prime and with little sense of mission for meeting the old person's distinctive needs. Kind and sensitive treatment is not unknown under these conditions; there are always some people who transcend the circumstances. Structurally, however, the mental hospital is an exceedingly poor alternative for the old person, as well as one that greatly increases stigma. In our society it is bad enough to be old, and worse to be institutionalized—but in a *mental* hospital?

At least one other problem should be mentioned. If *holistic medicine* has any meaning at all, it is in geriatrics. Physical condition, psychological state, and social circumstances are inextricably entwined. A given symptom (e.g., confusion) can be a function of a progressive dementing process, a potentially reversible toxicity or drug reaction, temporary effects of a cerebrovascular accident, stressful life events, sensory deprivation, a strategic withdrawal from unacceptable circumstances, or any combination of the foregoing. Effective care requires expertise in differential diagnosis, a trenchant understanding of the totality of the person, and awareness of the many supports and interventions that could be offered at various levels (Kahn, 1981; Kastenbaum 1981). The old person who is in trouble requires the best assessment and intervention techniques available, contrary to the superficial impression that geriatrics is a rather simple and not very interesting field. Those who are called upon to provide care for the geriatric patient in a mental hospital seldom have strong qualifications for this task. Custodial services salted with frequent orders from the pharmacy too often comprise the entire care plan. If the old person is not a true mental case upon entering, his or her prospects for this status increase markedly as time goes on.

If I had to summarize what I have learned about the health needs of the old person, perhaps it would be sufficient to say that there is just less margin for error. Even the frail, impaired, and stressed old person often has considerable holistic resources that can be mustered. Personal strength of some type can be taken as a working assumption; otherwise, this old person probably would not have come so far through life's perils and afflictions. What this person often lacks, however, is that "extra," that psychobiological energy reserve through which a younger person might be extricated from adversity. The numbing environment of a nursing home or mental hospital can defeat a person who might otherwise still have valuable life to experience and to share.

ALTERNATIVE APPROACHES

Fortunately, there are alternative approaches. Although these differ in their details and angles of intervention, they share a more favorable image of the old person. Common to most of these approaches is the belief that men and women can continue to be valuable to themselves and others throughout a very long life if provided with reasonable support and protection. A few practical examples can be given for purposes of illustration.

THE HIGHLAND HEIGHTS EXPERIMENT

The *Highland Heights Experiment* is important not only for its results but for its demonstration that positive ideas can actually be put into effective practice. It is worth presenting this social-experimental case history in some detail to show that there is no necessary conflict between warmhearted and tough-minded orientations.

A specialized housing project was conceived for the city of Fall Rivers, Massachusetts. The city's Housing Authority, the municipal facility for the chronically ill (Hussey Hospital), and the social gerontology research unit of Boston's Hebrew Center for Rehabilitation of the Aged collaborated in this project with funding from HUD. In its physical aspects, Highland Heights is a low-income 14-story apartment house with approximately 200 apartments designed specifically for the physically impaired (usually elderly) adult who lives alone or with one other person. The architecture and design features were planned to maximize the ability of the physically impaired residents to function safely and independently. In addition to physical features, the program also mattered. Made available on the premises were physical and occupational therapy and other health-related services, as well as space for ancillary services to be developed as needed, meeting halls, congregate dining, and social activities. Highland Heights was constructed on the grounds of Hussey Hospital, which made the full services of this facility easily available when necessary.

Well before the facility opened, social gerontologists developed an evaluation plan, a screening instrument for use with applicants, and a method for determining the need for various services. The application forms provided base-line data for research as well as information necessary for screening. Each applicant was then interviewed by a member of the medical-social screening team, again with the information being obtained in a form suitable both for research and practical action. Applicants were rated on their need and suitability for residence at Highland Heights. Economic circumstances made it advisable to admit almost all of the first-wave applicants who were eligible, however, even though they differed among themselves in need and suitability. The randomized design intended to provide the best analysis of Highland Heights' impact could not be put into effect, so a series of research adjustments and controls was devised (Sherwood, Greer, Morris, & Mor, in press). Over a 5-year period, 228 residents were matched with a like number of applicants who were not admitted.

The pattern of results clearly demonstrated that intelligently planned independent housing for the elderly could be a viable alternative to institutionalization. Significantly fewer Highland Heights residents (compared to their controls) became institutionalized over the 5-year study period. The "experimentals" spent less than half as much time in long-term care facilities than did the elderly men and women who were not admitted to Highland Heights. Even more dramatic are the mortality rates. Fewer Highland Heights residents died, and the average number of days alive were significantly greater for the Highland Heights member of the matched pairs. The Highland Heights experience also proved successful for elders who were deinstitutionalized there from long-term care facilities. Many of these people proved able to live independently in Highland Heights, although they had been characterized as disabled and dependent while institutionalized. From the deinstitutionalized elders' self-report as well as objective indices, it was clear that their quality of life had improved. Observations and interviews suggested that the residents much appreciated the fact that they could exercise choice in their activities and relationships (cf. Langor & Rodin, 1976). Even people who made what seemed to be sparing use of the opportunities for social interaction provided by the facility considered it important that the option was always there. It was good to have the choice, "just like everybody else does."

What about the fiscal picture? Was the Highland Heights experiment a lavish demonstration of what could be accomplished with unlimited funding, but one that would not be feasible elsewhere? Not at all! A careful analysis was made of all expenses involved with the Highland Heights program as compared with expenses that would have been involved had the residents been living in other circumstances. This cost–benefit analysis was highly favorable: There was an average saving of about $1000 per year per individual. More independent living. Less fostering of dependence. Access to a broad range of social and health services. And all this for less money! Furthermore, the overall experience indicated that elderly people with health problems would not automatically "absorb" all of the available services, therefore running up huge expenses. Rather, the services were used in moderation. Perhaps just knowing that the services were readily available and being able to use them before problems reached a critical stage were the most important factors here. This study—which both in its overall planning and its fine details is an exceptional model of social science collaboration in service delivery—makes it hard for many bureaucrats to rationalize their current policies. Spending money on social and health care of the elderly can clearly be quite effective both from the human benefit and fiscal standpoints.

Will this favorable outcome lead to widespread emulation? Not necessarily. Between decision makers and social gerontologists there is a Not-So-Grand Canyon. It was bridged in this instance because of favorable circumstances and some deft maneuvering. New applications of this model will have to overcome more than inertia. There are many vested interests at stake, as well as the vested disinterest in reading the work of social scientists or listening to what they might say if asked. The local power mongers have their constituents to protect and advance, and they have their turf to safeguard. Research such as the Highland Heights study takes skill and effort enough—but it may take even more to gain the serious interest of decision makers. This is not necessarily an unfortunate or unfamiliar pursuit for the social scientist, who recognizes that personal and political factors operate even within the sacred groves of academe and the various research funding agencies. The difference between a study that barely registers and one that leads to action can be as simple as a legislator's recognition that a system such as Highland Heights might be just perfect for his or her own parents.

This writer has occasionally employed a tactic beyond personalizing and humanizing research findings. The decision maker usually recognizes (or can be helped to recognize) that information is power. And there always is the other side. Insecurity is at times both realistic and useful: "The other side will probably come at you with all kinds of figures that they have dredged up to support their case. How will you handle that?" The joy of superiority is its flipside: "This is a real study here. Solid. Brandish this study and you will not only confound them in this encounter but bolster your reputation as an erudite person with access to the best sources.'' (You know: Sometimes it even works!)

The Emergency Alarm and Response System

Consider now another approach to humane treatment of the elderly—one that is perhaps even more ambitious in that it aims at helping old people remain in their own homes. The *emergency alarm and response system* for the aged (Morris, Dibner, Gabovitch, & Lowy, 1980) addresses itself to both the fear and the reality of crisis situations for the individual who lives alone in the community or with another aged person. The program involves a little communication hardware and a 24-hour response network. The United States version of this program is less advanced in its communication technology than some that have operated successfully in Scandinavian nations, but this also indicates that even a relatively simple (and hence, less expensive) program can be effective. The background problems are clearly stated by the investigators (Morris et al., 1980):

> Many elderly persons prefer to live alone even in the face of severe functional impairments, medical problems, environmental stresses, and social losses, while other vulnerable elderly will have to live alone simply out of necessity. For some of these persons, regular social and supportive contacts will be a part of daily life, while for others they will not, and serious questions can be raised concerning the ability of these isolated and non-isolated vulnerable elderly to function in the community as new problems arise. Of particular concern is the ability of these persons to adequately respond to new emergencies. Can they summon help? Will someone come? And most importantly, does concern over their safety cause some of them to prematurely enter institutional settings, an event most do not want and one which is costly to society?

The demonstration project experience identified some problems in implementing a successful emergency alarm system but also found that it was a successful and feasible endeavor. Unfortunately, there was no funding available to continue the service beyond the demonstration period, but even so, many of the low-income elderly decided to maintain it from their own pocket because it brought them so much peace of mind and had demonstrated its reliability. It was clear much of the value of the emergency alarm system program to its participants was the secure feeling that help would be available if necessary. It was rare that one actually required help—but the peace of mind was constant. This is one more demonstration of a principle well known to care providers, although it is inconsistently applied: Anxiety and distress can be relieved by establishing realistic and positive expectations that the system works. Confident expectations of this type are hard to come by in the overall fragmented and confused service-delivery system for America's men and women.

The emergency alarm system is, of course, only one of the many techniques that could be used to reduce the vulnerability of isolated or partially disabled elderly people. It represents a type of service that is in short supply today—one that reinforces competence, independence, and continuation of one's preferred life style. These services are likely to be cost effective for society at large, but they face the problem that few agencies want the money to come out of their particular budgets. The let-somebody-else-pick-up-the-bills mentality is rampant. Instead of investing *X* dollars in a timely and imaginative program that will help elders maintain health and independence, there is a tendency to pass the problem along until a fully developed crisis requires expenditure of $X+$ funds (but from another agency's coffers).

Even in our present nascent state of service development, there are a variety of program models for maintaining the health and independence of the older person. There are, for example, adult day-care programs, multipurpose senior centers, nutrition programs, and some in-home services. It is obvious that many of these programs work, some better than others. Often enough, the programs do not require much that is "exotic" or costly. What they do require is a more positive image of the older person and the willingness to do what is actually needed rather than drag around an ever-lengthening chain of regulations and bureaucratic quirks. A cohesive overall social policy to respect the aged and meet their needs is obviously required as well, as Koff (1981) has spelled out in some detail.

The positive view is expressed by Gelfand and Olsen in their new and much-needed presentation of *The Aging Network: Programs and Services* (1980):

> Aging has been viewed in the past as a pathological condition with the elderly merely in a final suspended condition awaiting their imminent demise. Growing old was not considered part of any developmental scheme. The problems faced by many elderly were simply attibuted to "old age." This pronouncement was used by many professions as if it were a clinical diagnosis. While aging affects our entire physiology the tendency to view these changes as irreversible has led to the use of labels as a substitute for diagnosis or treatment. Fortunately, this situation has begun to change, and these changes are reflected in new approaches to developing and evaluating programs and services for the aged. Recent efforts to develop an approach to providing aging services as a continuum of care assume that the elderly have varying degrees of need which must be matched to appropriate services. . . . The acceptance of a continuum model requires abandoning arguments over whether one service is "better" than another. The major question instead becomes: Is one service more appropriate than another for an individual with specific needs? [pp. ix–x].

Ideas and expertise are rapdily developing. Still needed is a social consensus for bringing appropriate services to elderly people who are at any point of the continuum from intact but limited to severely debilitated.

HOW CAN SOCIAL AND BEHAVIORAL SCIENTISTS CONTRIBUTE?

Social and behavioral scientists have already made many contributions to the understanding and care of the aged. Here are a few of the areas in which further contributions could be particularly valuable:

1. Attitude change. Negative attitudes toward old people—and toward the old person within oneself—remain common. The skills of many social and behavioral scientists could be directed here. We need to learn more about the roots of *gerontophobia,* and we need educational and other types of programs to reduce this self-destructive orientation. Simulation experiences in which young people have the opportunity to feel what it might be like to be old comprise one promising avenue. Pastalan, Mautz, and Merrill (1973), for example, have fitted young adults with glasses that present the visual world the way it appears to people who have had age-related changes in their eyes. Kastenbaum (1971) has explored social simulation games in which, for example, young people find themselves in the role of possessing outdated information or being forced to respond at an uncomfortably rapid tempo. The developmental psychology of attitude formation and the art of attitude change await systematic attention from social psychologists who are interested in reducing negative response sets toward the aged.

2. Health education. Not many of us have been prepared for maintaining our health and general well-being throughout the entire life span. A holistic approach to life span health requires collaboration from social and behavioral scientists, along with many others. The target population is not just the elderly but, at least, their middle-aged children as well. Intergenerational health education with the total family as a unit has a potential that has scarcely been tapped.

3. Life span conceptualization. The importance of a life span perspective is not limited to the health field. Developmental psychology is still confined to the stage of infancy and childhood in many colleges. Courses in other areas also have traditionally neglected the older adult (often enough, the middle-aged adult as well). Those who teach courses in learning, perception, motivation, personality assessment and theory, physiology, industrial psychology, psychotherapy, and a number of other subjects would be doing everybody a service if the situation of the elderly person was carefully examined. More courses in aging per se would also be helpful, although I personally favor an emphasis on incorporating life span adult/aging phenomena into a variety of existing courses.

4. Theories that do something. Most of the conceptualizations on which the social and behavioral sciences were founded gave little or no attention to aging. Later generations have not improved upon matters much. Disengagement theory (Cumming & Henry, 1961), the first age-relevant formulation to make an impression, had a stimulating effect on research and went in all directions, but not as far as practical implications were concerned. We need theories of a basic kind that have clear implications for action.

I have made some efforts along this line, including applications of developmental-field theory to social (Kastenbaum, 1972) and psychobiological (Kastenbaum, 1980) benefits from the moderate use of alcoholic beverages within specified contexts. A theoretical approach was proposed in which *aging* could be conceptualized as *old behavior* and then experimentally manipulated and simulated (Kastenbaum, 1968, 1971). Old behavior includes characteristics such as psychomotor retardation, reduced manifest behavioral repertoire, low energy, memory and attentional defects, and reluctance to deal with novel situations. When the broad concept of aging is replaced by specific and observable characteristics, it is possible under some circumstances to modify these characteristics and, thus, in a sense reduce oldness. More recently, another string was added to the developmental-field harp with the introduction of the *habituation* model in which negative old age is conceptualized as a form of hyperhabituation (Kastenbaum, 1981). Dishabituation techniques might be developed with the aim of helping the individual again become open to fresh experience. Specific possibilities for dishabituation include biochemical substances that temporarily reduce the control of higher neural centers and thereby facilitate new learning experiences. A substance as familiar yet as complex as wine is one specific possibility here. Dishabituation can be attempted by the use of specially designed learning and environmental situations as well. Habituation theory suggests that much of what is interpreted as the inevitable outcome of aging is more appropriately understood as the consequences of a psychological process in which habituation has become too dominant. Work along this line is in a very early phase at present and could benefit from the contributions of social psychologists.

Learned helplessness theory (Seligman, 1975) is another conceptual approach that has many potential applications to the welfare of the elderly. Schulz (1976), for example, has found that the physical and psychological well-being of institutionalized elders was improved when they had the opportunity to control the frequency and duration of visits by outsiders. Of particular interest, Schulz (1976) notes: "The manipulation of control and predictability had meaningful generalized effects on the well-being of the institutionalized aged subjects of this study [p. 571]." Quite possibly, any sense of control over any aspect of life enables the institutionalized elder to feel better about his or her total situation. Similar results were obtained by Langer and Rodin (1976) for those nursing home residents who were given both the expectation and opportunity to exercise their own behavioral options. Langer and Rodin (1976) appropriately conclude that: "Inducing a greater sense of personal responsibility in people who may have virtually relinquished decision making, either by choice or necessity, produces improvement [p. 197]." Both studies were able to demonstrate this effect by concentrating on small, everyday aspects of life in a nursing home. Here, then, is a promising example of a fairly general theory that can be put to good use in a practical setting.

5. *Sophisticated evaluation.* Decisions about health care and other programs for the elderly should be based on need, effectiveness, and cost. One would like to believe that such decisions will make appropriate use of evaluation research. Seldom an easy endeavor, evaluation research must cope with special problems and complexities in the field of aging. Poorly designed evaluation is worse than none. First-rate social and behavioral scientists are needed to raise the standard of evaluation research in geriatrics. The researchers should also be articulate communicators in order to increase the chances for their work to make its timely impact.

A CONCLUDING NOTE

The healing arts and the social/behavioral sciences have much to offer the elderly person. Pessimism either about the efficacy of services or their expense is based more upon our residual ignorance and anxieties than upon documented fact. There are already numerous examples of effective community-based and institutional programs. "It can't be done!" is a whimper we need not adopt as a motto. A lot more wisdom and a little more support today, and tomorrow "healthy, wealthy, and wise" may be an ideal that is much closer to reality.

REFERENCES

Butler, R. N. *Why survive? Being old in America.* New York: Harper & Row, 1975.

Cumming, E., & Henry, W. *Growing old.* New York: Basic Books, 1961.

Feifel, H. *The meaning of death.* New York: McGraw-Hill, 1959.

Frankfather, D. *The aged in the community.* New York: Praeger, 1977.

Gelfand, E. E., & Olsen, J. K. *The aging network. Programs and services.* New York: Springer, 1980.

Hudson, R. B. The "graying" of the federal budget and its consequences for old-age policy. *The Gerontologist* 1978, *18*, 428–440.

Kahn, R. L. *Services and settings.* Working paper from the Conference on Training Psychologists for Work in Aging, (Boulder, Colo., June, 1981.

Kastenbaum, R. Time and death in adolescence. In H. Feifel (Ed.), *The meaning of death.* New York: McGraw-Hill, 1959.

Kastenbaum, R. Perspectives on the development and modification of behavior in the aged: A developmental perspective. *The Gerontologist,* 1968, *8*, 280–284.

Kastenbaum, R. Getting there ahead of time. *Psychology Today.* December 1971, pp. 31–35.

Kastenbaum, R. Beer, wine, and mutual gratification in the gerontopolis. In D. P. Kent, R. Kastenbaum, & S. Sherwood (Eds.), *Research, planning, and action for the elderly.* New York: Behavioral Publications, 1972.

Kastenbaum, R. Exit and existence: Society's unwritten script for old age and death. In D. D. Van Tassel (Ed.), *Aging, death, and the completion of being.* Cleveland, Oh.: Case Western University Press, 1979. (a)

Kastenbaum, R. "Healthy dying": A paradoxical question continues. *Journal of Social Issues,* 1979, *35,* 185–206. (b)

Kastenbaum, R. The effects of wine on elderly people who are self-sufficient: A theory and its research findings. In B. L. Mishara & R. Kastenbaum (Eds.), *Alcohol and old age.* New York: Grune & Stratton, 1980.

Kastenbaum, R. Habituation as a model of human aging. *International Journal of Aging & Human Development,* 1981, 12, 159–170.

Kastenbaum, R. *Clinical psychology and the elderly: A Bolder model.* Working paper from the Conference on Training Psychologists for Work in Aging, Boulder, Colo. June, 1981.

Kastenbaum, R., & Candy, S. The 4% fallacy: A methodological and empirical critique of use of population statistics in gerontology. *International Journal of Aging & Human Development,* 1973, *4,* 15–22.

Kastenbaum, R., Derbin, V., Sabatini, P., & Artt, S. "The ages of me": Toward personal and interpersonal definitions of functioning aging. *International Journal of Aging & Human Development,* 1972, *3,* 197–212.

Koff, T. H. *Long term care: An approach to serving the frail elderly.* Cambridge, Mass.: Winthrop, 1981.

Langer, E. J., & Rodin, J. The effects of choice and enhanced personal responsibility for the aged: A field experiment in an institutional setting. *Journal of Personality and Social Psychology,* 1976, *34,* 191–198.

Markson, E. W. Referral for death: Low status of the aged and referral for psychiatric hospitalization. *International Journal of Aging & Human Development,* 1970, *1,* 261–272.

Markson, E. W., & Butra, G. R. *Public policies for an aging population.* Lexington, Mass.: Lexington Books, 1980.

Morris, J. N., Dibner, A. S., Gabovitch, R. M., & Lowy, L. *A report of the operation of an emergency alarm system for the aged.* Unpublished report. Boston: Department of Social Gerontological Research, Hebrew Rehabilitation Center for the Aged, 1980.

Pastalan, L. A., Mautz, R. K., & Merrill, J. The simulation of age related losses: A new approach to the study of environmental barriers. In W. F. E. Preiser (Ed.), *Environmental design research,* (Vol. 1). Stroudsberg, Pa.: Powden, Hutchinson & Ross, 1973.

Roosevelt, F. D. *Public papers and addresses.* New York: Random House, 1938.

Schulz, R. Effects of control and predictability on the physical and psychological well-being of the institutionalized aged. *Journal of Personality and Social Psychology,* 1976, *33,* 563–573.

Schulz, R., & Brenner, G. F. Relocation of the aged: A review and theoretical analysis. *Journal of Gerontology,* 1977, *32,* 323–333.

Seligman, M. E. P. *Helplessness.* San Francisco: Freeman, 1975.

Sherwood, S., Greer, D. S., Morris, J. N., & Mor, V. *The Highland Heights Experiment.* Cambridge, Mass.: Ballinger Press, in press.

Wershow, H. The four percent fallacy. *The Gerontologist,* 1976, *16* (Pt. 1), 52–55.

Author Index

H

L

T

Subject Index

A,B,C

D,G,H,I

L,M,N

R,S

T,U